Specialist Training in:
GASTROENTEROLOGY AND LIVER DISEASE

Commissioning Editor: Timothy Horne
Project Development Manager: Hannah Kenner
Project Manager: Frances Affleck
Design Direction: George Ajayi
Illustrator: Graeme Chambers

Specialist Training in Gastroenterology and Liver Disease

Edited by

Richard G. Long MD FRCP

Consultant Physician and Gastroenterologist
City Hospital, Nottingham, UK

Brian B. Scott MD FRCP

Consultant Physician
Lincoln County Hospital, Lincoln, UK

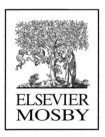

ELSEVIER
MOSBY

Edinburgh London New York Oxford Philadelphia St Louis Sydney Toronto 2005

ELSEVIER
MOSBY

First published 2005

ISBN 0 7234 3252 X

British Library Cataloguing in Publication Data
A catalogue record for this book is available from the British Library

Library of Congress Cataloging in Publication Data
A catalog record for this book is available from the Library of Congress

Notice
Medical knowledge is constantly changing. Standard safety precautions must be followed, but as new research and clinical experience broaden our knowledge, changes in treatment and drug therapy may become necessary or appropriate. Readers are advised to check the most current product information provided by the manufacturer of each drug to be administered to verify the recommended dose, the method and duration of administration, and contraindications. It is the responsibility of the practitioner, relying on experience and knowledge of the patient, to determine dosages and the best treatment for each individual patient. Neither the Publisher nor the editors assume any liability for any injury and/or damage to persons or property arising from this publication.
The Publisher

Printed in China

Contributors

Guruprasad P. Aithal MD PhD FRCP
Consultant Hepatobiliary Physician
Queen's Medical Centre
University Hospital
Nottingham, UK

Robert N. Cunliffe BSc DM MRCP
Specialist Registrar
Wolfson Digestive Diseases Centre
University Hospital
Nottingham, UK

Andrew F. Goddard MA MD MRCP
Consultant Gastroenterologist
Derby City General Hospital
Derby, UK

William P. Goddard DM FRCP
Consultant Gastroenterologist
Nottingham City Hospital
Nottingham, UK

Martin W. James BMedSci BM MRCP
MRC Clinical Research Fellow
Wolfson Digestive Diseases Centre
University Hospital
Nottingham, UK

Timothy M. Jobson BM PhD MRCP
Consultant Physician and Gastroenterologist
Taunton and Somerset Hospital
Taunton, UK

John Jones MA BM PhD MRCP
Specialist Registrar
Division of Gastroenterology
Queen's Medical Centre
University Hospital
Nottingham, UK

Brian McKaig MB PhD MRCP
Consultant Gastroenterologist
The Royal Wolverhampton Hospital
Wolverhampton, UK

Krish Ragunath MPhil MD MRCP
Senior Lecturer in Endoscopy and Consultant
Gastroenterologist
Wolfson Digestive Diseases Centre
University Hospital
Nottingham, UK

Stephen D. Ryder DM FRCP
Consultant Hepatologist
Queens Medical Centre
University Hospital
Nottingham, UK

Kathy Teahon MD FRCP
Consultant Gastroenterologist
Nottingham City Hospital
Nottingham, UK

Preface

This book is written as a practical guide to the diagnosis and management of gastrointestinal disease, including the liver and pancreas. It is aimed particularly at the doctor starting specialist registrar training in gastroenterology and should also be a valuable resource for house officers, senior house officers, specialist nurses and anyone looking for guidance in hospital gastroenterology. All the main disease groups are discussed, but the book is not meant to be comprehensive – rare conditions, scientific explanations of pathophysiology and extensive references are widely available in large textbooks of gastroenterology. Symptoms, diagnostic methods, pathology and treatment are linked. There are also sections on the changing situation in endoscopy units and on the interpretation of data to help in assessing the literature and applying it to clinical practice and to research projects.

Over the last 20 years, Mid-Trent (Nottingham, Derby, Lincoln and Mansfield) has developed an enviable reputation for the quality of its training and its trainees. Our contributors are all either trainers or past or present trainees on the Mid-Trent Rotation. All the contributors have a research background, remain active in training and have a predominant interest in clinical gastroenterology as practised in the National Health Service.

We are grateful to our Nottingham University professorial colleagues (Chris Hawkey, Richard Logan, Robin Spiller, Yash Mahida and John Atherton) for keeping us in touch with scientific developments. We acknowledge the debt we owe to our own teachers, especially Dame Professor Sheila Sherlock and Professor Monty Losowsky.

We are very grateful to Timothy Horne and Hannah Kenner at Elsevier for commissioning this book and supporting us through its gestation.

Richard G. Long
Brian B. Scott

Contents

General management of gastroenterology patients

MANAGEMENT OF OUT-PATIENTS

Gastroenterology is largely an out-patient specialty – most gastroenterological problems can be dealt with in the out-patient clinic without the need for admission. The main exceptions are patients with severe attacks of inflammatory bowel disease (IBD), severe liver decompensation, acute upper gastrointestinal (GI) haemorrhage and acute infective diarrhoea. There is much scope for organizing out-patient management to provide an efficient service for our patients and their referring GPs.

Booking and patient numbers

Most gastroenterology clinics in the UK consist of a mixture of new and follow-up patients. The Royal College of Physicians (RCP) recommends six to eight new patients or 15–20 follow-up patients per clinic. However, the workload in most UK hospitals is such that many consultants would see six to eight new patients plus 15 follow-ups per clinic. This is unsatisfactory, not least because it is impossible to give each patient the attention they need. It is impossible to predict how long each patient will take. Allowing the maximum likely time will result in a reduction in the total number of patients seen and gaps in the clinic, which is inefficient use of clinic time. Allowing the minimum time means that many patients will be kept waiting. Furthermore, GPs reasonably, but unpredictably, request urgent appointments that have to be squeezed in. Given the great variation in the complexity of patients' problems (from simple reflux or classical gallstones to severe Crohn's disease or decompensated liver disease) and in the need for detailed explanation and reassurance (from peptic ulcer to functional GI disturbance) one cannot safely allocate a standard time for each new and follow-up consultation. This all creates frustration for the consultant, discontented patients and complaints by management. This situation is likely to continue until there has been a great expansion in consultant numbers allowing compliance with RCP guidelines.

The number of booked patients should be adjusted according to the presence of students, Senior House Officers (SHOs) and Specialist Registrars (SpRs). All these are in the clinic primarily to be taught rather than to be an extra pair of hands. For students and SHOs the number of patients should be reduced to allow adequate teaching. Experienced SpRs have an overall neutral effect – the time spent in teaching them will be compensated by the increased throughput as they see some patients by themselves.

Depending on patient numbers it may be most efficient to have some regular specialized clinics such as hepatitis C, IBD, coeliac disease and decompensated liver disease, interspersed among general clinics. This may allow the joint involvement of dietitians and nurse specialists. IBD is perhaps the single largest group of patients attending gastroenterology clinics and it may, therefore, not be appropriate for the general gastroenterologist to segregate such patients. In any case there are several IBD patients every week who need an urgent appointment with a relapse and need to be fitted into the next clinic. It is helpful to have access to a specialist gastrointestinal surgeon in an adjoining clinic to allow cross referral. Clearly, in hospitals, especially teaching hospitals, with subspecialization of consultants, many clinics will be appropriately specialized.

Grading

Ideally, all patients should be seen within 2 weeks. Even if the condition turns out to be non-serious most patients, understandably, remain anxious until they are seen in the clinic. This ideal is seldom achieved. Most experienced consultants are able to determine from the referral letter the level of urgency and give urgent problems an early appointment. Unfortunately, their ability to correctly grade patients has been undermined by the government's cancer 2 week wait initiatives. Patients whose GPs choose to refer patients under this initiative are nearly always guaranteed an appointment within 2 weeks. Slots for such new patients have to be saved, thus reducing the spaces for other patients whose condition may be more deserving of an early appointment. Severe diarrhoea, dysphagia and jaundice are examples of conditions usually requiring an urgent appointment. If the total referral numbers exceed the capacity of the clinic then the waiting list will grow and the non-urgent patients may not be seen at all unless there are slots provided in each clinic for less urgent problems or the hospital arranges additional waiting-list-reduction clinics.

Pre-investigations

Usual abbreviations or acronyms for common investigations are shown in Box 1.1. It can often save time if certain tests are arranged in advance of the appointment. This requires the consultant's careful reading of the referral letter, often in conjunction with the previous hospital notes. For instance, patients with iron-deficiency anaemia could have a barium enema or oesophagogastroduodenoscopy (OGD) and small-bowel biopsy booked before their appointment. Patients referred with a positive hepatitis C virus (HCV) antibody test could have the polymerase chain reaction (PCR) test for HCV RNA allowing more precise planning of management when the patient comes to the clinic. Patients with abnormal liver function tests (LFTs) could have the usual diagnostic serology done. All these preliminary tests can be simply arranged by filling in the appropriate request card and writing to the patient, with a copy to the GP. The patients may be made less anxious by the wait for their appointment if they realize that they are already being investigated.

Box 1.1: Acronyms of some common investigations

OGD:	Oesophago-gastro-duodenoscopy
LFTs:	Liver function tests
U&Es:	Urea and electrolytes
FBC:	Full blood count
PCR test:	Polymerase chain reaction test e.g. for:
HCV:	Hepatitis C virus
RNA:	Ribonucleic acid
DEXA:	Dual energy X-ray absorptiometry

For review patients it may also be useful to arrange investigations just before their review appointment, e.g. urea and electrolytes (U&Es) in cirrhotics on diuretics, LFTs in primary biliary cirrhosis and autoimmune hepatitis. This is easily done by giving the patient the test request card at the previous appointment and asking them to take it either to the hospital laboratory or their GP's surgery (by arrangement with the practice nurse) a week before the next appointment. This enables firm management decisions to be taken in the clinic and obviates the need to see the case notes again.

Patient information before first attendance

Many patients have strange preconceptions about what will happen in the clinic. Often a GP will have mentioned the possibility of an OGD and the patient will be expecting that to be done at their first attendance causing both unnecessary anxiety and disappointment. Unfortunately, it is too complicated to set up a system to explain to most patients what to expect. However, there are certain vulnerable groups who may benefit from coaxing by an informative letter. For instance, a letter may be sent out with the appointment for patients with hepatitis C (a group notorious for non-attendance) explaining what will happen in the clinic and that, for instance, they will not be having a liver biopsy at that first attendance.

One-stop management

It is most rewarding to be able to diagnose and initiate treatment at the very first visit. Some conditions require a number of blood tests, imaging, etc., which, realistically, cannot be completed at the first visit. Colitis, however, can often be completely diagnosed in the clinic by flexible sigmoidoscopy and sometimes rigid sigmoidoscopy, especially if the upper limit is detected. A negative complete flexible sigmoidoscopy may be all that is necessary for anal-canal type bleeding and patients with irritable bowel may benefit from a negative sigmoidoscopy. Such patients may be discharged at that stage without need of a further visit. This facility does need willing out-patient staff and a robust system of cleaning and disinfecting the scopes. If the endoscopy unit is not too far away, it is usually best to send them there for disinfecting.

Patients needing OGD can be offered that examination during their first visit with appropriate organization and prior information. However, some would prefer to spend two short spells at the hospital on separate occasions than having to give up a whole half, or even full day. In addition, some patients would prefer to avoid the uncertainty of whether or not they were going to have the OGD at the first visit.

Extent of examination

Most gastroenterologists are also general physicians and formerly a full physical examination was expected on all patients, as in the MRCP (UK) long case, to avoid missing any medical problem. The pressure of work is now such that it is probably not efficient to do this for gastroenterological symptoms. In practice, the physical examination is seldom rewarding for GI symptoms; the history is usually the most revealing part of the consultation. It seems reasonable to leave the management of coincidental problems, such as hypertension, airways disease and cardiac problems, to the GP. However, for patients proceeding to invasive investigations such as endoscopy, it is useful to have a baseline knowledge of basic heart and lung function. Urine stick testing is a useful routine that may reveal relevant glycosuria or haematuria.

Examination of the neck for lymph nodes and the abdomen for masses and enlarged organs is sufficient for most patients with GI symptoms. In those with discomfort or pain in the lower chest or upper abdomen, especially right or left upper quadrant pain, which does not fit any particular GI problem, it is important to systematically and firmly palpate the costal margin looking for a tender spot, pressure on which reproduces the symptoms. This is the painful rib syndrome, a common condition for which reassurance and explanation is usually sufficient without the need for investigation or a further visit.

Sigmoidoscopy/proctoscopy is usually indicated for diarrhoea, rectal symptoms and rectal bleeding and this is often preceded by digital rectal examination. Digital rectal examination is otherwise seldom useful, although often recommended. Many gastroenterologists consider the benefits of routine digital rectal examination is outweighed by the discomfort, embarrassment and inconvenience.

Patient information sheets

Patients are often given more information with regard to the nature of their problem and its treatment than they can retain. It is, therefore, important to give appropriate information sheets or booklets. There are many sources of useful disease booklets, some of which are shown in Table 1.1. It is best to keep a supply in the clinic. However, they soon run out or become outdated and the patient at least should be offered details of the source or the web site so that they can obtain the information for themselves. The professionally produced booklets may not quite agree with local practice, in which case local literature should be produced to avoid the confusion of contradictory advice or information. Production of patient information needs a lot of practise and input from lay friends so that jargon is avoided and simple language used.

Table 1.1 UK sources of useful patient information booklets

Source	Address	Web site / telephone	Particularly useful booklets
British Liver Trust	Ransomes Europark Ipswich IP3 9QG	www.britishlivertrust.org.uk Tel.: 01473 276326	*Hepatitis B and C* (among others)
The PBC Foundation	The Dean, Longniddry, East Lothian EH32 0PN	Tel.: 01875 853552	*Primary biliary cirrhosis*
The Haemochromatosis Society	Hollybush Mount, Hadley Green Road, Barnet EN5 5PR	www.ghsoc.org Tel.: 020 84491363	*Haemochromatosis - an iron overload disorder*
National Association for Colitis and Crohn's (NACC)	4 Beaumont House, Sutton Road, St Albans, Herts AL1 5HH	www.nacc.org.uk Tel.: 01727 844296	*Understanding colitis and Crohn's disease* (among others)
Digestive Disorders Foundation	PO Box 251, Edgware, Middlesex HA8 6HG	www.digestivedisorders. org.uk	*Irritable bowel syndrome* (among others)
Coeliac UK	PO Box 362, High Wycombe, Bucks HP11 2GW	Tel.: 01494 437278 Between 10 am and 4 pm	*New Members Pack* including *Food & Drink Directory* and *The Coeliac Handbook*

For many problems, such as aerophagy, globus syndrome and pruritus ani, there does not appear to be any professionally produced literature and, therefore, units should be prepared to produce their own.

Patients increasingly want to know about their drugs. Patient information sheets covering the most frequently used drugs should be available. Drug company inserts are not useful – in fact they are positively harmful, often deterring use of the drug by the unbalanced presentation of every possible side effect. The drugs used in IBD are perhaps the most important group because of the large number of patients and their long-term use, often during pregnancy. These include aminosalicylates, steroids, azathioprine/mercaptopurine, methotrexate, ciclosporin and infliximab. An example of such a sheet used in Lincoln is shown in Figure 1.1.

Communication skills

Many patients are anxious, especially at their first out-patient appointment and they need to be put at their ease. Joviality has its place, but a formal introduction is most appreciated. It is important both that patients know whom they are seeing and that the doctor is clear about the patient's identity. After an opening such as, 'Hello, I'm Dr Scott. I'm sorry to have kept you waiting. Are you Jane Smith?' It might be appropriate to say, 'Your GP has told me a lot about you, but, in your own words, would you describe what you have noticed wrong yourself .... What is the main thing that's been bothering you?' or, 'Your GP has sent you to see me because he found that your liver tests were slightly abnormal. Is that right?'. To focus further on symptoms it is usually best to ask precisely

United Lincolnshire Hospitals

Drugs used in ulcerative colitis and Crohn's disease

Patient Information Sheet No. 2:

Steroids (prednisolone tablets)

What are steroids?

Steroids (strictly, **corticosteroids**) are hormones produced naturally by the adrenal glands. They maintain health and have effects on blood pressure, salts in the blood and glucose. When the body is under stress (for example in illness, after trauma, and following surgery) the adrenal gland produces more corticosteroid. Corticosteroids also help to reduce inflammation in many parts of the body and this is the main reason for using artificial corticosteroids in diseases such as Crohn's disease and ulcerative colitis in which there is inflammation of the bowel wall.

There are other types of steroids such as anabolic steroids used illegally by sportsmen and also by body builders. These are not the ones used by doctors in patients with inflammatory bowel disease.

When steroids are prescribed they are usually in the form of tablets called **prednisolone**. Sometimes steroids need to be given by injection and then we use another preparation called **hydrocortisone**. Some patients with inflammation mainly affecting the back passage (rectum) may be given prednisolone or hydrocortisone in the form of a suppository or enema.

How do I take them?

Prednisolone is taken by mouth in one dose every morning, preferably after breakfast if breakfast is taken. The usual size of tablet is 5mg. In an attack of colitis or Crohn's disease it is usual to start with 12 tablets (60mg) or 8 tablets (40mg) every morning for five days before reducing every 5 days until finishing.

How effective are steroids?

They are the most powerful drugs we have for rapidly reducing inflammation in the bowel. Most patients feel better within a week. Unfortunately about one in five patients doesn't respond well, but there is no way of knowing this beforehand.

What are the side effects?

Many patients notice no side effects at all. The commonest effects are weight gain, puffy face and a spotty skin (particularly on the back).

Because they reduce inflammation they may make patients more susceptible to infections. If someone has had TB in the past it might become active again. Patients who have never had chickenpox may become severely ill if they come in contact with someone with chickenpox. Raised blood pressure, easy bruising and diabetes might also develop. Some people notice mood changes. All these effects disappear after the course of steroids is finished, although after a prolonged course the body's own production of steroid (by the adrenal glands) may be depressed for a while and the patient may become ill under stress (for example after a road traffic accident or an operation). You will therefore be given a **blue warning card** to carry with you at all times so that a boost of steroid can be given if you do become ill.

One of the more serious effects is thinning of the bone (**osteoporosis**) and this will make patients more susceptible to bone fractures later in life, even when the course of steroids has finished. To try and minimize this you will be given the lowest dose for as short a time as possible. You may be given a bone density scan (DEXA scan), and you may be advised to taken tablets of **calcium and vitamin D** (such as Calichew D3 Forte or Cacit D3) whenever you are taking steroids. If the bone density is low you may also be given a **bisphosphonate** drug (such as etidronate, alendronate and risedronate) to either improve bone density or to protect the bones from the damaging effect of steroids.

Your doctor will have weighed up the risk of all these and other side effects before advising this treatment and will have decided that the bowel inflammation is bad enough to need these powerful drugs.

Can these drugs be taken during pregnancy?

Yes. There is no evidence that these drugs can cause damage to an unborn child. During breastfeeding small amounts of steroid may appear in the milk but that is unlikely to cause a problem.

Are there alternatives?

In patients with Crohn's disease a special liquid **elemental diet** without any ordinary food for 2–3 weeks is as effective as steroids and can always be considered. Unfortunately, many patients cannot tolerate this. There is a special information sheet about this treatment.

For patients with Crohn's disease or ulcerative colitis who need more than one course of steroids in a year we usually recommend a drug called **azathioprine** which can be taken for many years without causing osteoporosis. Use of azathioprine usually reduces the chance of relapsing and therefore reduces the chance of needing further steroids. There is a separate information sheet about this drug.

BBS 24.10.02

Fig. 1.1
A patient information sheet for steroid treatment

directed closed questions such as, 'In the past month/year, what is the longest you've gone without your pain/diarrhoea. What is the longest the pain/diarrhoea has lasted? What is the shortest time? During your attacks of diarrhoea, what is the most number of times you've been to the toilet in 24 hours? What is the least number of times? In an attack, what is the longest the pain has lasted? What is the shortest?'

During explanation of the diagnosis and management it is important not to speak for too long without checking the patient's understanding and giving them chance to ask questions. Bombarding the patient with information is usually counterproductive. Non-essential information should be avoided unless requested. Writing down the important points or giving a previously prepared patient information sheet is appreciated (see later).

Dissatisfied patients

Some patients and their relatives become angry when the diagnosis or plan is not what they expected and may verbally attack the doctor. In this situation it is usually best to keep the dialogue going with empathy, allow them to express their concerns and respond sensitively. It should always be the doctor's intention for the patient to leave the consultation satisfied, if not happy. Patients with functional disturbances and those with medically unexplained symptoms are more likely to be dissatisfied. But, for all patients, if dissatisfaction is sensed it is best to keep the patient talking until the cause of dissatisfaction is understood and, hopefully, dealt with. Some patients have such bizarre perceptions and preconceived ideas that no amount of explanation will satisfy and the consultation may have to terminate firmly with the statement that an honest and thoughtful opinion has been given that will be conveyed to their GP. If a second opinion is requested in such situations it is usually best to ask the patient to discuss this with the GP. This gives the patient time to reflect and avoids overburdening colleagues.

Management plans

We should all aim to follow best practice in the management of all conditions. There are now authoritative evidence-based guidelines for most gastroenterological problems. The British Society of Gastroenterology (BSG) guidelines are particularly appropriate (website: *www.bsg.org.uk*). However, it is difficult to remember even the salient details and summaries should be readily available in the clinic as aide memoires. Surveillance intervals after colonic polypectomy, timing of DEXA scans in IBD, monitoring of HCV treatment, indications for infliximab in Crohn's disease, diagnostic serology in the investigation of abnormal LFTs are a few examples of topics for which such aides mémoire may be useful.

Pro formas can save a lot of time as well as directing us to the right management plan. The monitoring of treatment of hepatitis C with peginterferon and ribavirin and the serial weights, blood counts and biochemistry of patients with ascites, for instance, lend themselves to this approach.

Investigations

Serial or en bloc?

To save money on tests it is best to do one at a time. However, this may not be cost effective in the long run and will prolong investigation. Investigating abnormal LFTs is a good example. Should one await the result of the ferritin or the immunoglobulins and autoantibodies before requesting tests for hepatitis B and C? Much will depend on the cost and availability of the different tests as well as the pre test probability of the various conditions being sought. Most of us would arrange all the blood tests at the first visit and see the results before deciding on imaging or biopsy. In the investigation of malabsorptive diarrhoea, should one await the result of small-bowel biopsy (which can usually be done within a few days) or endomysial antibody test before initiating testing of pancreatic function?

Threshold for arranging tests with waiting lists

To a large extent, the delay between deciding on a test such as endoscopy and its performance is determined by the gastroenterologist. If endoscopy is booked for every patient that it might possibly help, no patient will have it promptly – a 6-month delay is not uncommon. However, if endoscopy is reserved for those who are most likely to benefit it may be possible to avoid any waiting list. By following this policy, the author has nearly always been able to offer endoscopy within 1 week, apart from during periods of leave. In units with many colleagues requesting endoscopy this policy would only work if all subscribed to it and were able to agree on thresholds.

Dealing with results

A large part of a gastroenterologist's work is receiving and responding to reports of investigations. Although one gets no credit for dealing with these outside the out-patient clinics, it is far more efficient and less trouble for patients to do so than to give all patients a routine follow-up appointment simply to see and convey the results. To deal with results outside the clinic it is necessary to see the results with the case notes – it is not sufficient to see case notes just on patients with abnormal results; normal results may need action (e.g. stopping iron if no longer anaemic, or reducing steroids if LFTs are normal in autoimmune hepatitis). Furthermore, we should not underestimate the anxiety of most patients whilst awaiting even the simplest blood test, let alone a scan or barium enema looking for cancer. It is, therefore, appropriate to communicate the results by post to the patient at the earliest opportunity, usually with a copy to the GP. Often, this means that the patient can be discharged without coming back to the clinic. If the test result doesn't give a clear diagnosis then further tests can be arranged without seeing the patient, but with a suitable explanation. Where a serious diagnosis is made it is usually best to bring the patient back to the clinic as soon as possible after the test. No patient would appreciate seeing their consultant at a planned appointment 2 months after a barium enema to be told that it shows cancer.

Because individual results often come at different times, the secretary will need guidelines on when to hand over the results. For instance, one might give instructions to bring all the results together on a patient with suspected IBD when the histology is available, or on a hepatitis C patient when the result of the PCR test for HCV RNA is available. This will depend on knowledge of how long the various tests take to be reported. There needs to be a fail safe mechanism to deal with tests that go astray. The secretary will, therefore, need instructions on when to bring the notes back even if all the results have not been reported.

Breaking bad news

Although many patients are relieved to be given a diagnosis and treatment plan, for some the realization that they have a serious disease (particularly cancer, but also IBD, cirrhosis, HCV infection, etc.) can be very stressful and distressing. Having assessed the patient previously in the clinic may give an indication of the likely response and appropriate action to take, e.g. inviting the spouse or close relative or friend to the consultation and arranging for the appropriate nurse specialist to be present. If referral to another specialist is planned, e.g. surgeon or oncologist, it is best to have arranged that appointment beforehand and not more than a few days later. This helps to reassure the patient that everything is being done expeditiously and that their problem is being taken seriously. It is also important to realize that in the situation of receiving bad news the details of the interview may not be remembered correctly. Writing down the diagnosis, the treatment options and details of the next move, possibly with an explanatory pamphlet, will be appreciated.

Follow-up appointments

The decision on the need for follow-up appointments is important. It should be realized that if more new patients are followed-up than follow-up patients are discharged, the number of patients attending the clinic will grow progressively. The need for follow-up should be considered carefully for all patients. It is not necessary to bring all new patients back to see how they are doing or to see and convey results of tests. This can mostly be done by correspondence with the patient and GP. Don't assume that all patients prefer to see you again. It is often a struggle for an elderly or disabled patient and many working patients find it inconvenient or a threat to their job security.

Some chronic gastroenterological problems will usually require long-term follow-up by a consultant because of the high level of expertise required. These would include chronic or frequently relapsing IBD, decompensated cirrhosis and hepatitis C. Depending on the co-operation and training of GPs many other problems can be delegated to the GP with appropriate arrangements for urgent consultant review as necessary. Stable IBD lends itself to such shared care. Unfortunately, one is not able to readily advise on changes of practice such as the recently introduced renal-function testing in patients on aminosalicylates or testing for and treatment of osteoporosis. Many coeliac patients seem to manage very well without hospital follow-up, although many consultants feel that regular, albeit infrequent follow-up helps to deter straying from the diet and to recognize worrying features such as weight loss, further GI symptoms and osteoporosis. The educational value to the consultant of regular follow-up, especially of IBD, should not be ignored. It helps to give a global view of IBD in all its variety, which is to the benefit of all IBD patients. A policy on these issues needs to be formulated with the help of GPs and colleagues, but the view of individual patients will also need to be taken into account.

Out-patient prescribing

From the outset it is important to decide on the appropriate role of a consultant. The consultant is not usually responsible for the total medical care of a patient. The patient nearly always remains firmly under the basic care of a GP. The word 'consultant' helps to remind many consultants that they are basically being consulted by a GP for their advice on the diagnosis and management of their patient. It will usually be appropriate for the consultant to arrange all the appropriate investigations, although where standard blood tests are all that are needed, it is often more convenient for them to be arranged at the GP's surgery. Certainly many patients express this preference, especially when there are long queues at the venesection clinics. As far as out-patient prescribing is concerned, it seems most appropriate to make recommendations to the GP rather than write the prescription. GPs may have their own preferences when there are a number of drugs in the class; they will also be surer of what other drugs are being prescribed and there will be no doubt about what the patient is taking should the patient report side effects. The exception is where the delay would be detrimental. This mainly applies to steroids for IBD. Although most hospital pharmacies prefer to limit prescriptions to 2 weeks, it is important that for such a drug as prednisolone, given in a reducing course, the whole course is given to avoid confusion, especially since it is inexpensive.

Shared care

Some GPs are unhappy at prescribing drugs for an unlicensed indication, even though it is standard treatment. An example is azathioprine for IBD. However, it is quite within a GP's capability to prescribe and monitor, with appropriate guidance from the consultant, in a shared-care arrangement. In fact, the additional workload of regular prescription and blood monitoring of hundreds of IBD patients is more than some clinics can manage. Although an IBD nurse specialist could be employed for this, their time might be better spent in counselling patients and advising them in relapses. Other considerations include the preference of patients, especially in rural areas, for local monitoring and prescribing by their GP and, should the patient report a side effect, the GP would be fully aware of what is being prescribed (not always the case when prescribing is done at a hospital clinic). It may be appropriate to follow the policy of saying that, if the GP is not prepared to take our recommendation on the prescription of azathioprine, the patient does not get it. However, in some other districts, long-established practice would make the transfer to such a policy difficult.

MANAGEMENT OF IN-PATIENTS

Type of gastrointestinal problems encountered on the wards

Only a small minority of gastroenterology patients ever require in-patient management. They include patients with severe IBD, acute GI bleeding, decompensated liver disease, acute infective gastroenteritis and, sometimes, patients with advanced metastatic cancer. Patients seldom require admission solely for investigation, that is most efficiently organized on an out-patient basis.

Written protocols

The above sorts of gastroenterology problems lend themselves to management by written protocols. This is especially important when junior staff are on short attachments or are frequently absent from their main ward to be on duty on the admission ward, when continuity of care may be jeopardized. The management of severe colitis (Fig. 1.2), ascites, encephalopathy, hepato-renal syndrome, alcoholic hepatitis, GI bleeding, variceal bleeding, paracetamol poisoning and alcohol-withdrawal syndrome can all be optimized by succinct, frequently updated protocols. Thus, all the staff can be fully conversant with the management plan for each patient.

Support from other disciplines

It is most helpful to have the opportunity to regularly discuss patients and policy with pharmacists, dietitians and IBD and liver nurse specialists, as well as the ward nursing staff.

Care of the dying patient

Dying patients and their relatives need to be handled very sensitively, with special consideration given to them. Going out of the way to deal with their needs is often very much appreciated and should not be done grudgingly. After all, there may not be anything more useful than this that can be offered. The doctor should be available to talk to relatives after the death, especially when death is sudden or unexpected.

Specialist areas within medical wards

The same gastroenterology problems also require specialized nursing. It is, therefore, desirable to have designated areas (perhaps a bay within a general medical ward), with some protection of the beds so that they are always available for patients with such problems, where expertise can be concentrated and where there can be joint care with surgeons. This is especially important for severe GI bleeding, severe colitis and severe small-intestinal (mainly Crohn's) disease.

Preparation for discharge

It is important for a diagnosis to be decided and recorded in notes by the consultant or specialist registrar before discharge. The need for follow-up, if at all, after discharge needs to be considered and the reason should be specified so that the doctor seeing the patient in the clinic can see at a glance what is required. Blood tests are often needed before the clinic appointment and it is usually best to give the patient the appropriate blood test

LINCOLN COUNTY HOSPITAL

Management of severe ulcerative colitis (and severe Crohn's colitis)
(Modified Truelove Regime)

1. Set up iv infusion. Correct dehydration and electrolyte losses.
   Correct significant anaemia with blood transfusion (usually aim to keep Hb above 10.0g/dl).

2. Maintain fluid and electrolyte balance and nutrition according to individual requirements.
   A typical daily regime is:
   > 1 litre 0.9% saline containing 20 mEq potassium chloride over 8 hours
   > 1 litre 5% dextrose containing 20 mEq potassium chloride over 8 hours
   > 1 litre 0.9% saline containing 20 mEq potassium chloride over 8 hours

3. Give hydrocortisone 100mg iv 6 hourly.

4. Give rectal steroid retention enema bd,e.g. Predsol (prednisolone 20mg in 100ml) over about 20 mins. (There is no conclusive evidence that this is necessary but it has formed part of the traditional successful regimes.) Avoid if patient finds it distressing.

5. Give nothing by mouth except clear fluids for the first 36 hours. Taking a normal diet after that doesn't appear to affect the outcome, but some patients feel better continuing with clear fluids. Depending on patient's preference, allow light diet or sip feeds such as Fortisip and Maxijul (the dietitian will advise). Consider parenteral nutrition if poorly nourished.

6. Give heparin 10 000 units bd subcutaneously. As well as helping prevent venous thrombosis, which is more common in colitis, there is some evidence it helps recovery.

The above regime should be continued for 5–7 days.

If, on Day 3 of treatment, BO >8 daily, or BO x 3–8 **plus** CRP >45, there is an 85% chance the patient will need colectomy. Thus, the use of **ciclosporin** commencing on Day 4 should be considered and discussed with patient. See separate **ciclosporin** information sheet.

If there is no improvement by 7 days, or deterioration before then, discuss emergency colectomy with colorectal surgeon. If surgery seems likely ask stoma-therapist (bleep) to explain the implications of life with an ileostomy.

If there is good improvement at 5–7 days, allow normal feeding, give prednisolone 40–60mg mane orally and a 5ASA preparation (e.g. sulfasalazine 1g bd, or Asacol 400mg tds). Prednisolone is usually reduced every 5–7 days (e.g. 60mg mane, 40mg mane, 30mg mane, 25mg mane, 20mg mane, 15mg mane, 10mg mane and 5mg mane). When patient goes home prescribe the **whole** prednisolone course from our pharmacy.

Investigations:
- Stool culture and examination for *Clostridium difficile* toxin
- Daily stool chart recording number of bowel motions, consistency and amount of blood
- FBC and U&Es, CRP daily
- LFTs before and after 5 days
- Plain x-ray of abdomen at onset and repeat daily *if* any suggestion of toxic dilatation either radiologically (e.g. the minimum diameter of the transverse colon >5cm) or clinically
- Examine abdomen daily looking for tenderness and distension
- Record abdominal girth daily

Fig. 1.2
Ward protocol for managing severe colitis

request form to take to their GP a few days before the clinic appointment. An offer to see certain patients again, if necessary at short notice, can provide support, especially for those with advanced cancer; they will need to be given a contact number.

Further Reading

RCP Report: Consultant Physician's Working for Patients. Royal College of Physicians, London, June 1999
Scott EM, Scott BB. Painful rib syndrome – a review of 76 cases. Gut 1993; 34: 1006–8.

Upper gastrointestinal disease

2

Diseases of the upper gastrointestinal (GI) tract are the bread and butter of all bar the most specialized gastroenterologist. As gastroscopy is usually the first endoscopic procedure learnt by trainees, it is also the area of gastroenterology trainees get the most exposure to (with or without supervision). It is also an area where huge uncertainties remain (e.g. how to manage Barrett's oesophagus, what is the best operation for gastric carcinoma) and where new endoscopic techniques are being introduced all the time.

This chapter will be divided into two sections. Section 1 will cover the background and management of the most commonly seen upper GI conditions. This will include summaries of available evidence and data to allow informed discussion with patients, and national (and international) guidelines where relevant. Section 2 will outline commonly used upper GI investigations. Attempts will be made to demystify some of the terminology used. Guidelines for upper GI endoscopy (e.g. anticoagulation and antibiotic prophylaxis) and upper GI bleeding are covered elsewhere in this book.

SECTION 1: DISEASES OF THE UPPER GASTROINTESTINAL TRACT

Dysphagia

How should we investigate patients with dysphagia?

Patients with dysphagia are referred to both gastroenterologists and ear, nose and throat (ENT) surgeons at the discretion of GPs. The sensation of 'something sticking in the throat' is probably best investigated by direct pharyngoscopy following careful palpation, usually in the realm of ENT specialists. If this is normal a barium swallow may reveal a pharyngeal pouch or swallow co-ordination problems. If there is a high suspicion of an oropharyngeal dysmotility (i.e. symptoms of aspiration, repeated swallow attempts, history of neurological disease), videofluoroscopy is the most useful investigation. The common and important causes of dysphagia are listed in Box 2.1.

Box 2.1 Causes of dysphagia

- Dysmotility
  - Achalasia
  - Primary oesophageal dysmotility
  - Secondary dysmotility
  - Cricopharyngeal spasm
- Benign strictures
  - Reflux induced
  - Collagen diseases (e.g. CREST)
  - Radiation
  - Post surgical
  - Oesophageal webs/Schatzki ring
- Malignant strictures
- Infection
  - Candidiasis
  - CMV
- Extrinsic compression
- Gastro-oesophageal reflux disease

Oesophageal dysphagia can be initially investigated either with barium (or other contrast) swallow or gastroscopy. Some people feel that 'high dysphagia' should always be investigated by contrast swallow prior to endoscopy, in case there is a pharyngeal pouch. However, provided visualization of all the pharyngeal structures is maintained at intubation and excessive force is avoided, perforation should be averted. The choice of which modality to use first in dysphagia is outlined in Table 2.1. In many cases, however, the choice is governed by waiting lists.

If a motility disorder is suspected, either on history or from investigations, barium swallow and oesophageal manometry should be performed. These require expert interpretation by the person performing the test, but key features of the commoner causes of dysmotility are outlined later in this chapter.

Dyspepsia

What is dyspepsia?

Dyspepsia can be defined as persistent or recurrent abdominal discomfort centred in the upper abdomen or epigastrium.

How should we investigate patients with dyspepsia?

Dyspepsia accounts for 10% of GP consultations. Ten per cent of these patients will be referred to gastroenterologists. Gastro-oesophageal reflux is extremely common, accounting for 60% of 'dyspepsia' and can usually be diagnosed on history alone (heartburn, oro-pharyngeal reflux, response to acid inhibition).

Table 2.1. Risks and benefits of investigations for dysphagia

	Contrast swallow	Endoscopy
Benefits	Avoids perforation Allows motility to be assessed Can demonstrate gastro-oesophageal reflux (GOR)	High sensitivity for mucosal disease Allows biopsies
Risks	Aspiration	Perforation Failure to intubate stomach

Below the age of 55 years, reflux symptoms **alone** are extremely unlikely to be due to a malignant cause. Such patients can be safely managed with acid inhibition and do not need endoscopy. The only possible benefits of endoscopy in such patients are the identification of patients with Barrett's oesophagus and the finding of incidental early neoplasms. Current waiting lists often prohibit this.

Patients with non-reflux dyspepsia under the age of 55 can be managed either with a trial of acid suppression (many of these will still have dyspepsia due to reflux without typical symptoms) or by testing and treating for *H. pylori*. This will resolve symptoms in between 5 and 10% of patients and is not without its risks.

Above the age of 55, cancer is still only present in 2% of patients with dyspepsia. Patients over 55 **without** alarm symptoms can probably be managed similarly. However, many are uncomfortable with this and endoscopy is probably appropriate.

In the UK there are national criteria for identifying those who need urgent investigation. These criteria are listed in Table 2.2.

National guidelines

There are numerous dyspepsia guidelines throughout the UK.

The British Society of Gastroenterology (BSG) has produced guidelines that are rational, but rather non-prescriptive. They suggest test and treating for *H. pylori* below the age of 55, prompt endoscopy in new-onset dyspepsia over the age of 55 and 'antisecretory' treatment in under 55 years.

The Scottish Intercollegiate Guidelines Network (SIGN) have also produced guidelines that are rather more dogmatic. The Scottish guidelines specifically do not include a proton pump inhibitor (PPI) trial and do suggest test and treating for *H. pylori* in all age groups. (The evidence for test and treating over the age of 55 is rather sparse.)

The National Institute for Clinical Excellence (NICE) produced *Dyspepsia – management of dsypepsia in adults in primary care* in August 2004.

Our local guideline is shown in Figure 2.1, which may be helpful.

Table 2.2 Two-week upper gastrointestinal cancer guidelines

Alarm symptoms	Approximate incidence of cancer*
Dysphagia – food sticking on swallowing (any age)	10–15%
Dyspepsia at any age combined with one or more of the following alarm symptoms:	
Weight loss	15–20%
Proven anaemia	20%
Vomiting	5%
Dyspepsia in a patient aged 55 years or more with at least one of the following 'high-risk' features:	
Onset of dyspepsia less than 1 year ago	10%
Continuous symptoms since onset	5–10%
Dyspepsia combined with at least one of the following known risk factors:	No local data
Family history of upper gastrointestinal cancer in more than two first-degree relatives	
Barrett's oesophagus	
Pernicious anaemia	
Peptic ulcer surgery over 20 years ago	
Known dysplasia, atrophic gastritis, intestinal metaplasia	
Jaundice	35%
Upper abdominal mass	30%

*Data from referrals to Derby hospitals 1999–2002.

Gastro-oesophageal reflux disease

Should we endoscope patients with reflux disease?

Ideally, yes. It may confirm the diagnosis and detect complications. It may also reveal incidental tumours of the upper GI tract. However, the UK is a resource-poor environment and it is impossible to endoscope everyone with reflux symptoms. Endoscopy is normal in 30–60% of cases and symptoms are a very poor measure of severity of oesophagitis. Twenty-five per cent of people with mild symptoms have severe reflux oesophagitis and 20% of people with GORD have no endoscopic evidence of oesophagitis. However, improvement in symptoms does correlate well with healing of oesophagitis.

Different types of gastro-oesophageal reflux disease

GORD can be categorized into three broad groups according to the findings at endoscopy, 24-h pH studies and relation of symptoms to reflux episodes.

Erosive gastro-oesophageal reflux disease

In this case there is endoscopic evidence of GORD with or without symptoms. However, it can also be due to duodenogastro-oesophageal reflux.

Non-erosive gastro-oesophageal reflux disease

This has a normal endoscopic appearance, but typical symptoms and evidence of abnormal acid exposure on 24-h pH studies.

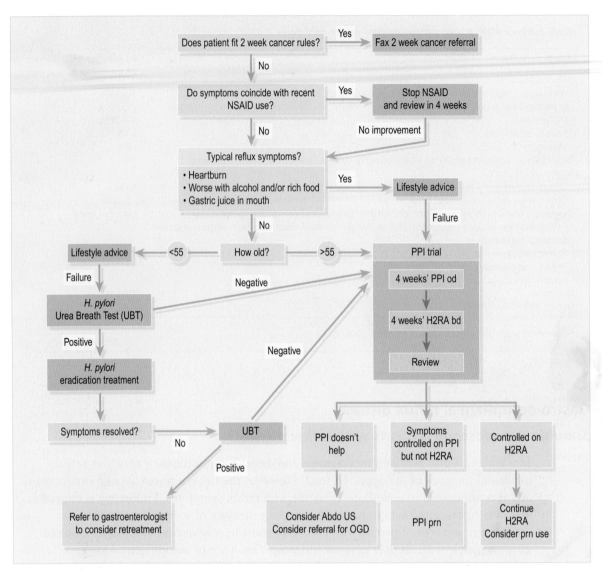

Fig. 2.1
A suggested dyspepsia guideline for primary care trusts. OGD, oesophago-gastro-duodenoscopy

Acid-sensitive, non-erosive gastro-oesophageal reflux disease

This has a normal endoscopic appearance, but typical symptoms with normal acid exposure on 24-h pH studies and correlation of symptoms with episodes of acid exposure.

These types are only useful insofar that the latter two only very rarely develop complications. The management of all types is the same.

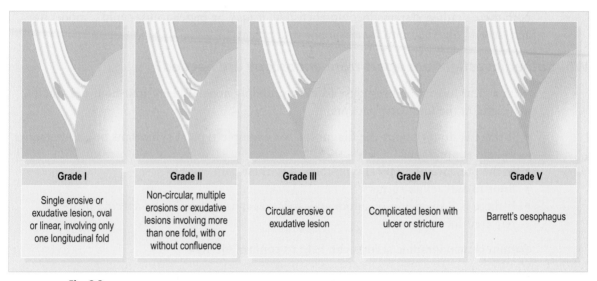

Fig. 2.2
Savary–Miller classification of reflux oesophagitis

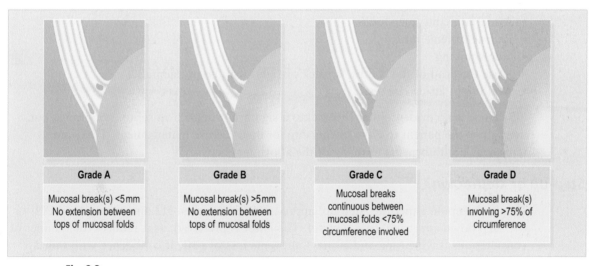

Fig. 2.3
Los Angeles classification of reflux oesophagitis

How do we classify endoscopic appearances of oesophagitis?

There are many ways of classifying oesophagitis (over 30 at the last count), the two commonest being the Savary-Miller and Los Angeles classifications. These are detailed in Figures 2.2 and 2.3. The Los Angeles system was developed by an international working group in an attempt to unify endoscopic grading. However, many patients and GPs find both these grading systems incomprehensible; it may be better to use 'mild', 'moderate' and 'severe' together with a measurement of extent.

What other investigations apart from endoscopy are needed?

With a clear history and response to PPIs, probably none. Twenty-four-hour pH studies are useful in the following patients:

- If there is doubt about the diagnosis, for example typical symptoms but no response to acid suppression.
- In the presence of atypical symptoms, e.g. chest pain.
- Prior to anti-reflux surgery.
- If there is a suspicion of duodenogastric-oesophageal reflux (a specific probe is required for this).

Barium or scintigraphic studies can help to confirm GORD.

What 'lifestyle manoeuvres' should be suggested to patients?

- Lose weight
- Eat smaller meals more regularly
- Don't eat late at night
- Avoid fatty and spicy foods
- Reduce caffeine intake
- Stop smoking
- Raise the head of the bed by 'a brick's height' (can be problematic)
- Avoid tight fitting clothes.

NB. There is no evidence that this makes a significant impact on reflux symptoms, but does allow the patient to have 'ownership' of their disease management. There are numerous health benefits to many of the above manoeuvres.

Step-up or step-down?

People champion either the 'step up' approach (antacid, then H2 antagonist, then PPI) or the 'step down approach' (the reverse). The latter is preferred, as it reduces the number of consultations (saving time and money), prevents loss of patient confidence with failed treatments and rapidly heals reflux oesophagitis. A useful way to give a trial of PPI is to prescribe a 4-week course of PPI followed by a 4-week course of H2RA before the patient is reviewed. Follow-up treatment after this is outlined in Figure 2.4.

Long-term proton pump inhibitor or anti-reflux surgery?

Many patients are utterly symptom free on PPIs, but are unable to come off them. This leaves young (i.e. less than 60) patients with the prospect of taking a PPI for over 20 years. There is little data on the long-term risks of PPIs, but it seems likely that they are safe at least over 5 years. The data there are suggest an increase in oesophageal carcinoma, but only in those with Barrett's oesophagus or complicated reflux disease. This is almost certainly related to the underlying oesophageal disease **rather** than the PPI.

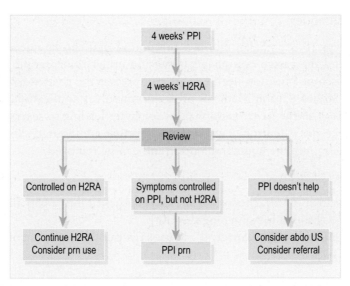

Fig. 2.4
Step-down management of gastro-oesophageal reflux disease

Concerns have been raised that PPIs drive *H. pylori* gastritis, leading to gastric atrophy and then possibly gastric carcinoma. This is all theoretical, but it may be worth eradicating *H. pylori* in patients with the prospect of taking long-term PPIs. However, there is also good evidence that this will increase the dose of PPI needed to control symptoms, which can itself lead to problems.

Techniques of anti-reflux surgery (ARS) are constantly improving. Open ARS has a mortality rate of at least 1:1000 and a morbidity rate of 10% (dysphagia, bloating, pain). Over 50% of patients who have had open ARS will still need to take a PPI to control their symptoms in the longer term. Open ARS does not reduce the incidence of Barrett's carcinoma or oesophageal carcinoma. Long-term results with laparoscopic ARS are awaited, but presumably will be similar.

What are the indications for anti-reflux surgery?

- Proven gastro-oesophageal reflux unresponsive to PPI (including 'volume reflux') without oesophageal dysmotility
- Intolerance to PPI
- Recurrent peptic strictures
- Patient preference (e.g. young patient on long-term PPI).

Are there any endoscopic treatments for gastro-oesophageal reflux disease?

There are several evolving endoscopic treatments for GORD. None have been extensively used in the UK and should be considered inferior to ARS until data otherwise exist. However, it seems likely that endoscopic fundoplication is here to stay and will improve considerably.

Non-suturing techniques

- Enteryx (Boston Scientific) is a compound that can be injected circumferentially around the gastro-oesophageal junction under fluoroscopic guidance via an endoscopic injection needle. This compresses the gastro-oesophageal junction (GOJ).
- The Stretta (Curon Medical) procedure involves application of radio-frequency ablation to the gastro-oesophageal sphincter leading to scarring.
- Gatekeeper (Medtronic) are small pellets that are inserted submucosally at the GOJ. These reduce the luminal diameter and can be removed.

Endoscopic fundoplication

- Endocinch (Bard). Mucosa at the GOJ is sucked into a cap allowing a suture to be placed through it, tightening the GOJ.
- The Plicator (NDO Surgical). Mucosa is pulled into a retroflexed plicator to tighten the GOJ.

What are the long-term complications of gastro-oesophageal reflux disease?

- Benign oesophageal stricture
- Barrett's oeosphagus
- Oesophageal carcinoma.

National Institute for Clinical Excellence guidelines for proton pump inhibitors (June 2000)

NICE has made several pronouncements on the use of PPIs in upper GI disease (Box 2.2). These guidelines are fairly free-ranging and will be subject to frequent review.

Benign oesophageal stricture

How can we confirm a stricture is benign?

The features shown in Box 2.3 suggest a stricture is benign.

However, all strictures should be biopsied at endoscopy (minimum of four biopsies). Unless the patient has severe dysphagia, it may be best to await the biopsy results before dilating the stricture as perforation is more common in malignant strictures (around 2%) and a perforated malignant stricture will necessitate stenting or even surgery.

How should benign strictures be dilated?

There are two methods of dilatation, balloon and bougie. Balloon dilatation is achieved with 'through the scope' (TTS) balloons. These can be of fixed diameter (e.g. 12, 14 and 16 mm) or of variable diameter (e.g. 12–15 mm, 15–18 mm). Some are reusable, others disposable. Some have the capacity to be passed over a guidewire. Numerous devices exist to inflate the balloons, depending on either volume or pressure to achieve the balloon diameter. The principle of balloon dilatation is that stricture fibres are disrupted by radial force. Bougie dilatation involved the passage of rigid dilators (bougies or 'olives') over a

Box 2.2 NICE recommendations on proton pump inhibitor use

- In patients with documented duodenal ulcer or gastric ulcer, a treatment strategy of testing for *H. pylori* and, where positive, eradicating the infection is recommended. Long-term acid-suppressing therapy should not be used. Those patients who are *H. pylori* negative or remain symptomatic after eradication therapy should be treated as described below.

- For patients with a documented non-steroidal anti-inflammatory-drug (NSAID)-induced ulcer, who must unavoidably continue with NSAID therapy (e.g. those with severe rheumatoid arthritis), an acid suppressor, **usually** a PPI, should be prescribed. After the ulcer has healed, the patient, where possible, should be stepped down to a maintenance dose of the acid suppressor.

- Patients who have severe GORD symptoms or who have a proven pathology (e.g. oesophageal ulceration, Barrett's oesophagus) should be treated with a healing dose of a PPI until symptoms have been controlled. After that has been achieved, the dose should be stepped down to the lowest dose that maintains control of the symptoms. A regular maintenance, low dose of most PPIs will prevent recurrent GORD symptoms in 70–80% of patients and should be used in preference to the higher healing dose. Where necessary, should symptoms reappear, the higher dose should be recommended. In complicated oesophagitis (stricture, ulcer, haemorrhage), the full dose should be maintained. Patients with mild GORD symptoms and/or those who do not have a proven pathology can frequently be managed by alternative therapies (at least in the first instance) including antacids, alginates or H2RAs (H2 receptor antagonists).

- Patients diagnosed with non-ulcer dyspepsia (NUD) may have symptoms caused by different aetiologies and should not be routinely treated with PPIs. Should the symptoms appear to be acid-related, an antacid or the lowest dose of an acid suppressor to control symptoms should be prescribed. If they do not appear to be acid-related, an alternative therapeutic strategy should be employed.

- Patients presenting in general practice with mild symptoms of dyspepsia may be treated on either a 'step-up' or a 'step-down' basis. Neither group should normally be treated with PPIs on a long-term basis without a confirmed clinical diagnosis being made.

- In circumstances where it is appropriate to use a PPI and where healing is required, the optimal dose to achieve this should be prescribed initially. Once healing has been achieved, or for conditions where it is not required, the lowest dose of the PPI that provides effective symptom relief should be used.

- The least expensive, appropriate PPI should be used.

- The use of PPIs in the paragraphs above refers, for each indication, only to those PPIs that have been licensed for that use.

- On present evidence, PPIs do not have any serious contraindications for the vast majority of users and have been in common use for some 8 or 9 years. While their use in sufficient dosage to cure, or to control symptoms is well warranted in terms of their clear benefits, any additional use cannot be recommended.

Box 2.3 Benign oesophageal stricture

- History of GORD
- Young age
- Absence of weight loss
- Short smooth 'pinhole' stricture with surrounding oesophagitis.

guidewire. Stricture fibres are disrupted by both radial and shear force. Bougie dilatation often produces longer lasting effects due to the greater forces involved, but may be more likely to perforate. Fluoroscopic placement of any guidewire may be necessary.

The approximate risks for dilating benign strictures are:

- perforation 0.5% (2% if caustic or radiation induced stricture)
- significant bleeding <1% (all will bleed a little).

Hints for dilating benign strictures without fluoroscopic guidance (see Figs 2.5a–d) include:

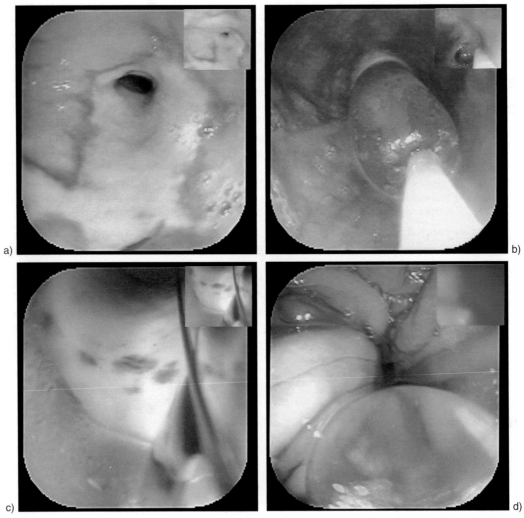

Fig. 2.5
Balloon dilatation of benign oesophageal stricture. (a) Stricture before dilatation. (b) Balloon across stricture. (c) Looking through balloon as it is pushed forwards. (d) View once stricture has been passed following (c)

- Use the endoscope with the largest channel you have.
- Lubricate the channel well prior to passing the balloon.
- Gently advance the balloon through the stricture. If it does not pass easily, *STOP* and rearrange the procedure for fluoroscopic guidance with a guidewire.
- Inflate the balloon to the desired volume/pressure and maintain this for 60 s. This can be very uncomfortable, so ensure the patient has adequate analgesia and/or sedation.
- After dilatation to the desired diameter, 'follow' the balloon through the stricture, by pulling the front of the balloon onto the scope and visualizing the stricture through the wall of the balloon. Then firmly push scope and balloon through the stricture.
- Inspect the dilatation site carefully for perforation.

Ensure the patient continues to take an adequate dose of PPI after the procedure. A dispersible formulation should be used if there is a history of tablet obstruction.

Barrett's oesophagus

What is Barrett's oesophagus?

Barrett's oesophagus (BO) can be used to describe several different entities:

- 'Endoscopic Barrett's' is the salmon-pink appearance of distal oesophageal mucosa that occurs as the result of gastric metaplasia of the squamous epithelium.
- 'True Barrett's' is the presence of both gastric metaplasia **and** specialized intestinal metaplasia (SIM) of biopsies shown histologically. There is reasonable evidence that only Barrett's mucosa including areas of SIM has pre-malignant potential.
- The original description by Barrett described what he thought was a 'congenitally short oesophagus'. His name has been subsequently used as above.

Care should be taken to ensure that a sliding hiatus hernia is not mistaken for BO (see Fig. 2.6). The true GOJ begins when the gastric folds finish. If there is doubt about the position of the hiatus, asking the patient to take a deep breath in will produce an indentation at the level of the diaphragm.

BO is arbitrarily divided into 'short-segment' (0–3 cm in length) and 'long-segment' (>3 cm in length). Most BO is 'short-segment'.

How should we manage Barrett's oesophagus?

BO is a common finding at endoscopy and how to manage it evokes great emotion amongst some gastroenterologists. The important facts to take into consideration when considering the importance of BO are as follows:

- BO is present in at least 5% of the population and 10% of those with reflux symptoms.
- Most patients are men over the age of 65.
- Over 95% of these will die from other causes apart from oesophageal cancer, especially ischaemic heart disease.

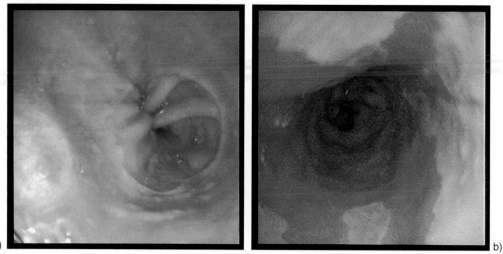

a)   b)

Fig. 2.6
Sliding hiatus hernia (a) and Barrett's oesophagus (b). Note the presence of gastric folds in sliding hiatus hernia. The gastro-oesophageal junction begins where these finish

- Two hundred to 400 'screening' endoscopies have to be performed to detect one cancer.
- Of the cancers detected, many will be inoperable, either because of stage of disease or fitness of the patient.
- 'Surveillance detected' cancers have a better prognosis than those diagnosed outwith surveillance.
- The mortality of oesophagectomy is around 5–10%.
- Carcinoma risk increases with length of Barrett's segment.
- Most cancers will occur in people with short-segment BO as this is far more common.
- Cost-effective analyses suggest only surveillance every 5 years is cost-effective, but many patients are unhappy with such a long interval between endoscopies.

The bottom-line is that Barrett's surveillance is not cost-effective, but it is all there is to offer to people with a pre-malignant condition. It seems reasonable to offer surveillance every 2 years to patients with long-segment Barrett's oeosphagus who are aware of the reasons behind surveillance. A suggested protocol is shown in Figure 2.7.

Treating high-grade dysplasia in Barrett's oesophagus

This is another contentious area. Useful facts in the debate are that:

- there is a large variability in grading of high-grade dysplasia (HGD) by histopathologists
- up to 30% of HGD will improve without intervention

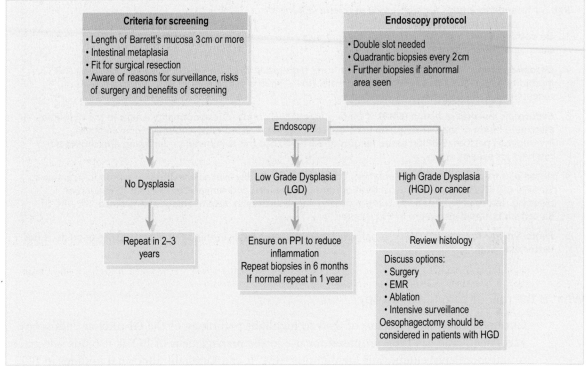

Fig. 2.7
A protocol for Barrett's surveillance

- co-existent carcinoma is present in up to 30% of patients with HGD
- all the treatment options have risks.

Modalities of treating HGD in Barrett's are shown in Box 2.4.

Argon plasma coagulation ablation for high-grade dysplasia (using Erbe machine)

- Sedate patient (midazolam and pethidine or equivalents).
- Use dual channel endoscope if possible (ease removal of spent argon and smoke).
- Erbe set to argon plasma coagulation (APC) at flow rate of 2 l/min and power setting to 'A65'.
- Treat semi-circumferential length of Barrett's (this reduces stricturing).
- Beware accumulation of argon and smoke in the stomach, frequent aspiration is required.
- Treat the opposite side at 4 weeks.
- Assess HGD by quadrantic biopsies at 2 cm intervals after a further 4 weeks.
- Maintain the patient on high-dose PPI (equivalent to omeprazole 20 mg bd).
- Repeat as needed.
- Once HGD ablated successfully, continue surveillance endoscopies every 6 months.

Box 2.4 Treatment options for high-grade dysplasia in Barrett's

1. **Do nothing.** Many advocate a close surveillance every 4–6 months, proceeding to oesophagectomy once carcinoma develops.

2. **Oesophagectomy.** This is the clearest way to 'cure' high-grade dysplasia (HGD). However, mortality and morbidity is high and this seems a little extreme. However, in a young patient with persistent HGD on repeated examinations it may be worthwhile.

3. **Endoscopic mucosal resection (EMR).** If there is an obvious endoscopic abnormality – akin to the dysplasia-associated lesion or mass of dysplasia in colitis – this can be resected endoscopically. Some Japanese investigators perform EMR on entire lengths of Barrett's, but this is quite an undertaking and should be reserved for experts only.

4. **Argon plasma coagulation (APC) ablation.** This is the most readily available technique. It probably removes 50–60% of HGD, but has a finite perforation rate (around 3%) and can lead to stricture formation or bleeding. Ten to 20% of patients will progress to adenocarcinoma despite ablation. A protocol for APC of Barrett's is outlined elsewhere in this chapter.

5. **Photodynamic therapy (PDT).** PDT is only available in a few centres in the UK. It is probably as good as, if not better than EMR.

What is the role of chromoendoscopy?

Chromoendoscopy is the use of dyes to highlight pathology of the GI tract at endoscopy. Methylene blue has been proposed for use in the management of BO as it binds selectively to intestinal epithelium, thus highlighting SIM. It can highlight abnormal nodules in BO, which may represent either HGD or intramucosal carcinoma. However, there is currently not enough evidence to say it improves the detection of HGD in BO screening (indeed, areas of HGD may lose their uptake of methylene blue).

A protocol for methylene blue staining of Barrett's is shown in Box 2.5.

Oesophageal carcinoma

Types of oesophageal carcinoma

The demographics of oesophageal cancer have changed considerably over the past 20 years. Most oesophageal cancers are now adenocarcinomas of the distal third.

Box 2.5 Methylene blue staining for Barrett's

- Sedate patient
- Endoscope patient with head end of trolley raised to 20–30°
- Wash Barrett's mucosa with nAcetyl cysteine (Parvolex – diluted to give 10% solution). This removes surface mucus
- Mix methylene blue with equal volume of normal saline
- Spray using spray catheter
- Wash with water
- Inspect mucosa for abnormal nodules

Squamous cell carcinomas account for only 30% of tumours. The reasons behind this shift are thought to be increased GORD and subsequent BO, changes in *H. pylori* prevalence and changes in diet.

Staging oesophageal carcinoma

Once histologically confirmed, tumours of the oesophagus need to be staged. This allows decisions about further treatment and assessment of prognosis to be made. Figure 2.8 outlines the TNM (extent of primary Tumour, local lymph Nodes, distant Metastases) oesophageal staging. The American Joint Committee on Cancer (AJCC) has produced a separate staging system based on the TNM classification (Box 2.6).

The three modalities used for oesophageal staging are:

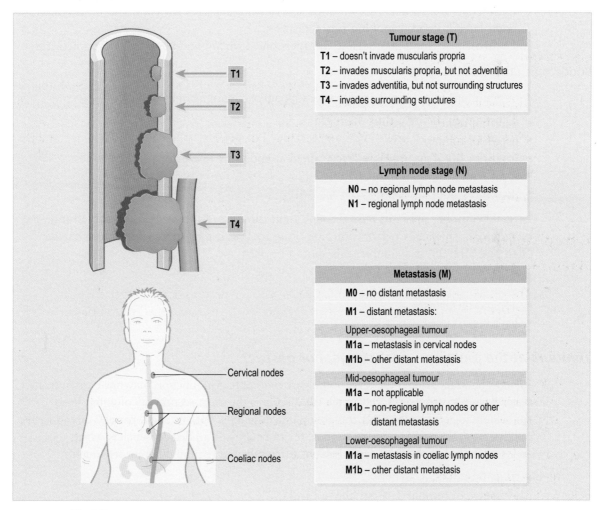

Tumour stage (T)

T1 – doesn't invade muscularis propria
T2 – invades muscularis propria, but not adventitia
T3 – invades adventitia, but not surrounding structures
T4 – invades surrounding structures

Lymph node stage (N)

N0 – no regional lymph node metastasis
N1 – regional lymph node metastasis

Metastasis (M)

M0 – no distant metastasis

M1 – distant metastasis:

Upper-oesophageal tumour
M1a – metastasis in cervical nodes
M1b – other distant metastasis

Mid-oesophageal tumour
M1a – not applicable
M1b – non-regional lymph nodes or other distant metastasis

Lower-oesophageal tumour
M1a – metastasis in coeliac lymph nodes
M1b – other distant metastasis

Cervical nodes

Regional nodes

Coeliac nodes

Fig. 2.8
TNM staging of oesophageal cancer

Box 2.6 American Joint Committee on Cancer oesophageal carcinoma staging system

• Stage 0	TisN0M0
• Stage I	T1N0M0
• Stage IIA	T2N0M0 or T3 N0M0
• Stage IIB	T1N1M0 or T2N1M0
• Stage III	T3N1M0 or T4 tumours
• Stage IVA	Any M1a tumour
• Stage IVB	Any M1b tumour

1. *CT chest and abdomen.* Good at assessing lung, liver and intraperitoneal spread. Poor at assessing depth of invasion.
2. *Endoscopic ultrasound (EUS).* Good at assessing depth of invasion and local lymph node spread. Poor at looking for metastases.
3. *Laparoscopy.* Good at assessing intraperitoneal spread and superficial liver metastases.

Endoscopic ultrasound staging

As a minimum EUS examination for oesophageal staging should include:

- depth of tumour (T stage)
- length of tumour
- length of BO if appropriate (ascertained at endscopy just prior to EUS)
- local nodes, size and number
- metastatic nodes, i.e. coeliac axis.

Large EUS probes may not pass through tight tumours. Balloon dilatation to 14 mm may be required. This has a perforation rate of up to 1%. If a tapered smaller probe (e.g. Olympus MH908) is available, this should be used.

EUS may also show:

- adrenal metastases
- liver metastases.

Tumours at the junction – oesophageal or gastric?

Adenocarcinoma around the level of the gastro-oesophageal junction may have arisen from either Barrett's oesophagus, the cardia (the cardia is the short section of columnar lined epithelium adjacent to the GOJ containing mucus glands, but not chief, parietal or endocrine cells) or from the gastric body or fundus. It can be difficult to decide which is which endoscopically, but the three types behave differently and require different treatment:

- Type I (oesophageal)
    - centre of tumour 1–5 cm above cardia
    - spreads to mediastinal and coeliac nodes
    - treat as oesophageal carcinoma

- Type II (cardia)
  - centre of tumour between 1 cm above and 2 cm below cardia
  - spreads to coeliac, splenic and para-aortic nodes
  - treat as gastric carcinoma
- Type III (gastric)
  - centre of tumour 2–5 cm below cardia
  - spreads to coeliac, splenic and para-aortic nodes
  - treat as gastric carcinoma.

Who should have surgery and/or chemotherapy?

All patients should be considered for surgery and discussed by a multi-disciplinary team, including oesophageal surgeon, gastroenterologist, radiologist, histopathologist and oncologist. It goes without saying that the patient (and usually their relatives) should be involved in the decision. 'Fitness' for operation is best assessed by an anaesthetist:

- Stage I tumours should be resected without neoadjuvant chemotherapy.
- Stage II tumours should have neoadjuvant chemotherapy.
- T3N1 tumours may benefit from neoadjuvant chemotherapy, although this is unproven.
- T4 and Stage IV tumours are inoperable, but could be considered for palliative chemoradiotherapy.

Twenty per cent of surgery is 'curative' and the operative mortality is between 5 and 10% in most centres.

How long have I got doctor?

Table 2.3 gives some data that may help answer this extremely common and difficult question.

Table 2.3 Survival in different categories of patients with oesophageal carcinoma

Stage/point of treatment	Median survival	5-year survival
Stage 0 – all patients		75%
Stage I – all patients		60%
Stage IIA – all patients		40%
Stage IIB – all patients		20%
Stage I-II – any undergoing surgery	13 months	
Stage I-II – any undergoing surgery with pre-op chemotherapy	16 months	
Stage III		15%
Stage IV		<5%
Inoperable tumour – chemoradiation given	12–15 months	
Inoperable tumour – stent placed	3 months	<5%

Which chemotherapy and what are the side effects?

Many different regimens are used and/or being assessed within trials. The rationale behind using neoadjuvant chemotherapy is based on the results of the MRC trial comparing surgery with and without pre-operative chemotherapy (also called OEO2). This trial used two 4-day cycles of 5-FU and cisplatin by infusion. This regimen has been adopted by many. It requires the placement of a Hickmann line and has the following side effects:

- Line complications including sepsis, thrombosis and blockage
- Nausea, vomiting
- Hair loss
- Pancytopenia, leading to bleeding and sepsis.

Endoscopic palliation of oesophageal carcinoma

There are numerous endoscopic methods for improving dysphagia in patients with oesophageal cancer:

- Stent insertion
- Thermal laser ablation
- Absolute alcohol injection
- Photodynamic therapy (PDT)
- Argon plasma coagulation (APC).

Each has its advantages and disadvantages. These are outlined in Table 2.4. It is a good idea to place stents under direct vision when patients are frail and a protocol for this is outlined below. In younger patients who can tolerate repeated procedures, a thermal laser may be used (Laserscope KPT/YAG).

Direct vision placement of oesophageal ultraflex stents

- Pass through tumour using either a nasal endoscope (6 mm diameter) or thinnest scope available with balloon dilatation (no more than 14 mm balloon). If balloon dilating, the balloon must pass easily. If not, **STOP** and arrange to place stent under fluoroscopic guidance.
- Position guidewire (floppy tip metal wire, e.g. Olympus 7028474 wire) in gastric antrum.
- Slowly withdraw scope, keeping wire in place.
- Measure length of tumour as you withdraw.
- Choose proximal releasing stent which is 2–3 cm longer than tumour
- Mark stent at level of proximal radio-opaque mark with Tippex or similar white marker making a circumferential 2–3 mm 'white band' (NB. newer stents may now include an external coloured marker as the direct vision technique has become established).
- Loosen two to three cotton ties.
- Lubricate stent with Aquagel or similar.

Table 2.4 Advantages and disadvantages of different modalities of oesophageal palliation

	Advantages	Disadvantages
Stent	Readily available Rapid resolution of dysphagia in 90% Various designs available	Perforation in 1–2% May need fluoroscopy Stent may block Risk of aspiration Semi-solid diet Pain is common after insertion – may need opiates
Thermal laser	Rapid result Easily repeated Can be used as bridge to stenting	Special equipment needed May need two to three treatments to achieve patency
Absolute alcohol	Readily available No special equipment needed Can be repeated	Mediastinitis if misplaced
Photodynamic therapy (PDT)	Patients may tolerate normal foods Ideal for high strictures Can be used for blocked stents	Photo-sensitivity (patients will need to wear full sunblock, hat, and gloves) Special equipment needed
Argon plasma coagulation (APC)	Relatively widely available Can be used to unblock stents	Multiple treatments needed to achieve patency

- Pass stent to approximate position (using distance markers on stent insertor).
- Re-endoscope such that the top of the tumour and stent are clearly seen.
- Position stent such that white mark is 1 cm above top of tumour and deploy stent under vision, adjusting position such that proximal wide part of stent sits on the tumour.
- Withdraw all endoscopic equipment and sit patient at 45°.
- Ensure adequate analgesia (opiates are often necessary for 24–48 h).

Other tips for stent management:

- If tumour is very high, fluoroscopic placement may be better.
- Uncovered stents are less likely to migrate, but have a high rate of tumour ingrowth.
- Covered stents should be used for fistulae.
- For high fistulae Diagmed-covered Choo stents are recommended, as these are covered across whole of length (many other types are only covered in the mid-portion).
- When placing stents under fluoroscopic guidance, Endoclips (Olympus) can be used to mark the upper and lower margins of the tumour. The old-fashioned approach of paper-clips stuck to the skin is out-dated and leads to frequent misplacement of stents.
- The patient can rarely drink too much carbonated fluid.

Dysmotility

What are the important causes of oesophageal dysmotility?

- Achalasia
- Diffuse oesophageal spasm
- Pseudoachalasia
- Presbyoesophagus.

What is the best test for achalasia?

Both endoscopy and barium radiography give typical appearances in late-stage achalasia:

- Smooth tapered 'stricture' – 'bird's beak' appearance on barium
- Dilated distal and proximal oesophagus containing stagnant food/fluid (see Fig. 2.10a)
- Loss of peristalsis
- Little resistance to passage of endoscope through 'stricture' and no bleeding.

However, early achalasia may not have these appearances and the best test is oesophageal manometry. Key features are:

- aperistalsis in distal oesophagus
- failure of lower oesophageal sphincter to relax on swallowing
- raised lower oesophageal resting pressure (it can, however, be normal)
- loss of amplitude and progression of peristalsis.

Pseudoachalasia (a submucosal tumour disrupting the myenteric plexus leading to appearances of achalasia) should be excluded. Endoscopic ultrasound is the most sensitive test for this, but most units rely on negative endoscopic biopsy.

What is the best treatment for achalasia?

Four options are available, surgery, balloon dilatation, botulinum toxin injection and calcium channel antagonists.

Surgery

Laparoscopic myotomy should be considered in all young healthy patients. It is highly effective giving relief in 90% of patients, has minimal risks and can be combined with an anti-reflux procedure. Open surgery has more peri-operative risks, but is equally effective.

Balloon dilatation

Balloon dilatation with either over-the-wire achalasia balloons or the over-the-scope 'Witzel' dilator is effective at relieving symptoms for 6 months in 70–80% of patients. There is a risk of perforation in around 2–5%.

Botulinum toxin injection

'Botox' injection has become popular recently for achalasia. However, it tends to last less well than balloon dilatation (3–6 months). There are also concerns that injection leads to scarring that may make future surgery more difficult. Botox may be reserved as a holding manoeuvre before surgery or in patients unfit for surgery.

How to give botulinum toxin injections   Two forms of botulinum toxin are available commercially, Botox (Allergan) and Dysport (Ipsen). There is far more clinical experience with Botox in achalasia and it is cheaper. Botox can, therefore, be used as follows:

- Ensure pseudoachalasia (carcinoma at the cardia) excluded
- Mix 100U of Botox in 5 ml sterile saline
- Endoscope patient with head of bed raised by 20° (to try and prevent the patient aspirating food/fluid in oesophagus)
- Use wide-channeled endoscope to allow suction of oesophageal contents
- Identify top of lower oesophageal sphincter
- Prime injection needle with 1 ml of Botox
- Make 1 ml deep injections at beginning of narrowed oesophagus at 12, 3, 6 and 9 o'clock
- Repeat at 6 months if successful.

Calcium channel blockers

Nifedipine 10–20 mg before meals may help patients with mild symptoms (10% of patients benefit).

What is the risk of oeosphageal carcinoma in achalasia?

The risk of oesophageal carcinoma in achalasia is probably overestimated due to the presence of pseudoachalasia, but there does seem to be an association with squamous cell carcinoma in 2–4% of patients.

The risk is greatest in untreated patients, then balloon-dilated patients and then lowest in patients who have had a myotomy. Surveillance is not currently advocated.

Other causes of oesophageal dysmotility

These can be divided into primary and secondary oesophageal dysmotility.

Primary causes include diffuse oesophageal spasm and nutcracker oesophagus.

Secondary causes include scleroderma, diabetes and presbyoesophagus (non-specific motility disorder in the elderly).

Manometric findings in these conditions are shown in Table 2.5.

Consider scleroderma oesophagus if:

- reflux oesophagitis and associated complications
- other features of scleroderma
- anti-centromere antibody positive.

Diffuse oesophageal spasm

Diffuse oesophageal spasm is thought to cause dysphagia and retrosternal pain. The dysphagia is usually intermittent, variable and non-progressive. It is not necessarily

Table 2.5 Manometric findings in oesophageal dysmotility disorders

Condition	Manometric findings
Diffuse oesophageal spasm	Episodes of normal peristalsis Simultaneous contractions in >30% swallows
Nutcracker oesophagus	Normal peristalsis High-amplitude contractions (>180 mmHg)
Presbyoesophagus	Failed peristalsis Decreased lower oesophageal relaxation Increased spontaneous contraction
Diabetes	Low-amplitude peristalsis Hypotensive lower oesophageal sphincter Failure of lower oesophageal sphincter relaxation

related to episodes of pain. The pain may last minutes or hours and usually radiates to the back. Swallowing is usually undisturbed during the pain.

It is usually sufficient to explain the nature of the problem and reassure the patient about its non-cardiac origin. In those requiring treatment it may be worth trying nifedipine or isosorbide dinitrate starting at 10 mg. For dysphagia the drug should be taken shortly before meals and, for pain, at the onset. For speed of action short-acting preparations should be used and absorption from the mouth encouraged by biting a capsule of nifedipine before swallowing or using isosorbide sublingually. Because of the risk of hypotension, patients should be advised to sit down when using these drugs, especially the first time.

Treatments for other oesophageal dysmotility disorders

Non-achalasia oesophageal dysmotility problems are notoriously difficult to treat.

Nifedipine 10–30 mg tds or isosorbide dinitrate 20 mg tds may help.

Prokinetics such as metoclopramide 5–10 mg tds (beware dystonic reactions) or domperidone 10–20 mg tds are often used.

Botulinum toxin injection has helped some patients with diffuse oesophageal spasm or nutcracker oesophagus.

Dietary modification is the most helpful treatment. Patients should be advised to:

- eat small regular meals
- sit or stand for 1–2 hours after meals
- thoroughly chew food
- avoid exercise after food.

Other diseases of the oesophagus

Schatzki ring

This is a web- or diaphragm-like constriction of the lower oesophagus that may be a chance finding at endoscopy or may cause dysphagia. They are said to be common, supposedly occurring in up to 15% of dysphagic patients (this is not born out in my practice). Two types are seen:

1. A ring
   - Muscular ring usually 2 cm above GOJ
   - Rare
   - Dysphagia unusual
2. B ring
   - Mucosal ring usually at squamocolumnar junction
   - Common
   - Dysphagia common once lumen diameter <13 mm
   - Upper surface is covered in squamous epithelium, lower surface in columnar epithelium
   - May be due to GORD or pill oesophagitis.

If symptomatic they can be dilated as for benign strictures. They are benign but often recur.

Candidal oesophagitis

Candida is a frequent commensal of the oesophagus. The demonstration of candida in smears and culture is not sufficient to make a diagnosis of candidiasis – it is usually necessary to demonstrate invasion of mucosa or ulcer slough with yeasts and hyphae. Oesophageal candidiasis is common in patients taking inhaled or oral steroids and in those immunosuppressed for other reasons (including AIDS) as well as in patients with oesophagitis from other causes and with other upper GI pathology.

Oesophageal candidiasis is often asymptomatic, but may cause dysphagia, chest pain and heartburn. Diagnosis is best confirmed by biopsy with periodic acid Schiff (PAS) staining.

Nystatin (e.g. pastilles or suspension 200 000 units five times daily for a week in the first instance) is both safe and relatively cheap and appropriate for those with normal immune status. Fluconazole tablets 50–100 mg daily for 1–2 weeks is more convenient, but more toxic; it is particularly indicated for patients with impaired immunity (at a dose of 100–200 mg daily). The choice of dose in each range is determined by age, weight and co-morbidity.

Other types of oesophagitis

These should be considered when the mucosa looks atypical for reflux oesophagitis or if the patient is immunocompromised.

- Viral oesophagitis:
  - herpes simplex virus (HSV)
  - cytomegalovirus (CMV)
  - Epstein–Barr virus (EBV)
  - Varicella zoster
  - human papilloma virus (HPV)
  - HIV.
- Tuberculous (TB) oesophagitis
- Cancer treatment
  - Radiation
  - Chemotherapy
  - Combined
  - graft versus host disease (GVHD)
- Crohn's disease
- Eosinophilic oesophagitis
- Pill oesophagitis
  - Doxycycline
  - Alendronate
  - non-steroidal anti-inflammatory drugs (NSAIDs)
- Behçets disease.

Gastritis

True gastritis is a histological diagnosis. However, gastritis is a term that is used to cover mild erythema of the antrum (with often disappointingly normal histology) to a widespread necrotic denuded mucosa seen in some chemotherapy patients. Most patients and junior doctors use the term to cover any episode of upper abdominal pain, whilst there is really little evidence to suggest inflammation of the gastric mucosa causes pain. It is, therefore, often a chance finding at endoscopy.

Gastritis has a complex classification system (the 'updated Sydney classification' – Table 2.6), but this does cover most of the causes.

How should gastritis be treated?

Usually treatment is not indicated. If you feel the gastritis is causing symptoms, or may cause future problems (for example the erosive gastritis seen with NSAIDs in some patients may be a prelude to true ulceration), treat as below:

- NSAIDs
  - Stop or consider COX-2 inhibitors or gastric protection with daily protease inhibitor (PPI) (omeprazole 20 mg od equivalent)
- *H. pylori*
  - Eradicate (see below)
- Duodeno-gastric reflux (biliary reflux)
  - Sucralfate 1 g tds (works less well if co-administered with PPI)
  - Aluminium hydroxide (beware constipation)
  - Colestyramine 4 g od-tds
  - Domperidone 10–20 mg tds
  - Surgery (in extreme cases).

Table 2.6 The 'updated' Sydney classification of gastritis

Type of gastritis	Subtype	Aetiology
Non-atrophic		H. pylori
Atrophic	Autoimmune	Autoimmunity
	Multifocal atrophic	H. pylori
		Dietary
		Environmental factors
Special forms	Chemical	Bile
		NSAIDs/aspirin
	Radiation	Radiation
	Lymphocytic	Cryptogenic
		Coeliac disease
		Drugs (ticlodipine)
		?H. pylori
	Non-infectious granulomatous	Crohn's disease
		Sarcoidosis
		Vasculitides
		Foreign substances
		Idiopathic
	Eosinophilic	Food sensitivity
		?other allergies
	Other infectious gastritides	Non-Helicobacter bacteria
		Viruses
		Fungi
		Parasites

Other drugs to be considered

Misoprostol 200–400 μg tds has been shown to be effective in reducing symptoms from chronic erosive gastritis (but not histological changes).

Peptic ulcer disease

The nature of gastric ulcers (GUs) and duodenal ulcers (DUs) has changed considerably over the past 10 years. *Helicobacter pylori (H. pylori)* is steadily being eradicated from the developed world, both by reduced transmission in childhood and increasing use of antimicrobial regimens. The use of aspirin and NSAIDs, however, has increased and is becoming the predominant cause of GU and DU (see Fig. 2.10c).

Differential diagnosis of gastric ulceration

- NSAID
- *H. pylori*
- Adenocarcinoma
- Lymphoma
- Stress (intensive-care patients, burns patients)
- Zollinger–Ellison syndrome (usually with co-existent DU and oesophagitis).

How should patients with gastric ulcer be managed?

- Take at least four biopsies from the edge of the ulcer
- *H. pylori* test from antrum
- Careful history for NSAID use. If present STOP
- If *H. pylori* present, treat
- PPI at high dose, equivalent to 20 mg bd omeprazole for 4–6 weeks
- Re-scope at 4–6 weeks whilst on PPI
- If GU still present, take further four to six biopsies (worry about malignancy)
- Check compliance with medication
- If compliant, consider increase PPI dose
- Continue to re-endoscope at 4–6 week intervals until ulcer is healed
- There is some debate as to when to treat *H. pylori* in patients on NSAIDs.

Ulcer healing may be impaired in *H. pylori*-negative individuals and PPIs work less well in *H. pylori*-negative individuals. The role of NSAIDs in the pathogenesis of ulcers is probably much greater than *H. pylori* in those with both aetiologies. However, delaying *H. pylori* treatment may lead to it being forgotten. *H. pylori* should be eradicated as soon as it is found when an ulcer is present.

The sensitivity for a single gastric biopsy to establish gastric cancer is 70%. This increases to 99% with seven biopsies.

How should patients with duodenal ulcer be managed?

- *H. pylori* test from antrum
- If multiple ulcers confined to duodenum, take histology (?Crohn's)
- If multiple ulcers in stomach and oesophagitis, check fasting gastrin
- Stop aspirin and/or NSAIDs
- Eradicate *H. pylori*
- Additional acid suppression only needed if:
  - multiple ulcers
  - NSAID/aspirin use
  - persistence of symptoms 4 weeks after eradication with negative urea breath test
  - complicated ulcer disease.

It is probably ideal practice to have a positive *H. pylori* test before eradication treatment in DU patients, but as 90–95% of DU are associated with *H. pylori* it is not unreasonable to treat blind. A follow-up test for *H. pylori* after eradication is only needed if there are symptoms, or the DU was complicated (e.g. bleed).

How should duodenitis be managed?

Erosive duodenitis is usually accompanied by similar symptoms to DU. If *H. pylori* is present, most experts would treat this as if it were a *H. pylori* associated DU.

The differential diagnosis of duodenitis includes:

- *H. pylori*
- NSAIDs/aspirin

- Crohn's
- Coeliac disease (unusual).

What is the best test for H. pylori?

All patients with an ulcer at endoscopy should have a biopsy to look for *H. pylori*. This may be either placed in a commercial agar based urease test (e.g. CLO-test, a name which stems from 'Campylobacter-like organism' as *H. pylori* was initially felt to be a *Campylobacter*), a local rapid urease test (it is easy to set up your own *H. pylori* test – see below) or, if neither of these are available, sent for histological assessment using specific stains. The best place to take the biopsy from is the antrum. If a PPI has been used it may be better to take an additional biopsy from the gastric body as *H. pylori* tends to migrate to the proximal stomach in the face of acid suppression.

If a biopsy is not taken (forgotten, too much blood) or is negative and suspicion remains high that *H. pylori* is present, a urea breath test, serology or the presence of faecal *H. pylori* antigen can be used. There are several versions of each available.

The pros and cons of each test are outlined in Table 2.7. The rationale behind all urea-based *H. pylori* tests is shown in Figure 2.9.

The most sensitive and specific (and thus leads to the lowest numbers of missed infected patients or mistreated uninfected patients) test is the urea breath test.

'Home-made rapid urea test'

- Capped Eppendorf vial
- 0.5 ml 10% urea (w/v) in deionized water at pH 6.8
- 2 drops 1% phenol red.

Help from your local clinical biochemist will be needed, but large numbers can be made at the same time and frozen. They can then be defrosted prior to an endoscopy list.

What is the best regimen for H. pylori treatment?

First-line treatment of *H. pylori* should be for 1 week with either:

- PPI bd + amoxycillin 1 g bd + clarithromycin 500 mg bd
- PPI bd + clarithomycin 500 mg bd + metronidazole 400 mg bd.

The doses of different PPIs are omeprazole 20 mg, lansoprazole 30 mg, rabeprazole 20 mg, pantoprazole 40 mg and esomeprazole 20 mg. Some PPI manufacturers have produced packs containing PPI and antibiotics in a well-labelled and packaged manner. Patients find these very helpful (Heliclear, Helimet).

These treatments will eradicate the infection in 80–90% of hospital patients. Compliance (i.e. taking all the tablets) is crucial to success. Side effects to be expected are taste disturbance, mild diarrhoea and nausea. Occasionally severe side effects may occur including oral ulceration and severe diarrhoea. In patients with the latter this usually settles spontaneously, but stools should be sent for *Clostridium difficile* toxin. Elderly

Table 2.7 Advantages and disadvantages of different H. pylori tests

Test	Cost	Advantages	Disadvantages
CLO test[†] (or similar commercial agar urease test)	£1.50*	Easy 90% sensitive	False-negatives with blood and proton pump inhibitor (PPI) Need to wait 24 h until result in some cases
'Home-made' rapid urea test	£0.10*	Cheap Result in 1–10 min	False-negatives with blood and PPI Needs preparation
Histology	£40* per biopsy	Allows assessment of mucosa (e.g. atrophy, dysplasia) Can give positive result when urease test negative	Expensive Special stains needed Pathologist needed 3 days to result
13-C urea breath test	£20–25	Highly sensitive and specific No radioactivity Easy for patients	Patient needs to stop PPI for 2–4 weeks Analysis equipment needed
Faecal antigen		Non-invasive	Patients not always keen on producing stool sample Low sensitivity
Serology	£2–3	Allows assessment in patients on PPI Non-invasive	No use for assessing eradication Relatively low sensitivity Microbiology lab needed
Near patient serology (e.g. Quick Vue)	£6	Rapid assessment (10 min) in clinic	Not accurate Leads to misdiagnosis

*Excludes the cost of the endoscopy and biopsy forceps.
[†]CLO test: this is the commercial name for a particular local rapid biopsy urease test. The name derives from 'Campylobacter Like Organism' because originally *Helicobacter pylori* was thought to be a Campylobacter.

patients are especially prone to this complication and should be warned of its possibility.

If first-line treatment fails, two options are available:

1. Blind treatment with either:
   * omeprazole 40 mg bd, De-Nol one tab qds, metronidazole 400 mg tds and tetracycline HCl 500 mg qds for 2 weeks (so-called OBMT treatment)
   or
   * pantoprazole 40 mg bd, amoxycillin 1 g bd and levofloxacin 500 mg bd for 10 days (so-called PAL treatment – this is still in the early stages of use and may be superceded)
2. Repeat endoscopy and collection of samples for *H. pylori* culture and sensitivity testing. Further treatment is then tailored to the patient. For example, someone with a metronidazole resistant and clarithromycin sensitive infection could have a PPI + amoxycillin + clarithromycin.

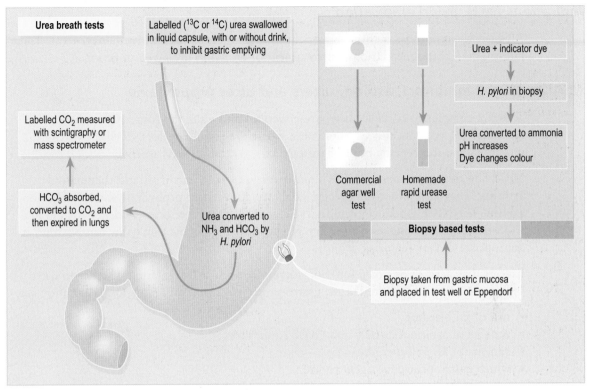

Fig. 2.9
Theory of urease-based tests for *Helicobacter pylori*

OBMT is complicated to take and often produces unpleasant side effects. However, it has the best track record for second-line treatments and can be expected to work in around 70–75% of patients. PAL is a much newer treatment that appears quite promising and has eradication rates in trials of around 70–80%. However, experience with this regimen is small.

Sensitivity testing of *H. pylori* is not available in every centre in the UK and culture of *H. pylori* can be difficult (possible in less than 80% of patients). Patients are often quite against the idea of further endoscopy, particularly if it turns out to be for unsuccessful culture. However, when eradication has failed and ulcer healing has not occurred, repeat endoscopy will be necessary anyway.

What to do if second-line treatment fails?

It is very unusual to successfully treat *H. pylori* on the third attempt. If patients have been non-compliant it may be worth admitting them for directly observed treatment (they would have to have a good indication for treatment though!). Most patients though will need to remain on PPIs long term. Surgery is rarely indicated.

Indications for H. pylori eradication

A consensus group has met in Maastricht to discuss *H. pylori* and its management. Their latest (2000) recommendations for treatment of *H. pylori* are given in Box 2.7.

NSAIDs, COX-2 inhibitors, aspirin, ulcers and ulcer prophylaxis

This is a complex area (hence a separate section) and often the source of confusion between GPs, patients and GI physicians. There are good data for NSAIDs and COX-2 inhibitors and the benefits of ulcer prophylaxis, but far less for aspirin.

NICE has given guidance on COX-2 inhibitor use in osteoarthritis and rheumatoid arthritis. They have **not** given specific guidance about ulcer prohylaxis with NSAIDs or aspirin. The NICE guidance includes the statement that there is no evidence for PPI and COX-2 inhibitors being used together. However, many people think this combination is appropriate in very high-risk groups.

Factors that need to be taken into consideration when contemplating whether to use aspirin, NSAIDs, COX-2 inhibitors, gastro-protective agents and *H. pylori* eradication are:

- risk of GI bleeding
- benefits of aspirin, NSAIDs and COX-2 inhibitors
- benefits of *H. pylori* eradication
- which gastro-protective agent to use.

What are the risks of gastrointestinal bleeding?

The risks of GI bleeding (and thus the need for ulcer prophylaxis) varies greatly between patients and the drugs they take. These are summarized in Table 2.8.

What are the benefits of aspirin?

- In patients with angina, aspirin reduces myocardial infarction (MI) by 1 per 100 patient years

---

Box 2.7 Treatment recommendations for H. pylori

- Treatment strongly recommended:
    - Duodenal or gastric ulcer (active or not, including complicated peptic ulcer disease)
    - Mucosa-associated lymphoid tissue (MALT) lymphoma
    - *Atrophic gastritis*
    - Recent resection of gastric cancer
    - First-degree relative of gastric cancer
    - Desire of patient (after full consultation with physician)

- Treatment advised:
    - *Functional dyspepsia*
    - *Gastro-oesophageal reflux disease (in patients requiring long-term profound acid suppression)*
    - *Use of NSAIDs*

The evidence for many of these recommendations is poor and many clinicians would not accept those shown in italics.

Table 2.8 The risks of gastrointestinal bleeding in different settings

	Approximate relative risk of bleeding
Patient-related factors	
Age >60 years	6.3
History of previous peptic ulcer	
Male gender	1.4
Drug-related factors	
NSAID/aspirin used:	
– Aspirin	1.6*
– Diclofenac	1.8*
– Naproxen	2.2*
– Meloxicam	0.8*
– Rofecoxib	0.4*
– Celecoxib	0.4*
Dose of NSAID used:	
– Concurrent use of steroids	2.8
– Concurrent use of anticoagulant	1.7

*Relative risk compared to ibuprofen.

- In patients with a history of mild cerebrovascular accident (CVA) or transient ischaemic attack (TIA), aspirin reduces further ischaemic events by 3 per 100 patient years
- In patients with a recent MI, aspirin prevents MI, stroke or vascular death in 3 per 100 patient years for up to 4 years
- There is risk reduction in patients with diabetes alone or with peripheral vascular disease
- Aspirin has other benefits such as risk reduction for oesophageal and colonic carcinoma.

Are COX-2 inhibitors 'better' than NSAIDs?

- With regards to pain relief, there is little difference in the analgesic effects of the two classes of drugs
- In comparative studies of NSAIDs and COX-2 inhibitors, there was an increase in ischaemic events in the COX-2 groups
- NSAIDs are protective against colonic carcinoma
- With respect to ulcer bleeding, yes. They reduce risk of bleeding by about 50–60%
- However, in patients with a high risk of cardiovascular disease, serious consideration should be given to giving the patient low-dose aspirin in combination with COX-2 inhibitors – this will undoubtedly increase GI bleeding, but is probably safer than aspirin + NSAID
- The dogma has always been that because COX-2 inhibitors are specific for COX-2 there is less gastric damage because COX-1 is preserved (the main isoform in gastric

45

mucosa responsible for mucosal defence). However, there are interesting data accumulating that the story is a lot more complex (local topical effects may be important). Certainly bleeding occurs in patients taking COX-2s and they are not the magic bullet they were once heralded as.

If starting aspirin or NSAIDs, when should H. pylori be eradicated?

- All patients with history of ulcer with or without bleeding
- All patients at high risk of ulcer complications:
  - over 65 years of age
  - on steroids
- Any patient expecting to take NSAIDs for more than 1–2 days
- It would probably be best to treat *H. pylori* in all patients taking long-term aspirin, although there is no evidence for this approach yet.

NICE guidelines on the use of COX-2 inhibitors for osteoarthritis and rheumatoid arthritis (issued July 2001)

'COX-2 inhibitors' covered were celecoxib, rofecoxib, meloxicam and etodolac:

- COX-2 selective inhibitors and other NSAIDs are indicated for pain and stiffness in inflammatory rheumatoid arthritis and for the short-term management of pain in osteoarthritis.
- All NSAIDs are associated with adverse events and should be prescribed only when there is a demonstrable clinical need and in accordance with their summary of product characteristics.
- Long-term use should be avoided without appropriate monitoring and re-evaluation of clinical need.
- COX-2 selective inhibitors are not recommended for routine use in patients with rheumatoid arthritis or osteoarthritis. They should be used in preference to standard NSAIDs in these conditions only in patients who may be at 'high risk' of developing serious GI adverse effects:
  - those of >65 years age
  - those using concomitant medications known to increase the likelihood of upper GI adverse events
  - those with serious co-morbidity or those requiring the prolonged use of maximum dose of standard NSAIDs
- The risk of NSAID induced complications is particularly increased in patients with a previous clinical history of GU/DU/GI bleeding/GI perforation. The use of COX-2 inhibitors should, therefore, be considered especially carefully in this situation.
- In all patients with cardiovascular disease there remains uncertainty over the use of COX-2 selective inhibitors and they should not be prescribed routinely in preference to standard NSAIDs where these are indicated.
- Furthermore, many patients with cardiovascular disease receive low-dose aspirin and this carries an increased risk of GI events. In patients taking low dose aspirin, the benefit of using COX-2 selective agents is reduced, so prescribing them is not currently justified.

- There is no evidence to justify the simultaneous prescription of gastro-protective agents with COX-2 selective inhibitors as a means of further reducing potential GI adverse events.

Which patients need ulcer prophylaxis?

If patients are considered according to the benefits of treatment and risks of bleeding the strategy shown in Table 2.9 can be adopted (after Hunt et al. 2002).

Non-ulcer dyspepsia

Non-ulcer dyspepsia (NUD) is a poorly defined and researched condition. It is a term used to put a label on upper GI pain with a normal endoscopy and abdominal ultrasound. Experts in the area have tried to refine NUD into different types. Functional dyspepsia is used interchangeably with NUD.

It is rare that treatment for NUD is hugely successful. Before labelling someone as having NUD, they probably ought to have had:

- *H. pylori* eradication if present (supposedly helps 1 in 15)
- a PPI trial (if successful suggests they have reflux disease)

Table 2.9a Ulcer prophylaxis in patients who have not received NSAID or COX-2 inhibitor

Risk of bleeding	Risk factors	Recommended prophylaxis
High	Previous gastrointestinal bleed Age >74 Concomitant steroid Concomitant anticoagulants	COX-2 inhibitor + PPI
Medium	No previous gastrointestinal bleed Age 60–75 years	COX-2 inhibitor alone
Low	No risk factors	NSAID or COX-2 inhibitor

Table 2.9b Ulcer prophylaxis in patients currently treated with NSAIDs/COX-2

Diagnosis	Recommended prophylaxis
Previous ulcer disease	COX-2 inhibitor Eradicate *H. pylori* if present
Previous complicated ulcer	COX-2 inhibitor + PPI Eradicate *H. pylori* if present
Mild/intermittent dyspepsia	H2RA or PPI
Moderate/non-responding dyspepsia	PPI
Current NSAID + PPI	Re-evaluate

- if biliary type symptoms:
  - cholescintigraphy or similar to detect sphincter of Oddi dysfunction
- if weight loss:
  - mesenteric ischaemia and pancreatic pathology excluded if possible.

Treatments for NUD include:

- Tricyclic antidepressants, e.g. amitriptyline 25 mg bd increasing as tolerated
- Prokinetics, e.g. domperidone 10–20 mg prior to meals.

Gastric cancer

Gastric adenocarcinoma is declining in incidence in the UK due to the reduction in *H. pylori* infection. However, it remains a devastating diagnosis and should not be missed in patients with upper GI symptoms. It is the second commonest cancer worldwide.

Strong risk factors for gastric adenocarcinoma are:

- *H. pylori* (2.5 increased risk)
- previous gastric surgery (leading to biliary reflux)
- family history. There is an autosomal dominant form of diffuse gastric cancer. It is rare (<1% cancers), but probably the cause of Napoleon Bonaparte's demise
- gastric atrophy.

How is gastric adenocarcinoma staged?

This is really quite confusing as there have been several redefinitions since the first TNM classification in 1966. The latest, in 1997, by the American Joint Committee on Cancer is outlined below in Box 2.8.

The main difference between this latest classification and previous ones is that the old classification N stage depended on site and distance of involved nodes from the tumour (notoriously difficult to measure accurately and poorly adhered to by surgeons).

Obviously, it is only possible to assess the true N stage of the tumour following resection and examination of all nodes histologically. The more nodes taken, the more likely a tumour will have a higher N stage (so-called 'stage migration'). The converse of this is that tumours that are a lower stage with >15 lymph nodes sampled have a greater survival than an equivalent stage tumour with <15 nodes sampled (when the tumour has been effectively understaged). The new classification has, therefore, been criticized because of this. However, overall it is more reliable than the old system.

Which operation?

The choice of surgery depends on the site of the tumour:

- Cardia tumours – oesophago-gastrectomy
- Body tumours – total gastrectomy
- Antral tumours – distal gastrectomy.

Box 2.8 American Joint Committee on Care gastric cancer staging system

Primary tumour (T)
- TX – tumour cannot be assessed
- T0 – no evidence of tumour
- Tis – (carcinoma in situ) tumour doesn't invade lamina propria
- T1 – invasion of lamina propria/submucosa
- T2 – invasion of muscularis propria/subserosa
- T3 – invasion of serosa
- T4 – invasion of surrounding structures

Regional lymph nodes
- NX – nodes cannot be assessed
- N0 – no nodal metastases
- N1 – 1–6 nodes involved
- N2 – 7–15 nodes involved
- N3 – >15 nodes involved

Distant metastasis
- MX – cannot be assessed
- M0 – no distant metastasis
- M1 – distant metastasis

Stage 0
- TisN0M0

Stage IA
- T1N0M0

Stage IB
- T1N1M0
- T2N0M0

Stage II
- T1N2M0
- T2N1M0
- T3N0M0

Stage IIIA
- T2N2M0
- T3N1M0
- T4N0M0

Stage IIIB
- T3N2M0

Stage IV
- T4N1M0 (some people believe this is Stage IIIB)
- T4N2M0
- Any M1 tumour
- Any N3 tumour

Standard teaching is to maintain a 5 cm resection margin proximally and distally (due to spread of tumour through small lymphatic vessels in the gastric wall).

As for staging, the terminology used in gastric cancer surgery causes confusion. Currently resection is classified as:

- R0 resection – complete resection, margins clear
- R1 resection – microscopic involvement of margins
- R2 resection – macroscopic tumour at margins (palliative operation).

However, these have also been used previously to define lymph-node resection:

- R0 – no lymph nodes removed
- R1 – local lymph nodes removed
- R2 – extended lymph node dissection.

The classification of lymph node resection have more recently been classified as:

- D1 – removal of N1 nodes (see below) and lesser and greater omenta
- D2 – D1 + removal of N2 nodes (see below), omental bursa, front leaf of the transverse mesocolon, spleen and tail of pancreas.

N1 nodes (not to be confused with TNM staging!) occur on the lesser and greater curvatures. N2 nodes occur along the left gastric, common hepatic, coeliac and splenic arteries. More distant nodes have been classified N3 and N4 by Japanese groups.

D1 or D2 resection

This is a 'hot topic' in GI surgery. The Japanese advocate the more aggressive D2 resection. A large randomized MRC study and one from the Netherlands comparing the two approaches, do not show a survival benefit though. This may well be due to the adverse effects of splenectomy and distal pancreatectomy. Despite this, the latest BSG guidelines recommend D2 resection in all patients with curable disease.

How long have I got doctor?

As for oesophageal cancer, an attempt has been made to give some data in Table 2.10 to answer this question. These data are for gastric adenocarcinoma only. There is a huge amount of data from the Far East on gastric adenocarcinoma. However, the disease behaves very differently there (much commoner, different risk factors, many more early cancers) and, therefore, the data in Table 2.10 are taken mostly from Western studies.

Is chemotherapy useful?

Probably yes, but in combination with radiotherapy. Palliative chemotherapy may be considered on a compassionate basis.

Table 2.10 Survival for different groups of patients with gastric cancer

Stage/point of treatment	Median survival	5-year survival
Stage 0 – post surgery		100%
Stage IA – post surgery		90%
Stage IB – post surgery		85%
Stage II – post surgery		50%
Stage IIIA – post surgery		25%
Stage IIIB – post surgery		10%
Stage III – undergoing curative resection		10–25%
Stage IV		6%
N1 disease (1–6 nodes)	36 months	
N2 disease (7–15 nodes)	20 months	
N3 disease (>15 nodes)	12 months	
All curative resections	27 months	
All curative resections + chemoradiotherapy	36 months	

Other tumours of the stomach and duodenum

Mucosa-associated lymphoid tissue (MALT) and other lymphomas

Lymphomas account for around 3% of gastric malignancies. Lymphoid tissue can be found in mucosae in many parts of the body. Gut-associated lymphoid tissue (GALT) occurs predominantly in the ileum and appendix, but is also found in the stomach following *H. pylori* infection. Neoplastic transformation of this gastric MALT can occur to form MALT lymphomas or 'MALTomas'. Thirty to 40% of gastric lymphomas are *H. pylori*-associated MALTomas. The rest are primary gastric lymphomas or extra-nodal lymphomas.

MALTomas are associated with *H. pylori* infection in 70–90% of cases (less so if the tumours are high grade). Treatment of *H. pylori* without other 'chemotherapy' is thought to successfully cure many of these lymphomas. However, close follow-up is advised with yearly endoscopies after treatment.

High-grade gastric lymphomas often require chemotherapy (such as CHOP) and/or radiotherapy. Chemotherapy often results in tumours 'melting away', which can cause bowel perforation necessitating surgery.

Gastrointestinal stromal tumours

GI stromal tumours (GISTs) are tumours of the subepithelial mesenchymal tissues and include tumours previously termed leiomyomas, leiomyosarcomas and leiomyoblastomas. The development of improved histochemical staining has shown these tumours are not tumours of the muscularis propria as previously thought.

GISTs are commonly found at endoscopy and can be easily identified at EUS (or indeed transabdominal ultrasound if large enough). Tumours tend to contain either spindle cells or epithelioid cells. Eighty-five per cent of GISTs contain cells with a mutation of the tyrosine kinase receptor C-KIT (or CD117). This mutation leads to uncontrolled cell growth. The other 15% often have mutations of the PDGFR (platelet-derived growth factor receptor) that also activates tyrosine kinase. These mutations are important as they act as targets for recently developed chemotherapy agents.

Imatinib (Glivec, Novartis) was developed for treating chronic myeloid leukaemia, but has been found to be highly active against C-KIT-positive GISTs. This drug can be given orally, is usually well tolerated (diarrhoea and oedema are common) and gives significant tumour response in over 50% of patients.

Which gastrointestinal stromal tumours should be removed, followed up or offered Imatinib?

The following features suggest a malignant (local invasion, metastasis) course:

- Size >5 cm
- Number of mitoses >10 per high-powered field
- Site (extra-gastric)
- C-KIT mutation
- EUS features including echogenic foci and cystic spaces.

Small GISTs with none of these features and no evidence of local spread can be observed (e.g. yearly ultrasound). Some people believe all GISTs have the potential to behave in an aggressive fashion. However, gastroenterologists have been ignoring small 'leiomyomas' for years without problem.

Indications for surgery include:

- Size >5 cm
- No CT evidence of invasion or metastases (especially liver)
- Complications, e.g. bleeding, dysphagia, outlet obstruction.

Indications for imatinib treatment include:

- CT evidence of local spread or metastasis
- Unfit for surgery with other indications for surgery.

Other diseases of the stomach and duodenum

Gastric antral vascular ectasia – 'water melon stomach'

This is a relatively uncommon condition, but one that causes recurrent admissions with anaemia. It is usually characterized by a severe antral gastritis with friable bleeding mucosa, emerging 'spoke-like' from the pylorus on the gastric folds (supposedly looking like a water-melon in cross section) (Fig. 2.10b). It is associated with:

- portal hypertension (30–40% of cases)
- scleroderma
- Sjogren's syndrome.

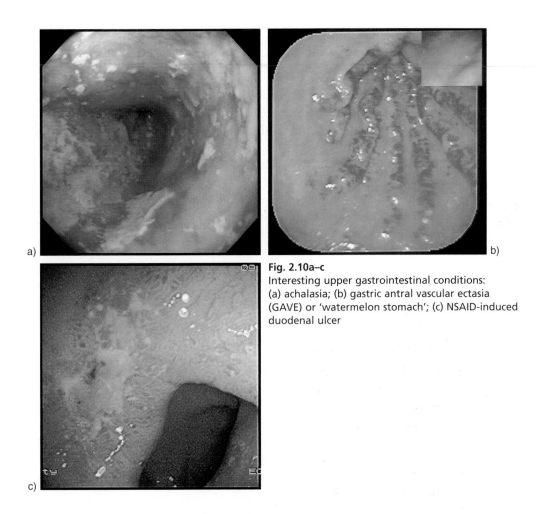

Fig. 2.10a–c
Interesting upper gastrointestinal conditions:
(a) achalasia; (b) gastric antral vascular ectasia
(GAVE) or 'watermelon stomach'; (c) NSAID-induced
duodenal ulcer

Most cases, though, are cryptogenic. Transfusion requirements can be high (1–2 units a week). It usually occurs in elderly women.

Treatments include:

- tranexamic acid 1 g tds (occasionally helps)
- PPI (high dose)
- argon plasma coagulation (works in 60–70%, but needs repeated treatments)
- NdYAG laser
- transjugular intrahepatic portosystemic shunt (may help in patients with established portal hypertension)
- surgery (antrectomy).

Gastroparesis

Gastric emptying is such a complex process that it will not be described in detail here. Over-simplified, three components must be thought about:

1. Proximal fundic tone
2. Propagating antral contractions, driven by the gastric pacemaker
3. Pyloric sphincter resistance.

Gastroparesis is a broad term for disorders of gastric motility, which usually become symptomatic once gastric emptying is impaired. Gastroparesis should be considered in patients with a large food and fluid residue at endoscopy without evidence of actual obstruction.

Tests for gastroparesis include:

- barium meal and follow-through (exclude small-bowel obstruction and look for evidence of conditions such as scleroderma)
- solid phase gastric emptying (see Section 2)
- electrogastrograph (akin to ECG – rarely available).

Causes of gastroparesis include:

- diabetes mellitus
- surgery (e.g. fundoplication)
- scleroderma.

Treatments include:

- prokinetics
  - metoclopramide 10 mg tds
  - domperidone 10–20 mg tds
  - cisapride 10–20 mg tds (named patient, beware diabetic with angina)
  - erythromycin 250–500 mg qds
- botulinum toxin injection – 100–200 units around pylorus every 6 months
- implantable gastric pacemaker.

SECTION 2: GASTROINTESTINAL INVESTIGATIONS

Upper gastrointestinal endoscopy

The equipment

Every good driver knows how his car works, so you should have at least some understanding behind the workings of the endoscopy system. Cotton and Williams book on Practical Endoscopy is strongly recommended for an explanation.

Anatomy of the oesophagus and stomach

The oesophagus is often divided into upper, middle and lower. For the purpose of TNM staging these have been defined as follows:

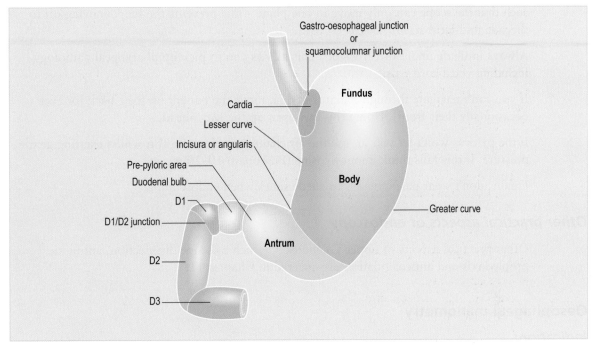

Fig. 2.11
Upper gastrointestinal anatomy for the endoscopist

- Upper – thoracic inlet to carina
- Middle – carina to midway point between carina and GOJ
- Lower – midway point between carina and GOJ to the GOJ.

The definition of these regions can be difficult clinically as without EUS it is impossible to accurately find the carina. Most endoscopists use the following distances:

- Upper – 18–24 cm
- Middle – 24–32 cm
- Lower – 32–40 cm.

There is much confusion (and debate) as to the anatomical landmarks of different regions of the stomach. Figure 2.11 is an attempt to simplify this.

Endoscopy technique

The explanation of how to endoscope a patient is outside the realms of this book. However, here are a few hints and tips which may help.

Before intubating, hold the scope such that the end drops vertically down. Ensure both large and small wheels are free and the scope is straight. Fix the small (left/right) wheel, such that the scope can only move in one plane – this prevents the scope moving off to the side mid-intubation.

Always intubate under direct vision. This allows you to pick up pharyngeal pathology including vocal cord palsy.

If you can't navigate through a hiatus hernia, move the patient on their back (or even occasionally their front). Doing this can open up the way ahead.

If the pylorus won't let you in, use the air channel to blow air at it whilst exerting gentle pressure. If this fails think about hyosine (Buscopan) 10–20 mg iv.

Finally, don't wear pale trousers or suede shoes when endoscoping.

Other practical aspects of endoscopy

Other practical aspects of upper GI endoscopy such as scope disinfection, antibiotic prophylaxis and anticoagulation are covered in Chapter 11.

Oesophageal manometry

Indications

- To establish a diagnosis and categorize oesophageal motility disorders
- To place pH electrodes for ambulatory pH monitoring.

The features of common motility disorders are described earlier.

Oesophageal pH studies

These are usually ambulatory, i.e. the patients are free to go about their normal daily activities and over a 24-h period. The most commonly used method involves a pH probe passed nasogastrically. However, capsule probes are now being developed that can be inserted endoscopically and left to record data for 48 h without the presence of a nasal wire (e.g. Bravo probe, Boston Scientific). There are several benefits to such a device.

Traditional probes are placed at 5 cm above the proximal border of the lower oesophageal sphincter. This is usually determined by oesophageal manometry, hence the two procedures are performed concurrently. Once connected to the recorder the patient documents the presence of symptoms by pushing a button on the recorder. The patient also records meals and when he or she is lying down. When the study is complete, the following parameters can be determined:

1. Percentage time below pH 4
2. Number of reflux episodes
3. Duration of reflux episodes
4. De Meester score
5. Symptom Index

6. Symptom Sensitivity Index
7. Symptom-associated probability.

Numbers one through to three are self explanatory.

The De Meester score uses six components of the recording (% total time pH<4, % upright time pH<4, % supine time pH<4, total number of reflux episodes, number of episodes >5 min and longest episode) and gives each component a score. Each score is weighted differently, e.g. supine reflux time is given a high score, such that the total score is representative of GORD.

A normal De Meester score is <14.7 (95% of the population). A score above this suggests significant GORD.

Numbers five through to seven are all ways of associating symptoms with reflux episodes. The following scores are considered to represent significant GORD:

Symptom index >50%
Symptom sensitivity index >10%
Symptom-associated probability >95%.

Scintigraphic studies

Gastric emptying studies

Radiolabelled meals can be given to confirm or refute gastroparesis.

Usually two different radio-isotopes are used with a liquid component (e.g. Indium111-labelled water) and solid component (e.g. Technetium99-labelled scrambled egg) to differentiate between the emptying of these two components.

Less than 10% of liquid and 50% of solid would normally be expected in the stomach 2 h after such a meal, but different nuclear medicine departments will have their own normal ranges depending on the meals used.

Oesophageal scintigraphy

Oesophageal scintigraphy can be used to assess either oesophageal motility or gastro-oesophageal reflux. To assess oesophageal motility, Technetium-99-sulphur-colloid-labelled water or bolus meals are used and images collected over up to 5 min. The oesophageal clearance can be obtained (usually >90%), but the technique also allows motility of the three to five separate regions of the oesophagus to be assessed.

To assess gastro-oesophageal reflux, 150 ml of Technetium-99-sulphur-colloid-labelled water, milk or orange juice is swallowed and the patient placed in the supine position. Various manouevres (Valsalva, abdominal pressure) are then used to try and encourage reflux. A normal study would usually have <4% of gastric contents refluxing into the oesophagus. Data about the extent of reflux, number and duration of reflux episodes can be obtained.

Further Reading

Barr H. Endoscopic surveillance of patients with Barrett's oesophagus. Gut 2002; 51: 313–4.

Delaney B, Moayyedi P, Deeks J et al. The management of dyspepsia: a systemic review. Health Technology Assessment 2000; 4: 1–197.

FitzGerald GA, Patrono C. The Coxibs, selective inhibitors of cyclooxygenase-2. N Engl J Med. 2001; 345: 433–42.

Goddard AF, Atherton JC. Gastritis, peptic ulceration and related conditions. In: Armstrong D, Cohen J, Powderly W et al (eds.) In: Infectious Diseases, 2nd Edn 2003. London, UK: Mosby, Chapter 42.

Graham DY. NSAIDs, Helicobacter pylori, and Pandora's Box. N Engl J Med 2002; 347: 2162–4.

Holloway, RH. Ed. Reflux disease. Bailliere's Best Practice and Research Clinical Gastroenterology 2000; 14: 681–879.

Leslie P, Carding PN, Wilson JA. Investigation and management of chronic dysphagia. BMJ 2003; 326: 433–6.

Miller LS, Szych GA, Kantor SB et al. Treatment of idiopathic gastroparesis with injection of botulinum toxin into the pyloric sphincter muscle. Am J Gastroenterol 2002; 97: 1653–60.

MRC Oesophageal Cancer Working Group. Surgical resection with or without preoperative chemotherapy in oesophageal cancer: a randomized controlled trial. Lancet 2002; 359: 1727–33.

Peterson WL. Improving the management of GERD: evidence-based therapeutic strategies. Continuing Medical Education: Consensus Opinion in Gastroenterology. American Gastroenterological Association 2002.

Spechler SJ. Barrett's Esophagus. N Engl J Med 2002; 346: 836–42.

Soykan I, Sarosiek I, McCallum RW. The effect of chronic oral domperidone therapy on gastrointestinal symptoms, gastric emptying, and quality of life in patients with gastroparesis. Am J Gastroenterol 1997; 92: 976–80.

Vaezi MF, Richter JE. Diagnosis and management of achalasia. Am J Gastroenterol 1999; 94: 3406–12.

Useful Websites

www.bsg.org.uk/clinical_prac/guidelines/oes_dil.htm (BSG oesophageal dilatation guidelines)

www.bsg.org.uk/pdf_word_doc/dyspepsia.doc (BSG dyspepsia guidelines)

www.bsg.org.uk/clinical_prac/guidelines/ogcancer.htm (BSG guidelines on oesophageal cancer)

www.cancer.gov/cancerinfo/pdq/treatment/esophageal/healthprofessional/ (US National Cancer Institute overview)

www.ncrn.org.uk (UK National Cancer Research Network – a useful site to find out what current studies are going on in Upper GI cancer)

www.medtronic.com/neuro/mfd/gastro/trainingarticle.html (DeMeester scoring for pH studies)

www.nice.org.uk/CG017NICEguideline

www.jr2.ox.ac.uk/bandolier/booth/Arthritis/aspNCP.html (Bandolier summary of ulcer prophylaxis)

Small-bowel disease

3

INTRODUCTION

The small intestine accounts for the largest portion of the gastrointestinal tract, both in length and surface area. However, it is often overlooked as it is the most inaccessible part of the gut to practising gastroenterologists. Owing to its important digestive, absorptive, immunological and endocrine functions, disorders of anatomy or function may result in disabling symptoms that often present a diagnostic challenge. This chapter aims to give an overview of important conditions affecting the small bowel, their investigation and rational management. Crohn's disease commonly affects the small intestine, but is discussed in Chapter 5.

STRUCTURE AND FUNCTION

The length of the small bowel depends on whether measurements are made in living subjects during endoscopy or surgery (mean length estimated at 280 cm) or at postmortem (mean length 600 cm) when length is increased owing to relaxation of the small-bowel musculature. Resection of the small bowel is often remarkably well tolerated, although a critical length needs to remain to allow adequate function, thought to be approximately 50 cm residual small bowel in the presence of an intact colon. The duodenum, named as it was thought to be 12 fingerbreadths in length, is mostly retroperitoneal and lies on the upper right side of the abdomen, encompassing the head of the pancreas. The embryonic foregut–midgut junction is between the first and second parts of the duodenum and can be seen endoscopically where the circumferential valvulae conniventes start. The rest of the small intestine is split into the jejunum (proximal 40%) and the ileum (distal 60%), although there is no distinct junction between the two. As one of the main functions of the small bowel is absorption, it is highly specialized in this regard. There are approximately 50 finger or leaf-shaped villi per mm^2 of small intestine (Fig. 3.1). These villi occupy approximately 60% of the full mucosal depth and become shorter towards the jejunum, before elongating again in the ileum. Cells lining the villi originate in the crypt and mature apically to become enterocytes, although mucus-secreting goblet cells are also present. The luminal enterocyte border has a highly

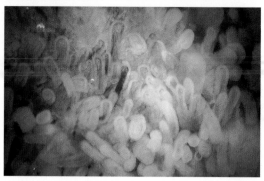

Fig. 3.1
The appearance of normal small-bowel mucosa using stereomicroscopy of a freshly taken biopsy. Finger-like villi containing vascular arcades are well shown

specialized ultra-structural surface consisting of microvilli, which further amplify the capacity for nutrient absorption.

As the gastrointestinal (GI) tract is bombarded daily with exogenous antigens and pathogens, immune surveillance and tolerance are important features of the normal small intestine. After ingested food has passed through the low pH conditions in the stomach, the small bowel is mostly sterile. However there are numerous organisms that readily and harmlessly colonize niches within the GI tract, predominantly strict or facultative anaerobes and predominantly in the distal small intestine (e.g. *Bacteroides* spp.). There are circumstances where pathogenic bacteria can colonize the small intestine, especially if there are structural abnormalities within the small bowel such as diverticulosis, or the presence of blind loops created either by fistulae or surgery (e.g. Roux-en-Y loops). The immune system within the intestine consists of intraepithelial and lamina propria lymphocytes and specialized 'Peyer's patches'. These are raised areas found mostly in the distal small-bowel mucosa as lymphoid aggregates and orchestrate the presentation of luminal antigens to B and T-lymphocytes. Activated lymphocytes migrate to the enteric surface, together with macrophages and other leukocytes, providing protection to the host from invading pathogens.

MALABSORPTION

Symptoms of malabsorption are perhaps the most common presenting complaint of small-bowel disease. There is usually diarrhoea, which may be steatorrhoeic or watery and is frequently associated with increased stool volume and weight. Weight loss results from inadequate absorption of dietary nutrients and the complications of malabsorption relate to the effects of vitamin or mineral deficiency. The pathophysiology of malabsorption is due to enterocyte damage or loss and has aetiologies ranging from autoimmune to infective causes. A spectrum of symptoms similar to malabsorption can result from maldigestion, where the small-bowel mucosa is often normal, but there is, for example, exocrine pancreatic insufficiency or altered bile salt secretion caused by biliary obstruction. Table 3.1 gives a broad classification of the causes of malabsorption. The more common causes originating in the small intestine will be dealt with in this chapter.

COELIAC DISEASE

Definition

Coeliac disease (CD) (or gluten-sensitive enteropathy) is an inflammatory condition predominantly affecting the proximal small bowel in genetically predisposed individuals. The toxic environmental triggers are the prolamins of wheat (i.e. the alcohol-soluble component, gliadin) or the corresponding portion of barley and rye. It appears that patients are less, or indeed not sensitive to oats, although the cultivation and processing of oats in the same location as wheat may allow minute, but significant, amounts of cross contamination. Symptoms and mucosal histology improve with the exclusion of dietary gluten and recur on gluten challenge. CD is a good example of an autoimmune condition where a single environmental trigger has been successfully identified.

Table 3.1 Classification of the causes of malabsorption

1. Mucosal lesions Coeliac disease Dermatitis herpetiformis Collagenous sprue Tropical sprue Hypogammaglobulinaemia	**5. Infection** Acute gastroenteritis Parasitic infection (e.g. giardiasis) Tuberculosis Whipple's disease Small bowel bacterial overgrowth
2. Structural lesions Intestinal lymphangiectasia Crohn's disease Lymphoma Amyloidosis Lymphatic obstruction Ischaemia Systemic mastocytosis Macroglobulinaemia Pneumatosis intestinalis Post-radiotherapy	**6. Maldigestion** Bile salt deficiency (e.g. obstructive jaundice) Pancreatic insufficiency **7. Short bowel syndrome (see Table 3.6)** **8. Biochemical abnormalities** Disaccharidase deficiencies (e.g. lactase deficiency) Abetalipoproteinaemia Zollinger–Ellison syndrome
3. Malignancy Carcinoma Neuroendocrine tumours Lymphoma	**9. Endocrine disorders** Hyper- and hypothyroidism Addison's disease Hyper- and hypoparathyroidism Diabetes mellitus
4. Pharmacological Drugs (e.g. NSAIDs, PPIs, antibiotics) Alcohol	

Epidemiology

CD predominantly affects northern Europeans with a prevalence in the UK of about 1%, as estimated by antibody screening. This is considerably higher than previously thought, although many individuals with a positive antibody test will be asymptomatic and may, indeed, have normal small-bowel histology. There is little sex difference and approximately 10–15% of first-degree relatives are affected. The concordance in monozygotic twin studies is approximately 70% and CD is closely associated with the possession of the extended haplotype HLA B8 DR3 DQ2. Over 90% of patients possess the DQ2 or DQ8 haplotype compared to 30% of the general population, suggesting a strong genetic influence.

Pathology

The small intestinal mucosa demonstrates the characteristic appearances of villous atrophy and crypt hyperplasia, with an increase in the intra-epithelial lymphocyte count (over 30 lymphocytes/100 enterocytes). The lamina propria becomes infiltrated with lymphocytes and plasma cells. In classical cases, the absorptive capacity of the intestine is markedly reduced resulting in malabsorption. The histopathological features of CD are usually most pronounced proximally in the small intestine, presumably due to an increased gluten load. There are considerable research efforts to determine the toxic peptides from gluten responsible for the induction of the inflammatory response and damage in the small bowel. In *in vitro* studies, amino acid sequences have been identified which appear to strongly induce a T-cell response. For these sequences to be generated, gliadin requires deamidation by tissue transglutaminase, a calcium-dependent enzyme that has also been identified in recent years as the antigen against which the endomysial antibody is directed.

Clinical features

There is a broad range of clinical presentations in adults. The classical presentation of weight loss, steatorrhoea, abdominal bloating and associated osteomalacia has become less common as greater awareness and simpler diagnostic modalities (e.g. antibody testing and endoscopic biopsy) have been developed. Patients commonly present with abdominal symptoms similar to the irritable bowel syndrome (IBS) with distension, bloating and diarrhoea, although constipation may occur in some. It is, therefore, appropriate to screen for CD in patients being investigated with IBS-type symptoms. Anaemia is a common presentation, either with associated symptoms such as lethargy, breathlessness and pallor, or as an incidental finding. The anaemia is multifactorial as there may be impaired iron and folate absorption in the jejunum together with increased iron loss from high enterocyte turnover or mucosal blood loss. Specific haematological findings are discussed below. Other symptoms include painful recurrent oral aphthous ulceration, ataxia, or symptoms of the associated conditions that are listed in Table 3.2.

Table 3.2 The prevalence of coeliac disease in other disorders

Disorder	Reported prevalence (%)
Hyposplenism	50–70
Bird fancier's lung	31
Unexplained ataxia	13–16
Primary Sjogren's	15
Primary biliary cirrhosis	6–7
Type 1 diabetes	5–6.1
Autoimmune thyroid disease	3.3–6
Cryptogenic hypertransaminasaemia	1.5–9
Recurrent aphthous ulcers	3.8–4

Diagnosis

Endoscopy with small-bowel biopsy

At endoscopy there is often a reduced number of duodenal folds and scalloping of the folds (probably a reflection of the flat mosaic pattern) in untreated disease (Fig. 3.2), but these cannot be relied upon in making a diagnosis. The presence of normal villi or the flat mosaic pattern of untreated disease can often be appreciated with newer (especially zoom) endoscopes or on stereomicroscopy of freshly taken biopsies (Figs 3.1, 3.3 & 3.4). Biopsy of the small intestine is important in establishing the diagnosis of CD. Taking endoscopic biopsies from the second or third part of duodenum is the usual method and has been well validated. As the distribution of histological abnormality can be patchy, taking at

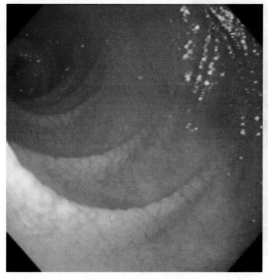

Fig. 3.2
Scalloping and reduction of duodenal folds seen at endoscopy in a patient with untreated coeliac disease

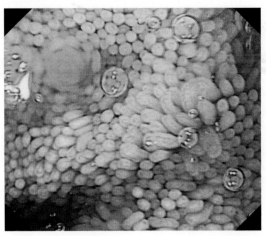

Fig. 3.3
Zoom endoscopy image demonstrating normal villi

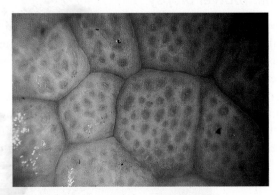

Fig. 3.4
The flat mosaic mucosal pattern of untreated coeliac disease. Stereomicroscopy of a freshly taken biopsy

least four biopsies is recommended. Although subtotal or total (synonymous terms) villous atrophy is the classical appearance in untreated CD, lesser degrees of abnormality are compatible with the diagnosis. There are many much rarer causes of villous atrophy (Table 3.3) and it is, therefore, necessary to also demonstrate a response (at least clinically) to a gluten-free diet (GFD), especially if the endomysial antibody test is negative.

Antibody testing

There have been several antibody tests used to aid the diagnosis of CD including anti-reticulin, anti-jejunal, anti-gliadin, anti-endomysial (EMA) and anti-tissue transglutaminase (tTG) antibodies. The EMA has a sensitivity of approximately 94% and specificity of 98% (and, therefore, a positive likelihood ratio (LR+) of 47) in published clinical studies and is the most accurate of those listed. It is an IgA class antibody detected by immunofluorescence using either primate oesophagus or human umbilical vein as the substrate. Approximately 2% of patients with CD have selective IgA deficiency (compared

Table 3.3 Some causes of subtotal villous atrophy

Without distinctive histological features	With distinctive histological features
Adults	
Coeliac disease	Giardiasis with hypogammaglobulinaemia
Soy protein sensitivity	T-cell lymphoma
Tropical sprue	Whipple's disease
Zollinger–Ellison syndrome	Crohn's disease
Hypothyroidism	Ischaemia
Macroamylasaemia	Radiotherapy
Drugs	Eosinophilic gastroenteritis
Tuberculosis	
Viral hepatitis	
Children	
Cow's milk protein sensitivity	
Fish, rice and chicken sensitivity	
Kwashiorkor	
Post-enteritis	

with 0.2% of the general population) and would be falsely negative. The anti-tTG antibody test is ELISA-based and is, therefore, objective and more convenient. It has been well validated with histology and EMA and may become the standard antibody test.

Whom to biopsy?

If the pre-test probability of a patient having CD is low (e.g. mild abdominal bloating with no other symptoms) antibody testing is advised, with a positive test directing the need for biopsy. A negative test effectively excludes the diagnosis. If the pre-test probability is high (e.g. a patient with iron deficiency anaemia and diarrhoea) no antibody testing is necessary and one should proceed directly to endoscopic biopsy. This is because even if such a patient had a negative antibody test, there is still a significant chance of having the disease.

Is it necessary to biopsy those with a positive anti-endomysial test?

Because of the accuracy of the EMA test, some consider biopsy to be unnecessary before treating a patient with a positive test. However, the following points should be taken into consideration:

- Without the objective baseline of abnormal histology, it will be difficult to judge villous response to treatment in those patients who don't seem to be responding symptomatically.
- It is not uncommon to find normal histology in patients with a positive EMA test. The significance of this is not fully understood, although some such patients develop typical histological abnormalities if biopsy is repeated after about 1 year.
- We would always recommend biopsy to confirm the diagnosis.

If histology were normal in a patient with a positive EMA test, we would usually continue a normal diet and repeat the biopsy after 1 year. However, if the patient has troublesome typical symptoms of CD, we would consider treatment with a GFD and carefully assess response according to symptoms and improvement in any abnormal blood tests. However, this is not ideal as there will always be doubt about the diagnosis and less commitment to a strict GFD for life.

Radiology

The well-described findings of proximal small-bowel dilatation, loss of valvulae conniventes and barium flocculation are often absent from small-bowel barium studies in patients with CD, especially in mild cases. Barium studies are not routinely performed, but may be useful to investigate patients who do not respond as expected to treatment, to detect strictures or ulceration that might indicate small-bowel lymphoma or ulcerative jejunitis, both of which may complicate CD.

Haematology

Patients with CD and anaemia are most commonly iron deficient due to the lack of absorption in the proximal small bowel, increased enterocyte turnover or mucosal bleeding, but may have a mixed deficiency, as folate is also absorbed in the jejunum. Vitamin B12 levels are low in approximately 15%. The mean cell volume is, therefore, commonly low, but may be high or even normal, but with a wide red cell distribution width (RDW) indicating the presence of two red-cell populations of differing size. The peripheral blood film may exhibit target cells, Howell–Jolly bodies (as splenic atrophy is common) and the features of a dimorphic anaemia. Bone-marrow examination may show a lack of stainable iron or features of megaloblastic erythropoiesis.

Biochemistry

Untreated patients often have mild hypocalcaemia and hypomagnesaemia, occasionally leading to tremor, tetany, personality change or the clinical features of osteomalacia. Persistent diarrhoea may cause hypokalaemia, although this is rare. Fat malabsorption is associated with deficiency of the fat-soluble vitamins A, D, E and K, which may exacerbate hypocalcaemia or lead to prolongation of the prothrombin time. Serum albumin may be low and can contribute to ascites or peripheral oedema.

Treatment

More than a century after the first accurate description of CD, treatment remains as first described by Samuel Gee in 1888 'by means of a diet'. A strict GFD, first publicly recommended by Dicke in 1950, reverses the small-bowel histological changes to normal. This has traditionally been tested for by repeat endoscopy and duodenal biopsy 4–12 months after the institution of a GFD. The reasons for repeating the biopsy are both to confirm the diagnosis and confirm a good response to treatment. However, the first reason is less important if the EMA test was positive and histological recovery can often be inferred from the clinical response. Secondary lactase deficiency due to severe villous atrophy may initially require a lactose-free diet until well established on a GFD with mucosal recovery. The titre of circulating antibodies often falls on treatment, although this is not a reliable method for assessing dietary compliance. Patients should be advised regarding the diet and initial input from a dietitian can be extremely helpful in this regard. The Coeliac Society (now Coeliac UK – see Table 1.1 for address) produces an invaluable 'Food and Drink Directory' that lists all the foods (by both brand names and supermarket suppliers) that are safe to eat. Many gluten-free items are also available on prescription. Symptoms usually respond within several weeks and subsequent weight gain is common. If there are any associated haematological or biochemical deficiencies these should be replaced (e.g. iron sulphate 200 mg bd for iron deficiency or calcium and vitamin D if osteomalacia is present). The importance of dietary compliance, both for symptomatic relief and the recovery of the small intestine should be regularly reinforced to the patient. Once on the GFD, patients often report increased sensitivity to the ingestion of gluten, with symptoms such as diarrhoea or oral ulceration being more severe than before the original diagnosis was made. The most common reason for treatment failure is taking a diet containing gluten, either intentionally or accidentally. If there is good compliance then alternative diagnoses should be considered and a plan for managing non-response is shown in Figure 3.5.

Latent and asymptomatic coeliac disease

It is unclear how best to manage asymptomatic patients with a positive EMA test and normal villous architecture on biopsy (so-called 'latent' CD). The risks of the complications of CD in this group are probably not significant, although there is no evidence on which to base management decisions. It would seem reasonable to keep such patients under review and repeat duodenal biopsies after 12 months or sooner if symptoms develop.

Complications

Cancer risk in coeliac disease

There is evidence from the UK and the USA that the relative risk of small-bowel carcinoma, lymphoma and other GI cancers are increased in patients with CD. However, these are uncommon tumours and the absolute risk for individual patients remains low. This risk has previously been used as an incentive to help ensure patient compliance with a GFD, but the mortality in treated patients is comparable to healthy controls.

Osteoporosis

Bone mineral densitometry (usually measured by DEXA scan of the femoral head and lumbar spine) is often reduced in patients at the time of diagnosis. This usually improves with treatment and recent population-based studies suggest that non-vertebral fracture risk is not substantial. DEXA scanning all patients at diagnosis or 1 year after starting a GFD may help to detect patients who need to be particularly vigilant with their diet. If

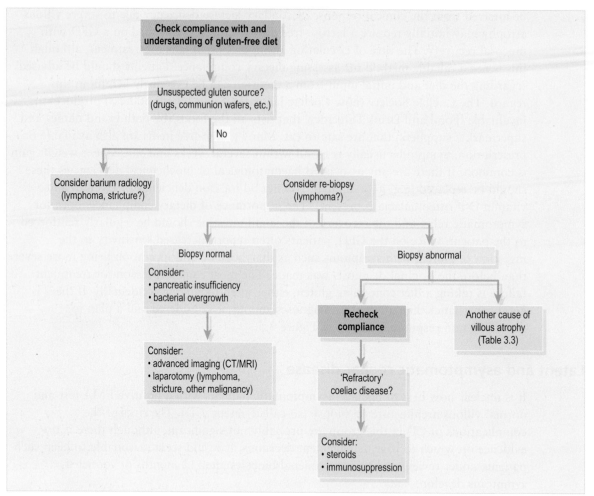

Fig. 3.5
Management of patients not responding to a gluten-free diet

DEXA scanning is not readily available it would be reasonable to restrict scanning to after the menopause only (or at an equivalent age in men, e.g. over 55 years), at an age when treatment with bisphosphonates would be indicated if osteoporosis was found.

Follow-up

Once the small intestinal mucosa has returned to normal and symptoms have resolved it is not essential to follow-up all patients in a specialist clinic. However, it can be useful to encourage adherence to the diet and to detect early sinister symptoms (e.g. weight loss, abdominal pain or diarrhoea) that may indicate small-bowel malignancy. This can then be looked for by repeat biopsy with T-cell marker studies or by barium radiology.

Association with dermatitis herpetiformis

Although few patients with CD have dermatitis herpetiformis (DH), 80% of patients with DH have CD, usually with lesser degrees of villous atrophy. DH is a pruritic blistering skin rash found mainly on the prominences, such as elbows, knees, shoulder blades and buttocks. Its diagnosis can be confirmed by the demonstration of granular deposits of IgA at the papillary tips on direct immunofluorescence of biopsies taken from uninvolved skin. It usually responds promptly to dapsone, but it also often settles after 1 year or so on a strict GFD and dapsone can then be stopped.

SMALL INTESTINAL INFECTIONS

Giardiasis

Giardia lamblia (or *duodenalis*, or *intestinalis*) is the commonest cause of small-bowel protozoal infection worldwide and in the UK. The prevalence of infection varies from approximately 5% in temperate countries to 30% in the tropics. Infection is, therefore, often suspected as a cause for diarrhoea in a returning traveller, although occasionally infection can be present without a history of travel. Infection is usually from a contaminated water supply.

Clinical features

Infection is commonest in young children and adults aged 20–40 years. There is a broad range of symptoms, from asymptomatic carriage to a severe malabsorption syndrome. As few as 10 ingested cysts (the infectious form of the organism) from contaminated water, food or by direct faeco-oral contact can establish infection. Transmission is facilitated by its ability to survive for weeks in cold water and its resistance to chlorination. Typically, after an incubation period of 1–3 weeks there is a sudden onset of watery diarrhoea with cramping abdominal pain, bloating, anorexia and nausea. Symptoms often abate over the course of a few weeks leaving persistent, mild diarrhoeal symptoms, although the passage of malabsorption-type pale, bulky, foul-smelling stools may follow. Not surprisingly, giardiasis is associated with immune deficiency states such as selective IgA deficiency, hypogammaglobulinaemia and HIV infection.

Investigations (Table 3.4)

Stool microscopy is the commonest technique for making a positive diagnosis. In formed stool, *Giardia* appears as cysts, with a faecal load of up to thousands of cysts per gram of stool. In diarrhoeal stools, trophozoites may be seen. One stool sample allows the diagnosis to be made in 60–80% of cases and if three samples are taken over 90% of cases will be detected. An ELISA faecal antigen test is available, but probably doesn't improve diagnosis significantly. It can be useful for examining large numbers of stool samples in an outbreak. In duodenal biopsies, the organism may be seen in clusters within the lumen or adjacent to the epithelial surface as sickle-shaped, basophilic structures. It

Table 3.4 Protocol for diagnosing giardiasis

1. Microscopy of three stool samples
2. If negative, take four small-bowel biopsies for histological examination for trophozoites
3. Make a smear from the luminal surface of two of the biopsies before fixation. Air dry the slides, fix in methanol, stain with Giemsa[1] and scan for the trophozoites (see Fig. 3.6)
4. If small-bowel biopsies are being taken anyway, stool examination may be omitted since mucosal smear is the most reliable test[2]

[1]Ament MA, Rubin CE. Relation of giardiasis to abnormal intestinal structure and function in gastrointestinal immunodeficiency syndromes. Gastroenterology 1972; 62: 216–226.
[2]Kamath KR, Murugasu R. A comparative study of four methods for detecting giardia lamblia in children with diarrheal disease and malabsorption. Gastroenterology 1974; 66: 16–21.

has a characteristic disc underneath used for epithelial cell attachment and under high-power flagella may be identified. Usually there are no changes in the small intestinal mucosa, but there may be villous atrophy, particularly in IgA deficiency. Diagnosis can be improved by making a smear on a glass slide from the luminal surface of a duodenal biopsy. The presence of trophozoites can be recognized easily (Fig. 3.6).

Treatment

Nitroimidazoles have traditionally been the mainstay of treatment for giardiasis. A recent review of the efficacy of all drug regimens recommended metronidazole 250 mg tds for 5–7 days or a single dose of tinidazole 2 g. In the UK metronidazole is not available as 250 mg and, therefore, 400 mg tds for 5 days is recommended. These regimens cure over 90% of infected individuals with stool clearance of the parasite within 3–5 days and symptoms resolving within 5–7 days. The side effect profiles of these two drugs are

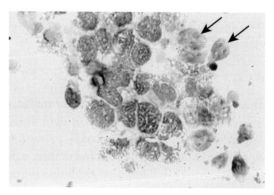

Fig. 3.6
Photomicrograph of a fixed and stained mucosal smear from a fresh small-bowel biopsy showing the trophozoites of *Giardia lamblia* (indicated by arrows)

similar and include headache and nausea. Other side effects such as reversible neutropenia, CNS toxicity and peripheral neuropathy are unlikely with a short course of treatment. Their potentially mutagenic properties make them unsuitable for use in early pregnancy, where paromomycin 500 mg qds for 7 days can be used.

Ascariasis

Ascaris lumbricoides (or the related pig roundworm *Ascaris suum*) is the most common and largest nematode to infect the human gastrointestinal tract, with a worldwide prevalence of over one billion people infected, especially in tropical and subtropical regions. Infection is common where there is poor sanitation, especially in areas where human faeces is used as fertilizer. Infection is caused by the ingestion of food contaminated with *Ascaris* ova, which hatch into larvae that penetrate the small intestine and are transported to the lung via the portal system and pulmonary arteries. This may cause transient respiratory symptoms with pulmonary infiltrates on chest radiograph and eosinophilia ('Loeffler's syndrome'). Migration to the pharynx is followed by ingestion and finally the adult worm develops in the small intestine, growing up to 30 cm in length. Infection is often asymptomatic, although vague abdominal discomfort may be present. If there is a worm bolus, especially in children, intestinal obstruction can occur. Other particular problems with *Ascaris* infection are migration of the worms into the biliary tree causing obstructive jaundice, cholangitis and occasionally hepatic abscesses, or into the pancreatic duct causing pancreatitis.

Diagnosis and treatment

Female worms produce up to 200 000 eggs per day, which can be detected by faecal smear. Occasionally, adult worms are passed spontaneously or can be seen on plain abdominal radiograph or barium studies. Treatment with mebendazole 100 mg bd for 3 days or a single dose of albendazole 400 mg are highly effective, with a 96% cure rate. Intestinal obstruction can sometimes be treated conservatively with naso-gastric suction, resuscitation and piperazine therapy, which paralyze the worms and aid their expulsion from the GI tract. However, laparotomy is frequently necessary to relieve the obstruction followed by anti-helminthic therapy.

Strongyloidiasis

Infection with the nematode *Strongyloides stercoralis* is common in the tropics and some temperate zones. Humans are the prime reservoir for infection, which may be dormant in the small intestine for several decades. Patients often have asymptomatic carriage or complain of mild diarrhoea, abdominal pain or pruritus ani. There may be a pathognomonic urticarial rash (larva currens) that migrates across the skin. There is frequently an eosinophilia on the peripheral blood film and the worm can be demonstrated by duodenal aspiration or biopsy and can cause variable villous atrophy. Hyperinfestation occurs in the setting of immunocompromise and is characterized by intestinal obstruction, pneumonia, meningitis and a mortality of over 50%.

Treatment

The parasite is relatively resistant to treatment. If albendazole 400 mg daily for 3 days or a single dose of ivermectin 0.2 mg/kg does not clear infection, a 4–week course of treatment is required. Prospective studies have found that up to 75% of treatment failures have HIV infection.

Whipple's disease

This uncommon multi-system disease was first described in 1907. The causative Gram-positive bacteria *Tropheryma whipplei* has proved extremely difficult to culture and was only isolated in 2000. The complete genome sequence has subsequently been published.

Clinical features

Infection is most common in middle-aged men causing malabsorption and joint disease in approximately 80% of cases. Presentation may be with general features of malaise, fever and weight loss or with anaemia, skin plaques, hypoproteinaemia and oedema. Almost any system can be affected including the cardiovascular system with pericarditis, endocarditis or cardiac conduction defects. Pleurisy or pulmonary infiltrates occur early in the disease.

Diagnosis

Whipple's disease is often fatal if untreated and the speed of diagnosis is often determined by the presenting symptoms. Endoscopic features are of patchy white or yellow plaques in the duodenum with a friable mucosa and duodenal histology demonstrates epithelial macrophages containing foamy magenta PAS-positive material. Light or electron microscopy can detect the rod-shaped organisms and PCR-based tests for microbial RNA have been developed.

Treatment

Antibiotic treatment cures the disease, with diarrhoeal symptom relief within a few weeks. Relapses can occur with short-course treatment, so a recommended regime is an initial 2 weeks intravenous therapy with ceftriaxone 2 g/day (or other antibiotic that readily crosses the blood–brain barrier as bacteria are often present within the CSF) followed by oral treatment for 1 year with trimethoprim/sulphamethoxazole 160/800 mg bd. Follow-up duodenal biopsies should be taken after 12 months and treatment can be stopped if there is no PAS-stained material present.

Tropical sprue

This cryptogenic malabsorption syndrome affects residents and visitors to tropical regions resulting in watery diarrhoea, abdominal bloating and nutritional deficiency. A map of endemic areas has been developed. The cause is unclear, but it may be that transient infection leads to enterocyte damage that persists in the absence of ongoing infection.

Some authors have suggested that there is actually persistent contamination of the small intestine, possibly with protozoa, although there is no clear consensus. Diarrhoea may be severe enough to cause dehydration and many of the deaths during epidemics are thought to be due to fluid and electrolyte abnormalities. In patients with an appropriate travel history, investigation relies on demonstrating malabsorption either by sudan staining for fat globules in faecal smears or by estimation of D-xylose absorption. Duodenal biopsy may show partial villous atrophy and other causes of malabsorption should be excluded.

Treatment

Treatment is directed at correcting fluid, electrolyte and nutritional deficiencies. Specific treatment with tetracycline 250 mg qds and folate 5 mg daily for 6 months has been used with success. Symptomatic control of diarrhoea can be achieved with loperamide 2–6 mg tds.

Small-bowel bacterial overgrowth

There are normally less than 10^4 (predominantly Gram-positive aerobic) bacteria in the jejunum, increasing to 10^5–10^8 mixed aerobic or anaerobic bacteria in the ileum. Bacterial overgrowth of the small intestine usually occurs on a background of small-bowel structural abnormality (e.g. gastrointestinal surgery involving the formation of a blind loop, small-bowel diverticulosis or Crohn's disease), disordered intestinal motility (including gastroparesis secondary to diabetes) or depressed immunity. Other risk factors for small-bowel bacterial overgrowth (SBBO) are increasing age, reduced gastric acid production (either by the presence of corpus-predominant *H. pylori* infection, proton pump inhibitor therapy or after gastric resection), chronic pancreatitis, cirrhosis and incompetence of the ileo-caecal valve. Conditions that can cause both structural abnormalities and altered GI motility, such as systemic sclerosis, are particularly associated with SBBO, especially as many patients will also be treated with acid suppression for gastro-oesophageal reflux disease. The small bowel becomes colonized with a predominantly Gram-negative flora that usually resides in the large bowel. Other organisms may be responsible in immunodeficiency, for example in HIV infection, where Gram-positive organisms or fungal pathogens may be prevalent.

Clinical features

SBBO is probably underdiagnosed and overlooked in clinical practice. There may be no symptoms, or patients may classically present with weight loss, diarrhoea or vitamin B12 deficiency with a macrocytic anaemia. There may also be abdominal pain, distension and nausea. As there is a wide range of predisposing conditions, many of which cause diarrhoeal symptoms in their own right, a high level of clinical suspicion is required to make the diagnosis. A recent prospective study found that a large proportion (66%) of patients with CD compliant with a GFD and normal duodenal histology, but with persistent GI symptoms had SBBO and responded to treatment with antibiotics. Approximately 40% of patients with chronic pancreatitis also have SBBO, in some cases due to reduced intestinal motility with the use of opiate analgaesia. Features of severe malabsorption such as osteomalacia and impaired fat-soluble vitamin absorption leading to clotting abnormalities and impaired night vision can occur in advanced cases.

Pathophysiology

There is competition for luminal nutrients between the host and the colonizing organism in the small intestine. Bacterial metabolism of ingested nutrients leads to the production of toxic products resulting in injury to the enterocyte. SBBO may, therefore, lead to nutrient deficiency and wasting. Vitamin B12 is utilized by the bacteria and is often reduced and cannot be corrected by intrinsic factor. Bacteria in the small bowel synthesize folate, which is then available to the host for absorption. The direct damage by bacteria to the small intestinal epithelium can be severe enough to cause bleeding and subsequently iron deficiency anaemia. However, the typical blood film is of B12 deficiency and megaloblastic anaemia. Extensive enterocyte damage can also result in protein loss, causing oedema and hypoalbuminaemia. There may be a secondary lactase deficiency and this needs to be considered when treating such patients.

Investigation

Small bowel bacterial overgrowth is associated with excessive numbers of bacteria in the proximal small intestine. This can be detected either directly by quantitation of bacterial numbers in the small intestine or by indirect methods such as breath testing.

Bacterial counts

Aspiration and quantitation of bacterial counts from the duodenum or proximal jejunum is possible at endoscopy and has been used as the gold standard for the diagnosis of SBBO. Traditionally, a diagnosis is made if there are, in the duodenal aspirate, total bacterial counts of over 10^5 colony-forming units (CFU)/ml, aerobic bacterial counts over 10^4 CFU/ml, Gram-negative counts over 10^3 CFU/ml or counts of anaerobes over 10^2 CFU/ml. This procedure is technically demanding, requiring close co-operation with the microbiologist. It requires sterile and, ideally, anaerobic collection of jejunal or distal duodenal fluid for culture. It is, therefore, now rarely done in clinical practice and a therapeutic trial of antibiotics or a breath test is mainly used.

Breath tests

A variety of non-invasive breath tests have been available for over 30 years. These tests work on the principle that bacteria not normally present in the proximal small bowel metabolize and allow early absorption of an ingested radiolabelled substrate, which can then be detected in expired air. A summary of the operating characteristics of tests used for detecting SBBO is listed in Table 3.5.

Treatment

Avoidance or reversal of the predisposing factors leading to SBBO is an obvious and attractive target for prevention. Acid reduction surgery, either by vagotomy and

Table 3.5 *Comparison of tests available for diagnosing small-bowel bacterial overgrowth*

Test	Sensitivity	Specificity	Simplicity
Jejunal culture	Excellent	Excellent	Poor
^{14}C-xylose breath test	Good	Excellent	Fair
^{14}C-bile acid breath test	Fair	Poor	Fair
Lactulose-hydrogen breath test	Poor	Fair	Excellent
Glucose-hydrogen breath test	Fair	Fair	Excellent
Urinary indican	Poor	Poor	Excellent

pyloroplasty or antral gastrectomy with gastro-jejunal anastomosis is now rarely performed after the discovery of *Helicobacter pylori* as the main cause of peptic ulceration. This will substantially reduce the amount of SBBO encountered in clinical practice as a result of blind loop formation and impaired intestinal motility following such surgery. The judicious use of PPI therapy will also reduce hypochlorhydria in many patients, especially the elderly. However, there are many conditions where correction of the structural abnormality is unrealistic, such as jejunal diverticulosis. Antibiotic therapy is, therefore, the mainstay of treatment. If bacterial culture is obtained at endoscopy, the sensitivities of the bacterial flora can guide appropriate treatment. However, antibiotic treatment is often empirical, either as a diagnostic test or after positive breath testing. As there is mostly a mixed bacterial population causing overgrowth, the antibiotic selected must be effective against both aerobic and anaerobic organisms. There are several choices of antibiotic therapy that are often guided by local sensitivites. Tetracycline 250 mg qds or ciprofloxacin 500 mg bd are commonly used agents. Most patients respond promptly to a 10-day antibiotic course, but treatment may need to be cyclical with antibiotic use determined by symptoms, or even continuous in resistant cases. There has been some success with the addition of a prokinetic (e.g. cisapride, although this can only now be prescribed on a named patient basis and requires a screening ECG for QT abnormalities). If there is vitamin B12 or other nutritional deficiencies these should be replaced. In some patients with extensive enterocyte damage, the resulting secondary lactase deficiency is treated with temporary dietary exclusion of dairy products.

OTHER CAUSES OF MALABSORPTION

Enzyme deficiencies in the small intestine

Carbohydrate intolerance occurs when there is a deficiency of the enzyme required to digest and absorb dietary carbohydrate. Symptoms include nausea, bloating, abdominal pain and watery diarrhoea, which occur within several hours of ingesting the offending food. The most common deficiency encountered in clinical practice is lactase deficiency. Less common disaccharidase enzyme deficiencies are of sucrase-isomaltase leading to sucrose intolerance and trehalase deficiency resulting in intolerance to mushrooms.

days. Isotonic oral rehydration salts (such as Dioralyte®) are useful preparations to replace water and salt losses.

Maintenance treatment

This will preferably be by the enteral route, although if there is insufficient calorie or electrolyte intake, or increased losses, parenteral therapy is indicated.

Recommended diets   A high calorie diet (often 4000–6000 calories per day) is required as there is faecal loss of unabsorbed food. A low-fat (20–40 g/day), high-carbohydrate intake is recommended and can reduce steatorrhoea whilst increasing body mass. If there is high fluid output, for example from a high jejunostomy, oral rehydration salts are effective and several sachets per day are often required. Bile acid malabsorption from resection of the terminal ileum not only leads to fat malabsorption and steatorrhoea, but can also cause diarrhoea in its own right in patients with an intact colon. Fat-soluble vitamins (A, D, E and K) need to be replaced and there are often deficiencies in calcium, magnesium, zinc and other trace elements such as copper, selenium and chromium, which can be treated with higher than normal doses of mineral preparations such as *Forceval*® (2–4 capsules per day).

Parenteral nutrition   If patients do not absorb enough of their oral intake, then parenteral nutrition is indicated. This may be a temporary measure post-operatively while the intestine adapts to increasing its capacity for absorption, or it may be a permanent therapy where there is insufficient residual small intestine. Parenteral nutrition is usually administered through a tunnelled central venous catheter and patients can be trained to administer the preparations at home, with nutritional team support. There are significant complications of infection or thrombosis relating to the catheter, while the parenteral nutrition itself can increase the already substantial risk of gallstones and cause cholestatic liver biochemistry. Patients who cannot tolerate long-term parenteral therapy should be referred for assessment by specialists in intestinal failure, where autologous bowel reconstruction (such as reversal of intestinal segments) or small-bowel transplantation may be considered.

Management of diarrhoea

The main aim of medical treatment in patients with SBS is to control diarrhoea. This not only increases contact time for nutrient absorption, but also improves patients' social confidence and quality of life. Treatment with loperamide 2–6 mg tds is first choice as there is no dependency, although codeine phosphate also reduces transit time and ileostomy output. Stepwise treatment may include other opiates, which may need to be in a liquid preparation to allow adequate absorption. Colestyramine can bind bile acids and reduce diarrhoeal symptoms in patients with ileal resections and an intact colon, although steatorrhoea may be increased due to a reduced circulating bile acid pool, together with cholelithiasis. Synthetic analogues of somatostatin (e.g. octreotide 50–100 mcg tds subcutaneously) reduce diarrhoea and electrolyte loss, but may also increase the risk of gallstones and protein malabsorption. Gastric acid hypersecretion occurs in some patients after small-bowel resection and treatment with PPIs not only protects against peptic ulceration, but can also prevent diarrhoea by reducing acid inactivation of secreted pancreatic enzymes. Patients after small-bowel surgery, especially those who had ileo-caecal valve resection, are at risk of developing small-bowel bacterial overgrowth. This is often treated empirically, as breath testing can be difficult to interpret in patients with SBS.

Protein-losing enteropathy

Loss of plasma proteins into the gastrointestinal tract is associated with various inflammatory and neoplastic conditions affecting the small bowel (or other parts of the gut) and commonly presents with steatorrhoea. Lymphatic maldevelopment, obstruction or stasis can also cause severe protein loss (Table 3.7). Hypoproteinaemia, with a reduction in the plasma oncotic pressure, causes peripheral oedema, ascites or pleural effusions that may overshadow symptoms related to the GI tract. It is important to exclude other causes of hypoproteinaemia such as renal or hepatic disease.

Diagnosis

The measurement of radioactively labelled $^{51}CrCl_3$ (which attaches to all plasma proteins) in the stool for 4–10 days after intravenous injection, is no longer widely used due to the risk from radiation, commercial availability, the expense and the long collection periods required. The most accurate and acceptable approach is to measure the 72-h faecal excretion of α_1-antitrypsin (α_1-AT). This protein is synthesized in the liver, has a similar size to albumin (50 000 d) and normally low levels of α_1-AT are detected in stool. False-positive tests can occur in the presence of GI bleeding and false-negative tests if the α_1-AT is lost from the stomach, as it is degraded at pH<3. The reference range (normal <5 mg α_1-AT/g of dry stool) needs to be adjusted for individuals who are *PiMZ* or *PiMS* heterozygotes, having predictably lower plasma levels of α_1-AT. Once protein-losing enteropathy has been diagnosed, there needs to be rational investigation to find the

Table 3.7 Some causes of protein-losing enteropathy

Altered intestinal permeability	Lymph stasis
Ménétrier's disease	Intestinal lymphangiectasia
Inflammatory bowel disease	Congestive cardiac failure
Infection	Constrictive pericarditis
(e.g. giardiasis, bacterial overgrowth)	
Malignancy	Retroperitoneal fibrosis
(e.g. lymphoma)	
Coeliac disease	Pancreatitis
Autoimmune enteropathy	Strangulated hernia
(e.g. systemic lupus erythematosus)	
Tropical sprue	Lymphoma
Drugs	
(e.g. NSAIDs)	
Eosinophilic gastroenteritis	

Gastrointestinal stromal cell tumours (GISTs)

These are non-epithelial mesenchymal tumours that were previously considered to be spindle-cell tumours of either smooth muscle (leiomyoma) or neural origin. Molecular analysis and in particular positive staining with markers such as CD34 and CD117 (c-kit) have helped to redefine these tumours. GISTs represent 1% of all GI tumours and are most common in the stomach; in the small intestine the commonest sites are the ileum and duodenum. Recent studies have demonstrated that tumour size >5 cm, high cellularity and high mitotic activity are the best predictors of malignancy and, therefore, prognosis. Metastasis is usually haematogenous to the liver and lung. Imatinib mesylate (Glivec®) is a selective inhibitor of tyrosine kinases (including c-kit) and has achieved clinical benefit and significant antitumour responses in patients with advanced malignant GISTSs.

Further Reading

Bentley SD, Maiwald M, Murphy LD et al. Sequencing and analysis of the genome of the Whipple's disease bacterium *Tropheryma whipplei*. Lancet 2003; 361(9358): 637–44.

Cook GC. 'Tropical sprue': some early investigators favoured an infective cause, but was a coccidian protozoan involved? Gut 1997; 40(3): 428–9.

Gardner TB, Hill DR. Treatment of giardiasis. Clinical Microbiology Reviews 2001; 14(1): 114–28.

Gauger PG, Scheiman JM, Wamsteker EJ, Richards ML, Doherty GM, Thompson NW. Role of endoscopic ultrasonography in screening and treatment of pancreatic endocrine tumours in asymptomatic patients with multiple endocrine neoplasia type 1. Br J Surg 2003; 90(6): 748–54.

Howard L, Ashley C. Management of complications in patients receiving home parenteral nutrition. Gastroenterology 2003; 124(6): 1651–61.

Klipstein FA. Tropical sprue in travellers and expatriates living abroad. Gastroenterology 1981; 80(3): 590–600.

Legesse M, Erko B, Medhin G. Efficacy of alebendazole and mebendazole in the treatment of Ascaris and Trichuris infections. Ethiopian Med J 2002; 40(4): 335–43.

Marth T, Raoult D. Whipple's disease. Lancet 2003; 361(9353): 239–46.

Mulder CJJ. In: Report of a working group of the United European Gastroenterology Week in Amsterdam, 2001. When is a coeliac a coeliac? Eur J Gastroenterol Hepatol 2001; 13: 1123–8.

Terashima A, Alvarez H, Tello R, Infante R, Freedman DO, Gotuzzo E. Treatment failure in intestinal strongyloidiasis: an indicator of HTLV-I infection. Int J Infect Dis 2002; 6(1): 28–30.

Toskes PP. Bacterial overgrowth of the gastrointestinal tract. Adv Intern Med 1993; 38: 387–407.

Tursi A, Brandimarte G, Giorgetti G. High prevalence of small intestinal bacterial overgrowth in coeliac patients with persistence of gastrointestinal symptoms after gluten withdrawal. Am J Gastroenterol 2003; 98(4): 839–43.

West J, Logan RFA, Card TR, Smith C, Hubbard R. Fracture risk in people with coeliac disease: A population-based cohort study. Gastroenterology 2003; 125: 429–36.

Wilmore DW, Byrne TA, Persinger RL. Short bowel syndrome: new therapeutic approaches. Curr Probl Surg 1997; 34(5): 389–444.

Colorectal disease

4

INTRODUCTION

At first glance colorectal disease may be an aspect of gastroenterology that predominantly comes under the auspices of our colorectal surgical colleagues. In clinical practice, however, colorectal pathology represents a large amount of a gastroenterologist's workload and encompasses a wide range of conditions varying from the most seemingly benign, such as haemorrhoids, through to life-threatening inflammation or malignancy.

In practice colorectal diseases account for approximately 50–60% of new out-patient referrals to a general gastroenterologist and, therefore, a detailed knowledge of these conditions is essential. In this chapter the commonly encountered colorectal conditions will be discussed that are not alluded to in more detail in other dedicated chapters.

COLORECTAL PHYSIOLOGY

The main functions of the colon are absorption of water, sodium and other minerals and the transport of faecal material from the ileocaecal valve to the rectum and subsequent defecation.

By removal of around 90% of the fluid entering the colon, it converts 1–2 l of isotonic chyme from the ileum to 150–250 ml of semisolid faeces. The ability of the colon to absorb fluid is predominantly created by a balance between colonic absorption and secretion, but is also dependent on colonic motility. Na^+ is actively transported out of the colon with water following along the osmotic gradient created. As a result, there is normally a net secretion of K^+ and HCO_3^- into the colon hence the significant hypokalaemia often observed in severe diarrhoea.

Colonic motility has a significant influence over water absorption from the colon and the general rule is the more the movement, the greater the quantity of water reabsorbed. In many cases, loose stools are a result of relative colonic inactivity.

The three movements of the colon are:

- segmental contractions, which facilitate the mixing of colonic contents and aid absorption

- peristaltic waves, similar to those occurring in the small intestine, which propagate faeces along the length of the colon
- mass action contraction, often initiating defecation.

Colonic motility is predominantly controlled by the intrinsic enteric plexus (which if absent results in severe constipation and colonic dilatation as seen in Hirschsprung's disease and Chagas' disease). This nerve plexus is influenced by a number of circulating hormones (serotonin, cholecystokinin, motilin, vasoactive intestinal polypeptide and catecholamines) whose varying circulatory concentrations significantly affect the contractile activity. Recently, serotonin has received considerable interest in its ability to influence colonic motility and this research has led to the development of specific serotonin receptor agonists and antagonists for the treatment of colonic motility disorders.

COLORECTAL CANCER

Epidemiology

Colorectal cancer (CRC) is a common and lethal disease. The risk of developing colorectal cancer is influenced by both environmental and genetic factors. In the UK, CRC is the second most common cause for cancer-related death and the third most common cause of cancer, affecting more than 30 000 people each year (Box 4.1). The incidence is higher in patients with specific inherited conditions that predispose to the development of CRC and this will be discussed below. Compared with women, men have a slightly greater incidence of both proximal and distal cancers. Despite this, during the same time period the incidence rates for cancer of the ascending colon have increased, particularly in women.

Risk factors for colorectal cancer

Environmental and genetic factors can increase the likelihood of developing colorectal cancer. Although inherited susceptibility results in the most striking increases in risk, the majority of colorectal cancers are sporadic rather than familial. Risk factors can be

---

Box 4.1 Epidemiology of colorectal cancer in the UK

- Incidence in men: 58 per 100 000
- Incidence in women: 37 per 100 000
- 5-year survival: 40%
- Rare <40 years
- 90% aged >50 years

Box 4.2 Key risk factors for colorectal cancer

Disease groups
Previous colorectal cancer
Colonic adenomas
Inflammatory bowel disease
Acromegaly

Family groups
Familial adenomatous polyposis
Juvenile polyposis
HNPCC
Two first-degree relatives with colorectal cancer

subdivided into those with an acquired risk (disease groups) and those with a proven genetic or familial risk (Box 4.2).

Patients with a personal history of colorectal cancer or adenomatous polyps are at risk of developing future CRC. Large or multiple adenomatous polyps in the colon increase the risk of colorectal cancer by a relative risk of approximately 3.5–6.5. Family history is also an important risk factor in sporadic disease with a single affected first-degree relative increasing the risk 1.7-fold of that of the general population. This risk is further increased if two first-degree relatives have colon cancer or if the index case is diagnosed below 55 years of age. Patients with an increased risk of colorectal cancer are an appropriate group for surveillance and this will be discussed below.

In addition to these risk factors for colorectal cancer there are certain protective factors that have been identified. These include diets high in fruit and vegetables, regular physical activity, the regular use of aspirin, calcium supplements and hormone-replacement therapy in menopausal women.

Our understanding of the molecular pathogenesis of colorectal cancer is evolving rapidly and these findings have led to the identification of several specific genetic disorders, all of which are inherited in an autosomal-dominant fashion that are associated with a very high risk of developing colon cancer. Familial adenomatous polyposis and hereditary non-polyposis colorectal cancer (HNPCC) are the most common of the familial colon cancer syndromes, but together these two conditions account for less than 5% of colorectal cancer cases. These specific syndromes will be discussed below.

Clinical presentation, diagnosis and staging of colorectal cancer

The majority of patients with colorectal cancer have at least one or more of the following:

- Rectal bleeding
- Abdominal pain
- Change in bowel habit
- Iron deficiency anaemia
- Weight loss.

Abdominal pain may be caused by partial obstruction, peritoneal dissemination or perforation and, in addition, tenesmus caused by rectal cancer may involve pelvic floor muscles and possibly involve pelvic nerves.

Overt blood loss is more frequently caused by a rectal or sigmoid tumour in contrast to iron-deficiency anaemia, which is most commonly associated with a right-sided tumour.

Investigation of suspected colorectal cancer

There are several modalities available to the modern-day clinician to allow visualization of the colon and those that are most familiar are colonoscopy and barium enema – these remain the mainstay of diagnosis of colorectal malignancy. The choice between these two investigations is often based on local availability. However, colonoscopy is probably the single best diagnostic test in symptomatic individuals, as it can localize lesions throughout the large bowel and allows biopsy of any lesions detected and also allows the ability to remove any polyps detected synchronously.

Colonoscopy, however, is not without risks and does not always provide a complete examination and the adjunctive use of a barium enema in this situation should not be underestimated. Virtual colonoscopy, using computerized tomography (CT) (CT colography) or magnetic resonance imaging (MRI) technology, can be used if the patient's condition does not allow an invasive procedure.

Staging

Once a diagnosis of colorectal cancer is established, the local and distant extent of the disease spread is best accomplished by physical examination with particular attention to hepatomegaly, ascites and lymphadenopathy further augmented by CT scanning of the abdomen and a chest X-ray. The final definitive staging is established at the time of operation.

The Duke's classification (Table 4.1) and the TNM (extent of primary Tumour, local lymph Nodes, distant Metastases) classification (Table 4.2) are used to stage colorectal cancers and are useful both in determining the most appropriate therapeutic strategy and also providing a relatively accurate prognosis. The TNM strategy has now gained greater acceptance in most parts of the world.

Tumour markers for colorectal cancer, such as carcinoembryonic antigen (CEA), are not recommended as a screening tool or for the diagnostic evaluation of patients with colorectal cancer. Their use is limited to track (in addition to clinical findings) recurrence of colorectal cancer or metastases following treatment.

Treatment for colorectal cancer

Surgical resection is the only curative treatment for localized colon cancer, although not all patients are cured by complete resection. The 5-year survival rates for surgically

Table 4.1 Duke's classification of colorectal cancer

Dukes A	Mucosal; above muscularis propria; no involvement of lymph nodes
Dukes B1	Into muscularis propria, but above pericolic fat; no lymph node involvement
Dukes B2	Into pericolic or perirectal fat; no involvement of lymph nodes
Dukes C1	Same penetration as B1 with nodal metastases
Dukes C2	Same involvement as B2 with nodal metastases
Dukes D	Distant metastases

Table 4.2 TNM classification of colorectal cancer

TNM staging system for colorectal cancer	
Primary tumour	
T is	Carinoma in situ; intraepithelial (with glandular basement membrane) or invasion of lamina propria (intramucosal)
T1	Tumour invades submucosa
T2	Tumour invades muscularis propria
T3	Tumour invades through the muscularis propria into the subserosa or into non-peritonealized pericolic or perirectal tissues
T4	Tumour directly invades other organs or structures and/or perforates visceral peritoneum
Regional lymph node (N)	
NX	Regional nodes cannot be assessed
N0	No regional nodal metastases
N1	Metastasis in one to three regional lymph nodes
N2	Metastasis in four or more regional lymph nodes
Distant metastasis (M)	
MX	Distant metastasis cannot be assessed
M0	No distant metastasis
M1	Distant metastasis

resected disease are stage-dependent (Table 4.3). The 5-year survival rates for rectal cancer are somewhat lower. About 90% of patients who develop metastases show signs of them within the first 5 years.

The basic principles of surgical resection are a thorough exploration of the intra-abdominal contents to rule out extra-colonic spread of the tumour, a complete resection of the involved bowel segment with negative proximal, distal and radial margins, and a wide lymphadenectomy to accomplish all draining lymph nodes for that segment of the bowel. Restoration of bowel continuity, when possible, is also an important goal.

Adjuvant therapy in colorectal cancer

In patients who have undergone potential curative surgery, disease relapse is thought to result from micrometastases that are clinically occult at the time of presentation. The goal

Table 4.3 5-year survival rates for CRC dependent on stage of disease

Stage	5-year survival rate (%)
Stage 0	100%
Stage 1	
T1	97%
T2	90%
Stage 2	
T3	78%
T4	63%
Stage 3	
Any T N1 (1–3 positive regional nodes), M0	56–66%
Any T N2 (4 or more positive regional nodes), M0	26–37%
Stage 4	
Any M1 (presence of distant metastases)	4%

of adjuvant therapy is to eradicate these foci of micro-metastatic disease thereby decreasing the recurrence rate and increasing the likelihood of cure.

Adjuvant therapy for CRC has been studied for at least 40 years and most initial regimens employed 5-fluorouracil monotherapy. With advances in chemotherapy it is now standard to combine 5-fluorouracil with a further chemotherapeutic agent such as levamisole or leucovorin. Such adjuvant chemotherapy is recommended to improve the overall survival of patients with stage 3 colon cancer, i.e node positive disease. The role of adjuvant therapy for patients with stage 2 cancer is still unclear and should be considered on an individual basis.

Adjuvant radiotherapy plus chemotherapy for resected colon cancer

The potential benefit of adding radiation to adjuvant chemotherapy for patients with resected colon cancer is unclear. This is in contrast to patients with resected rectal cancer in whom effective adjuvant therapy consists of a combination of chemotherapy and radiation.

Palliative therapy for colorectal cancer

In unresectable cancer, palliative therapy can be considered for those with significant symptoms. These patients tend to have low rectal tumours that cause significant discomfort and discharge. This type of tumour can be treated with radio- and chemotherapy and also can benefit from local ablation via endoscopic therapy with either argon plasma coagulation or, if obstructive symptoms are predominant, insertion of an expanding colonic stent can be beneficial.

COLONIC POLYPS

The term colonic polyp refers to a protuberance into the lumen from a normally flat colonic mucosa. Polyps are usually asymptomatic, but may present with altered bowel habit, ulceration and bleeding and, if very large, produce intestinal obstruction. Colonic polyps are usually classified as:

- adenomatous
- non-adenomatous (hyperplastic, inflammatory, hamartomatous and submucosal).

Adenomas are also observed (often in very large numbers) in specific polyposis syndromes, which have a strong genetic basis and have a high predisposition to malignant change. These syndromes (FAP, HNPCC) are discussed below.

Adenomatous polyps

Adenomatous polyps are the most common type of polyp in the colon and two-thirds of all colonic polyps are adenomas. These are very common in the general population and have malignant potential, although only a very small minority of adenomas progress to cancer. Approximately 30% of the population over the age of 50 have one or more adenomas, whereas the cumulative colorectal cancer risk is approximately 5%. Adenomas are histologically classified as tubular or villous or a mixture of the two. A villous component to an adenoma suggests a higher malignant potential. In addition to histology, other features that suggest a higher malignant potential of polyps is their size and number of polyps found in the colon. The larger the number the greater the risk of developing colorectal cancer. The risk of high-grade dysplasia in relation to features of adenomatous polyps is shown in Table 4.4.

Familial adenomatous polyposis

Familial adenomatous polyposis (FAP) and its variants (Gardner's and Turcot's syndromes, see Box 4.3) account for less than 1% of colorectal cancers. In typical FAP numerous colonic adenomas appear during childhood. Symptoms appear at an average age of 16 and colonic cancer occurs in 90% of untreated individuals by age 45. FAP is

Table 4.4 Polyp features and the frequency of high-grade dysplasia

Polyp	Frequency of high-grade dysplasia (%)
Tubular	2
Villous	31
Small adenoma (<5 mm)	1
Medium-sized adenoma (6–10 mm)	5
Large adenoma (>10 mm)	21

Box 4.3

Gardner's syndrome
This is characterized by autosomally dominant, inherited adenomatous polyposis of the colon, colon carcinoma and certain extra-colonic lesions (multiple osteomas, dental abnormalities, multiple epidermoid cysts and soft fibromas of the skin, desmoid tumours and mesenteric fibromatosis).

Turcot's syndrome
This is characterized by multiple colonic adenomatous polyps, central-nervous-system tumours (usually gliomas), café-au-lait spots, cutaneous port-wine stains and focal nodular hyperplasia.

caused by germ-line mutations in the APC gene that is located on chromosome 5. Treatment involves early prophylactic colectomy.

Hereditary non-polyposis colorectal cancer (HNPCC)

Although multiple polyps are unusual in HNPCC, discrete polyps may precede the development of cancer. HNPCC is an autosomal dominant syndrome that is more common than FAP and accounts for approximately 2–6% of all colonic adenocarcinomas. HNPCC is currently divided into two sub groups:

1. Hereditary site specific colon cancer (Lynch syndrome 1)
2. Cancer family syndrome (Lynch syndrome 2).

Both of these conditions have similar colonic cancer manifestations characterized by the early age of onset and the predominant involvement of the right colon. The mean age in initial diagnosis in these patients is around 50, but some patients can present in their early 20s. Lynch syndrome 2 is differentiated by a high risk of extra colonic tumours, the most common of which is endometrial cancer, which develops in up to 40% of female gene carriers and affected families.

Non-adenomatous polyps

Non-adenomatous polyps may be grouped into several distinct categories:

- hyperplastic polyps, which are usually small (less than 5 mm) nodules, do not exhibit dysplasia and do not require any intervention
- inflammatory polyps, which are often associated with active inflammatory bowel disease
- juvenile polyps, which are hamartomatous lesions that have very little malignant potential, are often removed because of a high likelihood of bleeding. Multiple juvenile polyps in the colon can rarely occur as part of the familial disease, familiar juvenile polyposis
- submucosal polyps, which includes a variety of lesions including lipomas, leiomyomas, hemangiomas and fibromas.

Management of adenomatous polyps

Adenomatous polyps are normally detected either coincidentally during investigation of other diseases or, occasionally, as a result of rectal bleeding and/or change in bowel habit. Colonoscopy is considered the optimal examination for the detection of polyps, particularly in view of the ability to provide therapeutic polypectomy in conjunction with diagnosis. Colonoscopy is superior to barium enema, particularly in detecting small polyps, although colonoscopy is not perfect. One report found that colonoscopic miss rate, determined by two same-day endoscopic examinations, was 27% for adenomas less than 5 mm, 13% for those 6–9 mm and 6% for adenomas greater than 1 cm.

There are a number of techniques used during colonoscopy to remove polyps, the most widely accepted and safest is snare excision, which offers the most complete removal of adenomatous tissue with the least likelihood of bleeding. Large polyps may be removed by piece-meal excision and more recent technological advances have allowed the development of endoscopic mucosal resection that has been advocated as the treatment of choice for the removal of amenable large broad-based colonic lesions. The endoscopic removal of large polyps is associated with a relatively high complication rate of perforation and should only be attempted by an experienced operator. Follow-up of patients found to have colonic adenomas is discussed below.

SURVEILLANCE AND SCREENING FOR COLORECTAL CANCER

CRC has a high incidence and poor survival rates. However, there are potentially curable precursors of colorectal cancer that make this condition a very attractive proposition for surveillance and screening.

There is little doubt that surveillance of patients at high risk of colorectal cancer will improve their survival and reduce the chances of developing colorectal cancer. The British Society of Gastroenterology and the Association of Coloproctology for Great Britain and Ireland have recently published guidelines for the surveillance of colorectal cancer in high-risk groups.

These groups include:

- patients who have had resection for colorectal cancer
- patients with colorectal adenomatous polyps
- patients with inflammatory bowel disease
- patients with acromegaly
- patients who have had a ureterosigmoidostomy
- family groups of patients including those with family history of CRC as well as those with hereditary polyposis conditions.

These recommendations are shown in Table 4.5 and Figure 4.1.

Table 4.5 Recommendations for colonoscopic screening of high-risk groups

Disease groups	Screening procedure	Time of initial screen	Screening procedure and interval	Annual procedures 300 000 population
Colorectal cancer	Consultations, LFTs and colonoscopy	Colonoscopy within 6 months of resection only if colon evaluation pre-op incomplete	Liver scan within 2 months post-op Colonoscopy 5 yearly until 70 years of age	175
Colonic adenomas				
Low risk 1–2 adenomas, both <1 cm	Colonoscopy	No surveillance or 5 years	Cease follow-up after negative colonoscopy	
Intermediate risk 3–4 adenomas, OR at least one adenoma ≥1 cm	Colonoscopy	3 years	Every 3 years until two consecutive negative colonoscopies, then no further surveillance	
High risk ≥5 adenomas or ≥3 with at least one ≥1 cm	Colonoscopy	1 year	Annual colonoscopy until out of this risk group then interval colonoscopy as per Intermediate risk group	
Large sessile adenomas removed piecemeal	Colonoscopy or flexi-sig (depending on polyp location)	3 monthly until no residual polyp; consider surgery		
Ulcerative colitis and Crohn's colitis	Colonscopy + biopsies every 10 cm	pan-colitis 8 years; left-sided colitis 15 years from onset of symptoms	Colonoscopy 3 yearly in second decade, 2 yearly in third decade, subsequently annually	46
IBD + primary sclerosing cholangitis +/– OLT	Colonoscopy	At diagnosis of PSC	Annual colonoscopy with biopsy every 10 cm	6
Uretero-sigmoidostomy	Flexi Sig	10 years after surgery	Flexi Sig annually	3
Acromegaly	Colonoscopy	At 40 years	Colonoscopy 5 yearly	1

Table 4.5 Recommendations for colonoscopic screening of high-risk groups (cont'd)

Family groups	Lifetime risk of death from CRC	Screening procedure	Age at initial screen (y)	Screening procedure and interval	Annual procedures/ 300 000 population
Familial adenomatous Polyposis (FAP) and variants (refer to clinical geneticist)	1 in 2.5	Genetic testing Flexi Sig + OGD	Puberty	Flexi Sig 12 monthly Colectomy if +ve	6
Juvenile polyposis and Peutz-Jegher (refer to clinical geneticist)	1 in 3	Genetic testing Colonoscopy + OGD	Puberty	Flexi Sig 12 monthly. Colectomy if +ve	6
At risk HNPCC*, or more than 2 FDR (refer to clinical geneticist). Also documented MMR gene carriers	1 in 2	Colonoscopy +/– OGD	Aged 25 or 5 years before earliest CRC in family. Gastroscopy at age 50 or 5 years before earliest gastric cancer in family	2 yearly colonoscopy and gastroscopy	48
2 FDR with colorectal cancer	1 in 6	Colonoscopy	At first consultation or at age 35–40 years whichever is the later	If initial colonoscopy clear then repeat at age 55 years	23
1 FDR <45 years with colorectal cancer	1 in 10	Colonoscopy	At first consultation or at age 35–40 years whichever is the later	If initial colonoscopy clear then repeat at age 55 years	12

Reproduced with permission from the BMJ Publishing Group; Gut 2002; 51(Suppl v):v28, Table.
OLT, orthoptic liver transplant; IBD, inflammatory bowel disease; FAP, familial adenomatosis polyposis; HNPCC, hereditary non-polyposis colorectal cancer; FDR, first degree relative (sibling, parent or child) with colorectal cancer; OGD, oesophago-gastroduodenoscopy.
*The Amsterdam criteria for identifying HNPCC are: three or more relatives with colorectal cancer; one patient a first degree relative of another; two generations with cancer; and one cancer diagnosed below the age of 50.
The above family groups are for a minimum number of affected relatives – life-time risk rises with additional affected relatives in other generations and with younger onset of disease.
These Guidelines assume complete colonoscopy, if incomplete then either immediate DCBE or planned repeat colonoscopy.
N.B. Family history may be falsely negative.
People with symptoms suggestive of colorectal cancer or polyps should be appropriately investigated; they are not candidates for screening.
This summary has been compiled by S Cairns and J H Scholefield.

DIVERTICULAR DISEASE

Colonic diverticular disease is common. The prevalence is age-dependent, increasing from less than 5% at aged 40, to 30% by age 60 and to 65% by age 85. Among all patients with diverticular disease 70% remain asymptomatic, 15–25% develop problems with diverticulitis and 5–15% develop some form of diverticular bleeding.

Whether or not diverticular disease causes significant symptoms in the absence of diverticular complications is unproven. Certainly many patients with symptoms of cramping, bloating, flatulence and irregular defecation have these symptoms ascribed to diverticular disease, but whether these are attributable to underlying diverticular disease or to the almost invariably coexistent irritable bowel syndrome remains largely unresolved.

Complications of diverticular disease

Diverticulitis

Aetiology

Diverticulitis represents perforation of a diverticulum. The primary process is thought to be erosion of the diverticular wall by increased intraluminal pressure or inspissated food particles. Inflammation and focal necrosis ensue, resulting in localized abscess formation, or free perforation and peritonitis.

Presentation (Box 4.6)

The diagnosis of acute diverticulitis is often made on history and clinical examination alone. However, further imaging of the abdomen is often indicated and CT scanning has become the optimal method of investigation of these patients. It is useful for diagnosis, assessment of severity, potential therapeutic intervention and for identifying further complications such as fistulae, abscesses or obstruction. CT has effectively superseded contrast enemas and ultrasound scanning.

Management

Conservative treatment, with nil by mouth and 7–10 days of antibiotics to cover Gram-negative rods and anaerobes (e.g. cefuroxime 750 mg tds iv plus metronidazole 500 mg tds iv; or ciprofloxacin 500 mg bd orally plus metronidazole 400 mg tds orally) is

---

Box 4.6

Symptoms
- Left iliac fossa pain (often recurrent)
- Alteration in bowel habit
- Fever

Signs
- Tenderness over left iliac fossa
- Palpable mass (20%).

successful in 70–100% of patients. Failure of patients to settle with conservative treatment or the presence or development of further complications (abscesses, fistulae, perforation and peritonitis and obstruction) may necessitate either radiological drainage of abscesses or surgery.

The longer term management of these patients has not been studied in well-designed randomized control trials. However, patients are generally advised to consume a high-fibre diet with the suggestion that this may reduce the incidence of recurrent episodes of diverticulitis. This has only been confirmed in small non-controlled studies.

Diverticular bleeding

Diverticular bleeding is thought to arise from rupture of a colonic intramural artery related to the neck of a diverticulum, in the absence of significant inflammation (Box 4.7).

Endoscopic examination of these patients whilst they are actively bleeding is often unfruitful due to poor luminal views. However, once bleeding has settled, colonoscopy will confirm the presence of diverticular disease and, in the absence of other pathology, a diverticular bleed is the most likely diagnosis. Less than 1% of diverticular bleeds require surgical intervention.

COLONIC ISCHAEMIA

The diagnosis and treatment of chronic ischaemia can be challenging since it often occurs in patients who are debilitated and have multiple medical problems (Box 4.8). Colonic ischaemia is usually the result of a sudden and temporary reduction in blood flow that is insufficient to meet the metabolic demands of discrete regions of the colon. Blood flow can be compromised by changes in the systemic circulation or by anatomical or functional changes in the local mesenteric vasculature (Box 4.9). In the majority of patients a specific occluding lesion cannot be identified on angiography and these patients are referred to as having non-occlusive ischaemia. Non-occlusive ischaemia most commonly affects the 'watershed' areas of the colon that have limited collateral blood supply such as the splenic flexure, right colon and rectosigmoid junction – of these, the splenic flexure is affected most commonly (75% of cases).

Box 4.7 Clinical features of diverticular bleeding

- Painless fresh rectal bleeding
- Most patients have minor bleeding
- Abdominal discomfort is *not* usually present
- Physical examination is generally unremarkable
- Vast majority of patients settle without treatment.

Box 4.8 Colonic ischaemia

- Ischaemic colitis is the most frequent form of mesenteric ischaemia.

- Predominantly affects the elderly.

- The majority (85%) of patients develop non-gangrenous ischaemia, which is usually transient and tends to resolve.

- A minority of these patients develop long-term complications that include persistent segmental colitis and the development of a stricture.

- Approximately 15% of patients with colonic ischaemia develop gangrene which is life threatening.

Box 4.9 Causes of ischaemic colitis

Major vascular occlusion
Mesenteric artery thrombosis
Cholesterol emboli
Colectomy with IMA ligation
Aortic dissection
Aortic reconstruction

Mesenteric venous thrombosis
Hypercoagulable state
Lymphocytic phlebitis
Portal hypertension
Pancreatitis

Small vessel disease
Diabetes
Vasculitis
- polyarteritis nodosa
- lupus erythematosus
- Takayusu's arteritis
- Wegener's granulomatosis
- anticentromere antibodies
- Buerger's disease
Antiphospholipid antibodies
Amyloidosis
Rheumatoid arthritis
Radiation

Shock
Cardiac failure
Haemodialysis
Pancreatitis
Anaphylaxis

Mechanical obstruction
Strangulated hernia
Colon cancer
Adhesions
Rectal prolapse
Faecal impaction or pseudoobstruction

Blood dyscrasia
Hypercoagulable state
Sickle-cell disease

Iatrogenic
Surgical
Aortoiliac reconstruction
Cardiopulmonary bypass
Renal transplant
Colonoscopy
Barium enema

Drugs
Alosetron
Digoxin
Diuretics
Cocaine
Oestrogens
Danazol
NSAIDs
Vasoactive substances
Paclitaxel and carboplatin
Sumatriptan

Others
Long-distance running
Dialysis
Neurogenic
Spontaneous in young adults
Infections (CMV, *E. coli* 0157:H7)
Aeroplane flight

Clinical features

Patients with acute colonic ischaemia usually present with:

- Rapid onset of abdominal pain
- Tenderness over the affected bowel (usually the left colon)
- Moderate amounts of rectal bleeding or bloody diarrhoea within the first 24 h
- Pain usually diminishes, becoming more continuous and diffuse throughout the abdomen.

If not clinically suspected (and mesenteric ischaemia is allowed to continue), fluid, protein and electrolytes start to leak through the damaged gangrenous mucosa leading to dehydration, sepsis and shock. The diagnosis requires a high clinical suspicion as physical examination and plain abdominal radiology are often not very helpful. Laboratory features that should heighten one's clinical suspicion are:

- raised serum lactate
- high white cell count ($>20\,000$ per mm^3)
- raised C-reactive protein (>100 IU/ml)
- metabolic acidosis.

If the patient's clinical condition allows a CT scan is the investigation of choice. A typical finding is thickening of the bowel wall in a segmental pattern, with pneumatosis and gas in the mesenteric veins as the ischaemia becomes more advanced. In patients in whom the diagnosis is unclear, colonoscopy can assist in diagnosis with specific features including a pale mucosa with petechial bleeding. Bluish haemorrhagic nodules may also be present and represent submucosal bleeding.

Treatment of acute colonic ischaemia

Treatment of colonic ischaemia is dependent upon its severity and the clinical setting. As a general rule, embolectomy, bypass grafting or endarterectomy are only very rarely used to treat colonic ischaemia as large artery obstruction is hardly ever the cause of the ischaemia.

Supportive care with intravenous fluid and empiric broad spectrum antibiotics is appropriate in the absence of colonic gangrene or perforation. Any medications that may promote ischaemia should be stopped. Local infusion of vasodilators (such as papaverine) has unproven benefit in humans and is not routinely practised.

Patients must be monitored closely as clinical deterioration is likely to necessitate surgery. Colonic infarction can rapidly progress to sepsis, peritonitis and perforation and should be regarded as a surgical emergency and such patients require urgent surgical intervention.

Although used for other forms of vascular disease, antiplatelet agents have not been well studied in this setting and are generally not used. However, anticoagulant therapy is usually necessary in patients who develop ischaemia due to mesenteric venous thrombosis or cardiac embolization.

Prognosis

Recurrence of ischaemic colitis is unlikely if predisposing conditions can be prevented. The prognosis of patients with ischaemic colitis depends upon disease severity and comorbidity. Patients who have non-occlusive ischaemia without colonic infarction will normally settle within 1–2 days and the affected colon normally returns to normal within 1–2 weeks; however, in a small percentage of patients the ischaemic areas may ulcerate and eventually form strictures. As a general rule, non-gangrenous colonic ischaemia is associated with a low mortality (approximately 6%) in contrast to gangrenous ischaemia, which is associated with a mortality as high as 75% (with surgical resection) and is almost always fatal if treated conservatively.

MICROSCOPIC COLITIS

Microscopic colitis is characterized by chronic watery diarrhoea without bleeding. It usually occurs in middle-aged patients (with a female preponderance), but can affect children. The colon appears normal by colonoscopy or barium enema and the diagnosis is established by biopsy of the colonic mucosa, which reveals colitis, but not mucosal ulcerations.

There are two predominant different types of microscopic colitis:

1. Lymphocytic colitis
2. Collagenous colitis.

Lymphocytic colitis is characterized by sub-epithelial lymphocytic infiltrate in the colonic mucosa, whereas collagenous colitis is characterized by a thickened sub-epithelial collagenous band in the colonic mucosa. The differentiation of microscopic colitis is somewhat arbitrary in that both types of microscopic colitis produce a similar clinical picture characterized by non-bloody chronic watery diarrhoea and are managed in a similar way.

A misdiagnosis of diarrhoea-predominant irritable bowel syndrome can easily be made unless the colonic mucosal pathology is examined. This reinforces the importance of taking a rectal biopsy in patients with diarrhoea despite a normal looking rectal mucosa. The majority of patients follow a chronic intermittent course during which general health and laboratory measurements remain unaffected.

An association between microscopic colitis and coeliac disease has been observed. Furthermore, collagenous colitis may represent a diffuse manifestation of gluten sensitivity and, therefore, it is sensible to seek a diagnosis of coeliac disease by at least the endomysial antibody if not by small-bowel biopsy.

Treatment

Large randomized controlled trials do not exist for the treatment of collagenous or lymphocytic colitis and, therefore, therapeutic options are based mainly upon reports of small numbers of patients and an appreciation of the natural history (Box 4.10). The

> **Box 4.10 Recommended treatment options for microscopic colitis**
>
> - Stopping NSAIDs, which are possibly implicated in the aetiology
> - Anti-diarrhoeal therapy such as regular loperamide (e.g. 2–4 mg on waking or tds before meals)
> - Aminosalicylates can be tried as for ulcerative colitis, but they are usually disappointing
> - Colestyramine could be tried next because of its relative safety over budesonide, especially in long term treatment – starting at one sachet tds increasing gradually to two sachets tds
> - If colestyramine is ineffective or poorly tolerated, budesonide should be tried at a dose of 9 mg mane for 4 weeks, 6 mg mane for 2 weeks and 3 mg mane for 2 weeks. If there is initial improvement, but relapse on reducing the dose or stopping, the lowest dose which appeared to control symptoms should be considered long term (with occasional trials of stopping).

usual drugs for inflammatory bowel disease are often tried but without convincing benefit. Bismuth subsalicylate and colestyramine have given favourable results in uncontrolled studies and budesonide has been shown to be effective in a placebo-controlled trial. Several other treatments (metronidazole, octreotide, verapamil and the immunomodulators, methotrexate, mercaptopurine and azathioprine) have been used, however, the studies are too small to determine if these have had any specific benefit.

ANAL ABSCESSES AND FISTULAE

Anal abscesses and fistulae are the acute and chronic manifestations of the same peri-rectal process. An anal abscess is an infection in one or more of the anal spaces and an anal fistula is a connection between two epithelial lined spaces, one of which is the anus or rectum.

Abscesses

The majority of anal abscesses originate from infected anal glands. Anal abscesses can involve different planes in the anorectum that may have distinct presentations and require specific therapy.

Clinical features

- severe pain in the anal area
- may have constitutional symptoms including fever and malaise
- purulent rectal drainage may be noted if the abscess has begun to drain spontaneously.

There are several types of anal abscess:

- perianal
- ischiorectal
- intersphincteric
- supralevator
- horse-shoe deep postanal abscess.

101

Prior to embarking on surgical therapy for anal abscesses, it is important to accurately delineate which type of abscess is present and the use of endoanal ultrasound and MRI scanning of the pelvis can now give very clear resolution.

Treatment for anal abscesses is predominantly surgical drainage. Antibiotics may have a role in special circumstances including immunosuppression, extensive cellulitis or valvular heart disease.

The risk of developing a chronic fistula as a result of an anal abscess is around 50%.

Fistulae

Anal fistulae are uncommon in the general population with an incidence of approximately 8 per 100 000 and in 90% of cases there is no underlying aetiology identified.

Four general types of anorectal fistula have been recognized:

1. Intersphincteric
2. Transsphincteric
3. Suprasphincteric
4. Extrasphincteric.

Fistulae can have complicated anatomy with one or more extensions and accessory tracks.

Anorectal fistulae usually present with a non-healing anorectal abscess following drainage or with chronic drainage and a fluctuant lesion in the perianal skin or buttocks. Patients may have pain during defecation (which is much less severe than in patients with fissures) and the perianal skin may be excoriated and itchy.

Perianal fistulae are recognized as a common complication of Crohn's disease. However, it is unusual for this to be the presenting feature of Crohn's disease and over 90% of perianal fistulae are not associated with additional pathology.

Treatment

Optimal treatment of perianal fistulae depends on correctly classifying the fistula, which requires careful investigation, such as endoanal ultrasound, MRI or, occasionally, examination under anaesthesia.

Surgical treatment is usually required in patients with symptomatic anorectal fistulae, although patients with Crohn's disease can be an exception to this. The goals of surgical therapy are to eradicate the fistula while preserving faecal continence.

ANAL FISSURES

An anal fissure is a tear in the lining of the anal canal distal to the dentate line. This most commonly occurs in the posterior mid line. The majority of anal fissures are caused by local trauma to the anal canal, such as after passage of a hard stool. However, they can also be seen in patients with conditions such as Crohn's disease.

Following a tear the exposed internal sphincter muscle beneath the tear goes into spasm. In addition to causing severe pain, the spasm pulls the edges of the fissure apart, which impairs healing of the wound. This cycle may lead to the development of a chronic anal fissure and it has also been proposed that ischaemia may contribute to the development of this problem as blood flow in the posterior mid line is poor.

Anal fissures can usually be diagnosed from the history. Affected patients describe a tearing pain with the passage of bowel movements and the passage of stool may be accompanied by bright red rectal bleeding. The best way to diagnose an anal fissure during physical examination is to spread the buttocks apart gently looking carefully in the posterior mid line. Often patients are too uncomfortable to tolerate digital rectal examination or proctoscopy.

Treatment

The goals of therapy are to break the cycle of sphincter spasm and tearing of the anal mucosa and to promote healing of the fissure. Medical therapy is successful in the majority of patients with surgery being reserved for refractory cases. Medical therapy has traditionally consisted of three components:

1. Relaxation of the internal sphincter
2. Institution and maintenance of atraumatic passage of stool
3. Pain relief.

These goals can normally be accomplished with treatment with fibre to keep the stools soft and formed and with topical anaesthetic creams (e.g. Anusol) to soothe the inflamed anoderm.

With the observation that ischaemia may be an important factor, topical nitroglycerin has been used to increase the blood flow in this area and has been evaluated in multiple series and in controlled trials, which have shown a beneficial effect compared with placebo. Topical treatment with 0.2% glyceryl trinitrate ointment has healing rates of the order of 70% and is now generally used as first-line therapy. The major side effect of this therapy is headache, which only very rarely requires cessation of the drug. The median time to healing is 6 weeks.

Surgical therapy is reserved for patients in whom an anal fissure has failed to heal despite adequate medical therapy; the goal of surgical treatment is to relax the internal anal sphincter, which is most often accomplished by a lateral internal sphincterotomy.

HAEMORRHOIDS

The anal canal is lined by three fibrovascular cushions that are suspended in the anal canal. In health, vascular structures within the cushions can be engorged to provide fine continence control. Haemorrhoids develop as a result of pathological changes in the anatomy of prolapsed anal cushions and this process is promoted by age and straining at hard stool. Haemorrhoids are classified as internal or external in relation to the dentate line and internal haemorrhoids are further classified as first (bleeding but no prolapse), second (with prolapse but reducing spontaneously), third (with prolapse requiring manual reduction) and fourth degree (prolapsed and incarcerated).

The predominant features of haemorrhoidal disease include:

- fresh rectal bleeding on the paper or in the toilet bowl
- anal pruritus
- prolapse
- pain due to thrombosis.

Although these symptoms strongly suggest a diagnosis, this should be confirmed by digital rectal examination and proctoscopy. Additional pathology (malignancy and inflammation) should be borne in mind particularly in those patients in whom underlying disease may be more prevalent.

Treatment

Dietary and lifestyle modification

- increased fibre intake (e.g. Fybogel one sachet at night)
- avoid straining on defecation
- prolonged defecation should be avoided.

Medical management

Several ointments including local analgesics (e.g. Anusol) and steroids may be used to provide short-term relief of symptoms, but are limited by their propensity to sensitize the anoderm and cause dermatitis.

Interventional procedures

If conservative management has failed, out-patient treatment with rubber-band ligation of haemorrhoids lying above the dentate line is a pain-free and effective treatment and, if tolerated, up to three bands can be applied at one visit. This technique will cure 80% of patients with first- to third-degree piles.

Injection sclerotherapy is an alternative to band ligation, but benefit tends to be short lived with up to 70% of patients relapsing within 6 months.

Surgery

Surgery is recommended for symptomatic third-degree haemorrhoids not responding to banding and for fourth-degree haemorrhoids. Surgical options include haemorrhoidectomy and stapled haemorrhoidopexy. Limited open haemorrhoidectomy is currently the gold standard for treatment in the UK and, with necessary infrastructure and patient education, can be performed safely as a day-case procedure in the majority of patients.

PRURITUS ANI

Dietary factors and faecal soilage account for the majority of patients with pruritus ani. Most of these patients probably do not come to medical attention; however, there are a variety of disorders that can contribute to or underlie the development of pruritus including haemorrhoids, anal fissures, rectal and anal cancers and underlying dermatological diseases (psoriasis, contact dermatitis and atopic dermatitis).

Treatment

- The treatment of anal pruritus should be aimed at the underlying cause. Conservative treatment and reassurance is successful in approximately 90% of patients.
- Fibre supplementation can help bulk stools and prevent faecal leakage in patients who have a degree of faecal incontinence of partially formed stools.
- Patients should be instructed about appropriate anodermal care. The anoderm should be kept clean and dry, but without excessive wiping or the use of astringent cleaners. Proprietary moist tissues can be very helpful when away from home, but bathing following defecation (especially using a bidet) is ideal.
- Topical therapy with a 1% hydrocortisone cream applied twice daily can relieve pruritus and promote healing. However, it should not be used for more than 2 weeks.
- Capsaicin 0.06% has recently been shown to be effective in intractable pruritus ani.

SOLITARY RECTAL ULCER SYNDROME

Solitary rectal ulcer syndrome is an uncommon condition for which the diagnosis and treatment can be challenging.

Clinical features

- bleeding
- passage of mucus rectally
- straining during defecation
- sense of incomplete evacuation.

The lesions are normally located in the anterior rectal wall within 10 cm of the anal verge and endoscopic findings may vary, including mucosal ulcerations, polypoid lesions or simply erythema. As a result misdiagnosis is common.

The pathogenesis of solitary rectal ulcer is incompletely understood. It is thought that rectal prolapse and paradoxical contraction of the puborectalis muscle, which can result in rectal trauma, is the most likely mechanism.

The diagnosis is usually based upon clinical symptoms combined with endoscopic and histological findings. The differential diagnosis should include Crohn's disease, ulcerative colitis, chronic ischaemic colitis and malignancy.

The treatment of solitary rectal ulcer disease is difficult and depends upon the symptoms and whether rectal prolapse is present or not. Observation alone or treatment with bulking laxatives and bowel retraining and reassurance are the normal approach; only in very rare cases, where there is definitive evidence of rectal prolapse, is surgery considered.

CONSTIPATION

Constipation is a symptom that can affect up to 25% of the population at any given time. Constipation can be defined in many different ways, but it is generally accepted under the Rome II Criteria for Constipation that adults should have two or more of the six features shown in Box 4.11 for at least 12 weeks in the preceding 12 months.

Bowel frequency is influenced by several factors including intake of dietary fibre, emotional make up and psychological morbidity.

Constipation can be subdivided into three specific types:

1. Normal-transit constipation
2. Slow-transit constipation
3. Disorders of defecation or rectal evacuation.

Normal-transit constipation is the more common form and is usually due to a perceived difficulty with evacuation or the presence of hard stools. This type of constipation will normally respond to an increase in dietary fibre or addition of an osmotic laxative.

Slow-transit constipation occurs most commonly in young women who have infrequent bowel movements, usually once a week or fewer. It is important in this group to distinguish whether or not the bowel is of normal diameter or dilated. With a non-dilated colon, slow-transit constipation is seen commonly in women of reproductive age and the key physiological abnormality is diminished colonic propulsive activity. Neural abnormalities can be shown within the colon. However, it is uncertain whether or not these are primary changes or secondary to chronic ingestion of laxatives.

Box 4.11 Features used in the Rome II Criteria for Constipation

- Straining during more than 25% of bowel movements
- Lumpy or hard stools for over 25% of bowel movements
- Sensation of incomplete evacuation for more than 25% of bowel movements
- Sensation of anal or rectal blockage for more than 25% of bowel movements
- Manual manoeuvres to facilitate more than 25% of bowel movements, e.g. digital evacuation
- <3 bowel movements per week.

Defecatory disorders are most commonly due to dysfunction of the pelvic floor or anal sphincter and occasionally can be associated with conditions causing anal pain, such as fissures or haemorrhoids, which result in prolonged avoidance of passing stool due to pain. Structural abnormalities would include rectal intussusception, rectoceles, sigmoidoceles and excessive perineal descent.

History and physical examination

A detailed history can usually exclude most secondary causes of constipation and there should be an emphasis on an accurate drug history, particularly over-the-counter opiates. Chronic constipation is often associated with psychological morbidity and in some patients is the key causative factor. Other factors include childhood problems, such as sexual or physical abuse, loss of a parent through death or separation, or disturbed toileting behaviour. Underlying depression is a further common cause. These psychological factors should be sought at the initial assessment, but not all patients should be assumed to have a psychological problem.

Physical examination is often unrewarding. However, a careful rectal examination should be performed to look for local disease such as fissures and fistulae. Patients should also be asked to bear down to assess the extent of perineal descent. Laboratory tests should include thyroid function, calcium, glucose, urea and electrolytes, which will exclude most metabolic causes of constipation.

In the absence of lower gastrointestinal alarm symptoms further imaging of the colon is rarely required. In patients who have resistant constipation further physiological examination may be appropriate, but should probably be reserved for tertiary referral centres. Further investigations that may prove to be beneficial in such centres include colonic transit time testing, anorectal manometry, balloon expulsion and defecating proctography.

Management of constipation

Basic advice such as increasing fluid intake and physical activity usually have a minimal effect on patients with chronic constipation, except in those who are obviously dehydrated.

Patients with normal- or slow-transit constipation should initially increase their dietary fibre intake either with changes in their diet or with fibre supplements such as Fybogel one sachet daily. Patients who do not respond to fibre treatment should then be treated with an osmotic laxative such as Milk of Magnesia or Lactulose 10 ml bd (the dose being increased until the stools are soft). Stimulant laxatives such as senna and bisacodyl are usually reserved for patients with more severe constipation who have not had a response to the above two measures (Table 4.6). Patients who fail to respond to oral laxative therapy and who still produce a hard stool can be advised to add a stool softener given rectally such as glycerol suppositories 1–2 daily, or arachis oil enemas.

There is currently development of newer prokinetic medications such as tegaserod (a

Table 4.6 Medications commonly used for constipation

Medication	Type of laxative	Maximal recommended dose
Fybogel (Ispaghula husk)	Bulk	One to two sachets daily
Normacol (Sterculia)	Bulk	One to two sachets once daily
Regulan (Ispaghula)	Bulk	One sachet one to three times daily
Lactulose	Osmotic	15 ml twice daily, increased as required
Movicol	Osmotic	One to three sachets daily
Magnesium hydroxide	Osmotic	25–50 ml daily
Senna	Stimulant	Two to four tablets, increased as required
Bisacodyl	Stimulant	5–10 mg at night
Docusate sodium	Stimulant	Up to 5 mg daily in divided doses
Sodium picosulphate	Stimulant	5–10 mg at night

partial 5 hydroxytryptamine 4 receptor agonist). This has been shown to be an effective treatment for patients, particularly women, with severe constipation. It is not yet licensed in the UK.

Patients who fail to respond to the above basic measures could be considered for biofeedback therapy in which patients receive both visual and auditory feedback on the functioning of the anal sphincter and pelvic floor muscles. This is a labour-intensive and time-consuming therapy and again should be reserved for tertiary referral centres. Biofeedback has, however, been shown to have a high success rate in the order of 60–70% and the effects of biofeedback do seem to be long lasting.

Surgery for refractory constipation should only be considered if the patient does not have a defecatory disorder and only after all medical therapies have failed. Colonic resection for intractable constipation is generally reserved for patients with slow-transit constipation.

MEGACOLON AND MEGARECTUM

Megacolon and megarectum are conditions in which the colon or rectum are dilated, often massively, in the absence of mechanical obstruction. In megacolon the diameter of the descending colon or sigmoid is >6.5 cm. They are very uncommon conditions and are usually managed in tertiary centres.

Idiopathic megacolon

Patients with idiopathic megacolon generally have onset of symptoms either in childhood or early adulthood. There is notable thickening of the muscularis externa and a decrease in the density of innervation of the longitudinal muscles supplying the colon. Management of these patients is difficult and drug treatment with combinations of laxatives and enemas is successful in around 75% of patients. Surgery is often required and is clearly indicated if there is evidence of volvulus. Colectomy and ileo-rectal anastomosis should be considered for those patients with disabling symptoms that do not respond to laxatives and enemas.

Idiopathic megarectum

Patients with idiopathic megarectum form a clinically distinct group. Patients generally present at a young age developing symptoms in childhood or adolescence. There is an association with intellectual impairment and/or psychiatric disease. However, whether these associations are due to shared abnormality of the brain and gut neurological development, or to the long-term use of psychotropic drugs or to the effects of suppressed defecation is unresolved.

Idiopathic megarectum appears to be an isolated abnormality with no upper gastrointestinal or proximal colonic abnormalities. Rectal sensation to distension is impaired, as is the response of the rectum to electrical stimulation, raising the possibility of abnormalities in extrinsic innervation. Again, these patients are often managed in tertiary centres and most will respond to oral laxatives and rectal enemas. Faecal incontinence due to rectal impaction of faeces is often a problem and can create significant psychological stress. Maintenance treatment for these patients is life long. Surgery is rarely required.

Further Reading

Atkin WS, Northover JMA, Macafee DAL, Scholefield JH. Debate: population-based endoscopic screening for colorectal cancer. Gut 2003; 52: 321–6.

Cairns S, Scholefield JH. Guidelines for colorectal cancer screening in high risk groups. Gut 2002; 51(Suppl V).

Casillas S, Pelley RJ, Milsom JW. Adjuvant therapy for colorectal cancer: present and future perspectives. Dis Colon Rectum 1997; 40: 977–92.

Debatin JF, Lauenstein TC. Virtual magnetic resonance colonography. Gut 2003; 52(Suppl IV): iv17–iv22.

Gattuso JM, Kamm MA. Clinical features of idiopathic megarectum and idiopathic megacolon. Gut 1997; 41: 93–9.

Gershon M. Importance of serotonergic mechanisms in gastrointestinal motility and sensation. In: Camillieri M, Spiller RC (eds) Irritable Bowel Syndrome: Diagnosis and Treatment: Elsevier, 2002; 95–115.

Kamm MA. Constipation and its management. BMJ 2003; 327: 459–60.

Lembo A, Camillieri M. Chronic constipation. N Engl J Med 2003; 349: 1360–8.

Lund JN, Scholefield JH. A randomised, prospective, double-blind, placebo-controlled trial of glyceryl trinitrate ointment in treatment of anal fissure. Lancet 1997; 349: 11–14.

Lysy J, Sistiery-Ittah M, Israelit Y et al. Topical capsaicin – a novel and effective treatment for idiopathic intractable pruritus ani: a randomised, placebo controlled, crossover study. Gut 2003; 52: 1323–6.

Stampfl DA, Friedman LS. Collagenous colitis. Pathophysiological considerations. Dig Dis Sci 1991; 36: 705–11.

UK Flexible Sigmoidoscopy Screening Trial Investigators. Single flexible sigmoidoscopy screening to prevent colorectal cancer; baseline findings of a UK multicentre randomised trial. Lancet 2002; 359: 1291–300.

US Preventitive Task Force. Screening for colorectal cancer: recommendations and rationale. Ann Intern Med 2002; 137: 129–31.

Vaizey CJ, van den Bogaerde JB, Emmanuel AV et al. Solitary rectal ulcer syndrome. Br J Surg 1998; 85: 1617–23.

Winauer SJ, Stewart ET, Zauer AG et al. A comparison of colonoscopy and double contrast barium enema for surveillance after polypectomy. N Engl J Med 2000; 342: 1766–72.

a variety of pro-inflammatory cytokines including tumour necrosis factor-alpha (TNF-α) that result in further activation of Th-1 cells and enhancement of the inflammatory response. If Th-1 responses against invading pathogens were to persist unchecked in the intestinal mucosa, then chronic intestinal inflammation would result. In the normal intestine, specialized subsets of T-helper-2 (Th-2) lymphocytes quickly downregulate the Th-1 response by producing anti-inflammatory cytokines such as interleukin-10 (IL-10) and TGF-β, which inhibit Th-1 responses and macrophage activation and promote mucosal healing. Furthermore, via the mechanism of oral tolerance, a state of immune non-responsiveness to luminal (orally derived) antigens, including the indigenous bacterial flora, is induced. The presentation of antigen in this manner also results in activation of T-cells that secrete inhibitory cytokines such as TGF-β, thus limiting development of an inflammatory response.

Current thinking suggests that in IBD there is a failure of this natural downregulation of the mucosal immune response. The reasons for this are likely multiple, including factors such as the dysfunctional NOD2 gene in CD. The end result is chronic uncontrolled inflammation with intestinal tissue damage. An understanding of the mechanisms involved in intestinal mucosal immune responses may lead to development of new therapeutic strategies for the management of IBD, a point well illustrated with the successful use of anti-TNFα antibodies in the treatment of CD.

Bacterial factors

Involvement of microbes in the pathogenesis of IBD has been suspected for many years. Members of the mycobacterial species (particularly *Mycobacterium paratuberculosis*) and the measles virus have been implicated as specific aetiological agents in CD. However, evidence from studies is conflicting and inconclusive. Furthermore, attempts to treat CD with antituberculous therapy have been disappointing.

It now seems likely that, in susceptible individuals, the host's own indigenous microbial flora play a role in initiation and perpetuation of the chronic inflammatory response seen in IBD. Compelling evidence for this comes from several observations. Many animal models of IBD exist and, in general, these animals only develop IBD in the presence of a luminal microbial flora; germ-free animals do not develop the condition. Diversion of the bacteria-laden faecal stream by means of an ileostomy in CD patients results in disease improvement distally. Pouchitis in UC patients with an ileo-anal pouch only develops on colonization of the pouch by enteric bacteria. Finally, treatment of IBD with antibiotics is beneficial in some circumstances, suggesting that alteration of the bacterial flora affects disease progression. Increasing awareness of the role indigenous bacteria play in the pathogenesis of IBD has led to the development of probiotic bacterial therapies, which is an area of considerable current interest.

Environmental factors

The fact that concordance rates for IBD in twin studies are not 100%, along with an increasing incidence during this century, suggests that environmental factors are important in development of these conditions. Many factors have been studied, but only a few seem to be consistently involved.

The relationship between smoking, CD and UC is intriguing. Cigarette smoking is a risk factor for the development of CD and continued smoking in CD patients worsens the disease course. Conversely, smoking is protective against development of UC and the development of UC may follow some months after stopping smoking. Treatment with nicotine patches has been shown to be of benefit in active UC, but not in maintenance of remission. The reason for the different effects of nicotine in UC and CD is unknown and serves to indicate that, whilst the two diseases have many similar features, they remain distinct.

The incidence of UC, but not CD, is lower in individuals who have had an appendectomy. Further analysis of this has shown that the beneficial effect of appendectomy on UC is only apparent if the surgery was undertaken before the age of 20 and only if it was for an inflammatory disease such as appendicitis or mesenteric adenitis. The protective effect against UC is not apparent if the appendix was removed incidentally, suggesting it is the inflammatory process occurring at a young age that protects against subsequent development of UC.

Finally, non-steroidal anti-inflammatory drugs (NSAIDS) have a detrimental effect in IBD, both precipitating disease relapse and worsening disease course.

DIAGNOSIS OF INFLAMMATORY BOWEL DISEASE

IBD is diagnosed using varying combinations of histological, clinical, endoscopic and radiographic evidence.

Histology

UC is characterized by inflammatory change extending proximally from the rectum to involve a variable extent of the colon. The proximal limit of inflammation is usually sharply defined macroscopically. UC may be classified according to extent of colonic inflammation (Table 5.1). Knowledge of UC extent is clinically useful for optimizing treatment and may determine future risk of colonic malignancy. Often in longstanding

Table 5.1 Classification of ulcerative colitis according to the extent of colonic inflammation

Classification	Proximal limit of inflammation
Proctitis	Rectum
Distal colitis	Sigmoid colon (proctosigmoiditis)
Left-sided colitis	Descending colon
Extensive colitis	Transverse colon
Pan or total colitis	Right colon and caecum. Backwash ileitis occurs in 20%

UC, inflammatory polyps may line the colonic lumen and these tend to indicate areas of past severe inflammation.

Histologically, active UC is characterized by an acute neutrophilic inflammatory infiltrate, crypt abscesses and goblet cell depletion. The inflammation is limited to the colonic mucosa and submucosa, but in severe colitis transmural inflammation due to wall ischaemia, with colonic dilatation, may occur. Distortion of the colonic crypts is seen, with crypt atrophy and branching.

In CD, the extent of inflammation is potentially greater than in UC and any part of the gastrointestinal (GI) tract may be affected. Inflammation often occurs in a patchy distribution, with normal mucosa in between ('skip lesions' seen on radiological contrast studies). The inflammation may extend across the entire bowel wall and the loops of bowel are often considerably thickened. If the disease is penetrating, then complicated CD may result with formation of enteric fistulae and abscesses. Chronically inflamed loops of bowel often undergo fibrosis and become stenotic.

The classical histological appearance in CD is patchy, transmural inflammation, with non-caseating granulomata. However, in many colonic biopsies the appearances may be identical to that of UC.

Clinical features

Clinical features in UC and CD reflect the nature and extent of intestinal inflammation. Diarrhoea is a common feature. In severe IBD, systemic symptoms such as fatigue, tachycardia and fever may be apparent. IBD is a remitting and relapsing condition, although attacks may be protracted over many months or even years.

Ulcerative colitis

Owing to superficial ulceration of the rectum and colon, passage of diarrhoea with blood is the predominant symptom. Urgency of defecation and incontinence are common and disabling. Severe disease is recognized by marked increase in frequency of defecation, including call to stool overnight.

Crohn's disease

Transmural inflammation in any part of the GI tract may occur. Pain is often a feature and may reflect the site of intestinal disease, for example terminal ileal disease causing right iliac fossa pain. When the small bowel is involved in CD, malabsorption and consequent weight loss are common. Penetrating tissue damage may result in complicated CD with the formation of abscesses and fistulae that may cause symptoms such as pain, increased frequency or change in the nature of diarrhoea and cutaneous discharge. Localized entero-enteric fistulae are often asymptomatic, but a fistula that bypasses a substantial length of small bowel can cause malnutrition and significant diarrhoea. Entero-vesical fistulae may present with frothy urine (pneumaturia). Stenotic intestinal disease may result in symptoms of subacute bowel obstruction. Perianal involvement with fissures and discharging sinuses and fistulae is common in CD, being seen in about 15% of patients. CD of the oesophagus, stomach and duodenum is rare, affecting fewer than 5% of patients. *Helicobacter pylori* negative gastritis is probably the commonest manifestation of CD in the upper intestinal tract. Aphthous mouth ulcers are common in CD and granulomatous swellings of the lips and gums are occasionally seen.

Physical examination

External examination of the patient may contribute little to diagnosis of the patient with IBD, although evidence of perianal disease or abdominal masses will point towards a diagnosis of CD. It is important to recognize signs of severe disease, such as tachycardia, pyrexia, abdominal tenderness and malnourishment; abdominal distension in a sick patient with colitis may indicate the development of toxic megacolon. Examination of the patient is completed by sigmoidoscopy with rectal biopsy. In UC and rectal CD, characteristic erythema, granularity, contact bleeding and ulceration of the mucosa may be seen.

A variety of extraintestinal manifestations of IBD are recognized and may present with characteristic symptoms and physical signs. These are shown in Table 5.2.

Investigations

Laboratory investigations

Routine blood count and biochemistry often provides evidence of ongoing inflammation in the form of an elevated white cell count, platelet count, C-reactive protein (CRP) and a

Table 5.2 Extraintestinal manifestations of inflammatory bowel disease

System	Manifestation	Comments
Rheumatological	Peripheral arthropathy	5–20%; HLA B27, B4 associated; treat active inflammatory bowel disease; also physical therapy and intra-articular steroids
	Sacroileitis	Often asymptomatic
	Ankylosing spondylitis	5–10%; HLA B27 associated; physical therapy; unrelated to activity of IBD
Skeletal	Osteoporosis	Common; exacerbated by corticosteroids
	Osteomalacia	Commoner in Crohn's disease (CD); vitamin D malabsorption
Dermatological	Erythema nodosum	10–20%; correlates with disease activity; treat active IBD
	Pyoderma gangrenosum	1–10%; commoner in ulcerative colitis (UC); may require immunosuppressants
	Metastatic CD	Rare; cutaneous ulcerating nodules
Ophthalmological	Uveitis	1–5%; sight threatening; requires topical/systemic corticosteroids
	Episcleritis	Treat active IBD
Renal	Nephrolithiasis	7–10%; uric acid and oxalate stones
	Amyloidosis	Rare; long-standing IBD
Hepatobiliary	Primary sclerosisng cholangitis (PSC)	2.4–7.5% (75% of patients with PSC also have IBD); may require liver transplant

low albumin level. Anaemia may be seen and this can be due to chronic intestinal blood loss or vitamin B12 and folate deficiency in patients with CD and ileal involvement and/or resection. There has been some interest in the use of serological markers in the diagnosis of IBD, particularly in differentiating UC from CD. These include perinuclear staining antineutrophil cytoplasmic antibodies and anti-*Saccharomyces cerevisiae* antibodies. Currently the sensitivity and specificity of these markers are inadequate and their use is not recommended.

If there is any suspicion of enteric infection, particularly in patients with symptoms of colitis and a short history, then it is important to obtain stool samples for microbiological analysis including an examination for *Clostridium difficile* toxin and also for intestinal parasites such as *Entamoeba histolytica*.

Endoscopy

Endoscopy is most useful in the investigation of patients with IBD, enabling both direct vision of the intestinal mucosa and mucosal biopsy sampling for a histological diagnosis. Characteristic confluent mucosal inflammation seen at sigmoidoscopy enables a reasonably confident diagnosis of UC to be made before biopsy results become available (Fig. 5.1). Colonoscopy is more useful, but not initially necessary, in defining disease extent in UC. Colonoscopy is valuable in the investigation of CD, enabling visualization and biopsy of patchily distributed colonic disease and often revealing characteristic terminal ileal involvement (Fig. 5.2). Colonoscopy is also used in the screening of IBD patients for colonic malignancy (see later).

Enteroscopy enables visualization and biopsy of the small intestine, but is time consuming and not widely available and so has not generally replaced small-bowel radiology in the

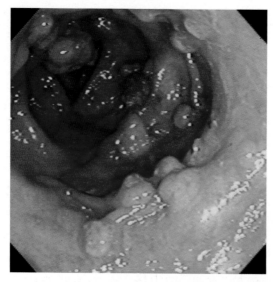

Fig. 5.1
Characteristic appearance of ulcerative colitis at sigmoidoscopy showing confluent inflammation with inflammatory polyps

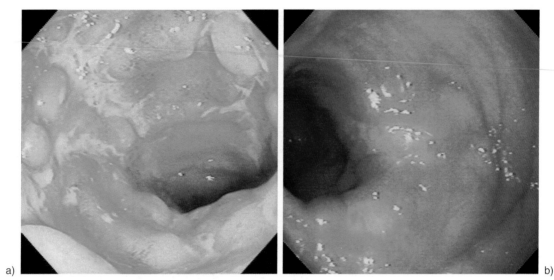

a) b)

Fig. 5.2
Ileocolonoscopic views of Crohn's disease affecting the terminal ileum in two different patients showing deep mucosal ulceration

investigation of CD. Capsule endoscopy may become useful in this context. Conventional upper GI endoscopy can be useful in CD patients with upper intestinal symptoms.

Radiology

Plain supine abdominal radiography often gives an indication of disease extent in UC and Crohn's colitis. It is also useful to identify proximal constipation in distal colitis and to monitor patients with fulminant colitis for the development of toxic megacolon.

Barium enema examination can be used to define disease extent in UC and Crohn's colitis. Often characteristic appearances for either disease may be seen; a featureless 'lead pipe' colon is seen in chronic pan UC (Fig. 5.3), whilst in Crohn's colitis the disease tends to be patchy, and deeper 'rosethorn' ulcers and fistulous connections may be seen. Colonoscopy is preferred to barium enema examinations, having the advantage that histological samples may also be taken. Occasionally, 'instant enemas' using safer water soluble contrast agents may be useful in the investigation of severe colitis of unknown type, where sigmoidoscopy is deemed too risky.

Barium studies remain useful in the investigation of suspected small-bowel CD (Fig. 5.4). Small-bowel barium follow-through examinations can identify ulcerated and stenosed segments of bowel and some idea of disease activity may also be obtained – in active disease bowel loops are often thickened with apparent separation.

Ultrasonography has value in the initial investigation of CD-related abscesses and inflammatory massess. It is also useful in identifying thickened, fluid-filled bowel loops, suggestive of active inflammation.

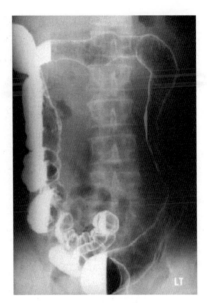

Fig. 5.3
Barium enema examination in a patient with chronic extensive ulcerative colitis, showing a featureless colon

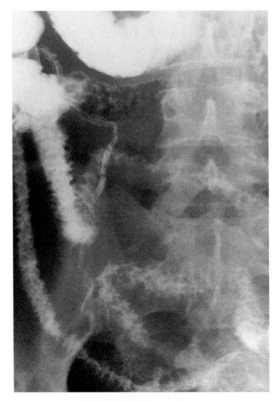

Fig. 5.4
Small bowel barium meal showing very extensive Crohn's disease of the ileum with ulceration and a long terminal ileal stricture

CT scanning is of little use in the investigation of UC, but is valuable in CD, particularly for the identification of extraluminal complications such as abscesses and fistulae. It is particularly useful for imaging the retroperitoneal tissues, for example when there is a suspicion of psoas abscess. CT colography is a newer technique used to provide detailed three-dimensional images of the colon. It currently remains inferior in quality to colonoscopy and is unlikely to replace it in the investigation of IBD, since histological samples cannot be obtained.

MRI scanning is an increasingly used technique and is now the investigation of choice for identification and mapping of fistulous and sinus tracts in perianal CD.

Nuclear medicine

Radioisotope-labelled leukocyte scans are used effectively in some centres in the investigation of IBD. They may be particularly useful when endoscopic investigation has proved difficult and when it is desirable to avoid excess exposure to X-rays. Labelled leukocyte scans may be used to give information on disease extent in UC and colonic CD and also to localize disease activity in cases of CD (Fig. 5.5). A positive-labelled leukocyte scan suggests disease activity and this may be useful in differentiating symptoms due to active small-bowel CD from those due to fibrostenotic obstructing disease. Labelled leukocyte scans are unlikely to be positive if the CRP is not raised.

Assessing disease activity in inflammatory bowel disease

A variety of clinical and endoscopic scoring systems are available for quantifying disease activity in IBD, for example the Crohn's Disease Activity Index (see Tables 5.3a–c). These are useful in clinical trials, where response to a therapy needs to be quantified and recorded, but in routine practice disease activity is normally estimated according to a combination of clinical, laboratory, endoscopic and radiographic features, in combination with the clinician's judgement.

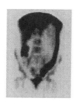

Erratum

Please note that Figure 5.5b on page 119 is incorrect. The correct Figure 5.5 is shown here.

Fig. 5.5 Labelled leukocyte scans showing Crohn's disease of the descending colon and caecum (left panel) and distal ileal CD (right panel)

Table 5.3a Simplified Crohn's Disease Activity Index (CDAI). The patient's symptoms on the preceding day only are evaluated

Symptoms in preceding day	Sum
A Number of liquid stools	–
B Abdominal pain	0 = none 1 = mild 2 = moderate 3 = severe
C General well being	0 = well 1 = slightly under par 2 = poor 3 = very poor 4 = terrible
D Number of six of following features present: 1. arthritis/arthralgia 2. iritis/uveitis 3. erythema nodosum; pyoderma gangrenosum; aphthous stomatitis 4. perianal disease 5. other fistula 6. fever	–
E Abdominal mass	0 = none 2 = questionable 5 = definite

The total score is calculated as according to the formula: Score = 20(A+2(B+C+D+E)). Score = <50: remission; 150–250: mild disease activity; 250–400: moderate disease activity; >400: severe disease activity

MANAGEMENT OF INFLAMMATORY BOWEL DISEASE

In this section, practical strategies for medical treatment of UC and CD will be outlined. In general, options for medical treatment of both conditions are similar. The mainstays of IBD treatment are corticosteroids, 5-aminosalicylates and immunomodulatory agents. Infliximab is a 'biologic' therapy that has proved effective; others are emerging. Antibiotics and dietary forms of treatment are used occasionally. The principles of treatment are based upon controlling active inflammation to induce remission, followed by prolonged maintenance of remission. IBD is a spontaneously remitting condition and data from early placebo-controlled trials suggest that up to 30% of patients may achieve some degree of remission without treatment. Medical treatment will fail a significant proportion of patients and surgical treatment will have to be considered. The medical management of severe acute UC requires special consideration and is dealt with separately. The main medical strategies for the treatment of IBD are summarized in Table 5.4.

Table 5.3b Harvey Bradshaw index for Crohn's-disease activity

A General well being	0 = well 1 = slightly under par 2 = poor 3 = very poor 4 = terrible
B Abdominal pain	0 = none 1 = mild 2 = moderate 3 = severe
C Number of liquid stools per day	–
D Abdominal mass	0 = none 1 = dubious 2 = definite 3 = definite and tender
E Complications	Score 1 for each of: Arthralgia Uveitis Erythema nodosum Pyoderma gangrenosum Aphthous ulcers Anal fissure New fistula Abscess

The total score (A+B+C+D+E) correlates well with the CDAI, e.g. a CDAI score of 100 approximates to a Harvey Bradshaw score of 2, and a CDAI score of 300 approximates to a Harvey Bradshaw score of 9

Table 5.3c Baron score for the severity of ulcerative colitis on sigmoidoscopic examination

Colitis grade	Sigmoidoscopic mucosal appearance
0	Normal
1	Non-haemorrhagic
2	Haemorrhagic; bleeding on light contact
3	Haemorrhagic; spontaneous bleeding proximal to the depth of insertion

Corticosteroids

Corticosteroids are useful in the treatment of IBD due to an inhibitory effect on the host immune response. This is incompletely understood but is probably effected via multiple actions, including inhibition of pro-inflammatory cytokine production and inhibition of leukocyte function.

Table 5.4 Established medications for the treatment of inflammatory bowel disease and their suitability for treatment across the spectrum of disease

Drug	Ulcerative colitis			Crohn's disease		
	Distal/left-sided colitis	Extensive/pan-colitis	Maintenance therapy	Ileo-colonic	Perianal and fistulating	Maintenance therapy
Sytemic steroid	+	+	–	+	–	–
Rectal steroid	+	–	–	+[1]	–	–
Oral 5-ASA	+	+	+	+	–	±
Rectal 5-ASA	+	–	+	+[1]	–	–
Azathioprine/6-MP	+	+	+	+	+	+
Methotrexate	–	–	–	+	?	+
Ciclosporin	+	+	–	+	+	–
Infliximab	?	?	?	+	+	+
Antibiotics	–	–	?	+	+	–

[1]Rectal corticosteroid and 5-ASA preparations are suitable for use in distal and left-sided colonic Crohn's disease

Indications

Corticosteroids are the main agents used to induce remission in moderate to severely active UC and ileo-colonic CD and response rates of 80% may be expected. They are usually ineffective for maintenance of disease remission.

Dosage and use

Oral prednisolone is usually prescribed at a dose of 0.5–1 mg/kg daily (generally 30–60 mg) for 7 days and then reduced by 5 mg every 5–7 days thereafter until the course is complete. Patients who are severely unwell may require hospital admission and administration of intravenous hydrocortisone, usually at a dose of 100 mg three to four times daily; the parenteral route of admission is probably more effective. Corticosteroids have a rapid onset of action and most patients usually respond within about 1 week.

Although corticosteroids are not considered effective in maintenance of remission of IBD, a minority of patients are intolerant of other preparations, unsuitable for surgical treatment and relapse rapidly on corticosteroid withdrawal. For such patients there is little alternative but maintenance on a small dose (up to 7.5 mg daily) of prednisolone.

Adverse effects

Corticosteroid preparations are generally well tolerated. Numerous side effects are associated with their use and are well known. Important side effects to consider include hypertension, glucose intolerance, adrenal suppression, mood swings and weight gain. It is important to remember that patients receiving high-dose corticosteroids are profoundly immunosuppressed and increased vigilance for infections should be maintained. IBD patients requiring multiple courses of corticosteroids are at increased risk of osteoporosis and subsequent fragility fracture. Concurrent use of vitamin D and calcium supplements (e.g. Calcichew D3 Forte, two tablets daily) during the corticosteroid course and

Table 5.5 Sulfasalazine and other 5-ASA oral preparations used in the treatment of inflammatory bowel disease

Drug (daily dose)		Target organ(s)
Sulfasalazine	(2–8 g)	Colon
Olsalazine	(1–3 g)	Colon
Balsalazide	(3-6.75 g)	Colon
Asacol®	(1.2–2.4 g)	Colon
Ipocol®	(1.2–2.4 g)	Colon
Salofalk®	(0.75–1.5 g)	Ileum and colon
Pentasa®	(1.5–4 g)	Jejunum, ileum and colon

monitoring for the development of osteoporosis by bone densitometry (preferably DEXA scanning) each year that a course is given may be beneficial. Those who do develop osteoporosis should be treated with a bisphosphonate. If the DEXA T score is less than −1.5, then a bisphosphonate should be given concurrently with corticosteroids. It is now generally recommended that all patients over 65 years receiving corticosteroids should be treated with a bisphosphonate also.

In an attempt to minimize the adverse systemic effects of corticosteroid therapy, novel agents have been developed. Budesonide, which is available in an oral formulation for treating ileal and right-sided colonic CD, is poorly absorbed from the intestine and has high first-pass metabolism. It is less effective than conventional corticosteroids and whilst classical side effects are less apparent in the short term, concerns remain over its safety in long-term use.

Aminosalicylate drugs

A variety of 5-aminosalicylate (5-ASA) preparations are available (Table 5.5). Sulfasalazine, olsalazine and balsalazide all incorporate an azo bond requiring metabolism by colonic bacteria to release the active 5-ASA molecule. Mesalazine is available in several preparations with resin-based coats that dissolve in a pH- and/or time-dependent manner and allow selective delivery of the drug to targeted regions of the bowel. An appropriate drug may, therefore, be chosen according to the site of disease. The mechanism of action of 5-ASA preparations is unclear, but probably includes reduction of inflammatory mediator production via inhibition of cyclooxygenase and 5-lipoxygenase pathways.

Indications

5-ASA drugs are used for induction of remission in mild to moderately active UC and improvement rates of up to 60% may be achieved. Similar, although not quite as effective results have been achieved in CD, particularly when there is a colonic component to the disease. 5-ASA drugs are also of benefit for maintenance of disease remission in UC and up to 75% of patients may remain relapse free. Evidence for their use as maintenance therapy in CD is less compelling.

Dosage and use

The highest recommended dose of 5-ASA drugs, if tolerated by the patient, is of most benefit in achieving disease remission. This dose should be continued for maintenance therapy long term if effective. Long-term use of 5-ASA drugs may have a beneficial effect in reducing the risk for development of colorectal cancer in UC.

Adverse effects

Dose-related side effects such as nausea, abdominal pain and headache are common (up to 50% of patients) with sulfasalazine and have been attributed to the sulfapyridine moiety. For this reason the drug is now less popular and alternative 5-ASA preparations, which are better tolerated, were developed. Rare side effects of 5-ASA drugs include blood dyscrasias (there is no good evidence that monitoring blood tests are necessary), hypersensitivity reactions, diarrhoea and a paradoxical exacerbation of colitis. Interstitial nephritis appears to be a rare, although serious, complication of treatment of IBD with mesalazine and it may be prudent to measure baseline creatinine before treatment initiation and on a periodic basis (e.g. annually) during maintenance therapy.

Local corticosteroid and 5-ASA preparations

Local corticosteroid and 5-ASA preparations are of benefit in inducing and maintaining remission in proctitis and distal and left-sided colitis due to UC or CD. Many patients prefer not to use these local preparations and, therefore, oral treatment should also be offered as an alternative. A variety of preparations in suppository (for proctitis) and foam or liquid retention enema (for distal and left-sided colitis) forms are available and choice of use depends partly on patient preference. Evidence in UC patients suggests that rectal 5-ASA preparations used at high dose (2 g of mesalazine daily) are more effective at inducing remission than rectal corticosteroid preparations. In difficult cases, benefit may be obtained by additional use of a corticosteroid preparation. In distal colitis where local therapies are not effective alone, the addition of oral 5-ASA drugs, corticosteroids and immunomodulators may be required in a stepwise fashion.

Immunomodulating agents

Azathioprine, 6-mercaptopurine (6-MP), methotrexate and ciclosporin are immunomodulating agents of established use in the treatment of selected IBD patients.

Azathioprine/6-MP

Azathioprine is a pro-drug that is metabolized to 6-MP; both agents are available in the UK. 6-MP is metabolized to 6-thioguanine (6-TG) purine analogues, which are the major active metabolites. The precise mode of action of 6-TG in IBD is unknown, but a T-cell suppressant action is probably one of the main mechanisms. Thiopurine methyltransferase (TPMT) is an enzyme that contributes to 6-MP inactivation. TPMT activity is genetically determined with low activity found in 0.3% of the Caucasian population, intermediate

---

Table 5.6 Three possible schemes for the initiation of azathioprine and 6-mercaptopurine treatment

Start with target dose and measure FBC at 2 weeks, 4 weeks, 3 months and thereafter every 3 months. If there are side effects, including a WBC <3.0, stop until side effects disappear, restart at 50 mg and then follow scheme 2.

This is the simplest scheme and will achieve the target dose soonest and has been used by many clinicians without serious problems.

Start with 50 mg daily and measure WBC at 2 weeks:

If WBC hasn't fallen by >25%* and if no side effects go straight to target dose
If WBC has fallen by >25%* increase dose by 25 mg every 2 weeks until side effects or WBC <3.0 or target dose reached
If WBC <3.0 abandon treatment

Although this will help to prevent complications it is time consuming and will delay achievement of the target dose.

Measure TPMT activity:

If very low abandon treatment
If normal follow scheme 1
If intermediate, follow scheme 2

Although perhaps the safest scheme, waiting for the TPMT result may delay treatment.

---

* This fairly arbitrary reduction threshold is chosen to detect those who may have low or intermediate TPMT activity and are therefore more sensitive to the effects of the drug

---

activity in 11% and normal activity in 89%. Individuals with low levels of TPMT are prone to accumulate high levels of 6-TG, which puts them at risk of bone-marrow suppression with profound leukopenia.

Indications

Azathioprine/6-MP is useful for treating chronically active UC and CD that is unresponsive to corticosteroid therapy or rapidly relapses on reducing the corticosteroid dose. Patients who cannot be maintained in remission on 5-ASA preparations and require two or more reducing courses of corticosteroids for disease flares in 1 year may also benefit from treatment with azathioprine/6-MP. Response rates of up to 75% may be expected. In contrast to corticosteroids and 5-ASA drugs, azathioprine/6-MP are also useful in healing fistulating CD. Once remission is induced, azathioprine/6-MP may be continued long term and is effective at maintaining disease remission, with relapse free rates of up to 65% over 5 years reported.

Dosage and use

The target dose of azathioprine for both induction and maintenance therapy is 2.5 mg/kg and that for 6-MP is 1.5 mg/kg. There is no consensus or firm evidence on which to base how to achieve or modify the target dose. There are many possible variations; three are outlined in Table 5.6. These agents have a delayed onset of action and a period of 2–4 months treatment is required before their full effect is achieved and disease activity is controlled. For this reason it is preferable to ensure that treatment initiation coincides with another therapy (e.g. prednisolone or ciclosporin). Rapid loading treatment with intravenous azathioprine is of no added benefit. Limited available evidence shows that a beneficial effect in preventing relapse is seen for up to 5 years. After this period little information is available and many clinicians would try withdrawing treatment at this stage if asymptomatic for a few years.

Adverse effects

From 5 to 10% of patients experience side effects such as nausea, vomiting, malaise, diarrhoea and arthralgia, which may be avoided if the dose is increased gradually to the target dose over a 2-week period. Dividing the daily dose and taking it with meals may also be helpful. Fifty per cent of patients who are unable to tolerate azathioprine because of such side effects, may tolerate a switch to 6-MP instead. Pancreatitis occurs in up to 3% and resolves on drug withdrawal, but recurs on retreatment with either agent. Abnormalities of liver function occur in up to 2% and usually resolve on drug withdrawal. Allergic reactions such as fever and rash and hypersensitivity reactions may also occur. Initial concerns about an increased risk of lymphoma and other malignancies amongst IBD patients on azathioprine/6-MP remain unconfirmed.

Bone-marrow suppression with leukopenia (leukocyte count $<3.0 \times 10^9/$ l) is the most serious side effect of treatment with these agents. It occurs in up to 4% of patients and its time of onset after treatment initiation is variable and unpredictable, but more cases probably occur within the first few weeks of treatment. Affected patients are at risk of overwhelming sepsis and death. Pancytopenia may occur, but is rarer. For this reason monitoring of the full blood count during treatment with azathioprine/6-MP is mandatory. It is recommended that monitoring is done at 2 weeks, 1 month and 3 months and thereafter every 3 months, checking that, in particular, the white-cell count does not fall below 3.0. The drug is usually stopped when the white-cell count falls below 3.0 and restarted at a lower dose when the white-cell count recovers. It should be noted that the mean corpuscular volume (MCV) almost always rises and the lymphocyte count falls on these drugs, but that doesn't seem to be of any clinical importance.

The risk of leukopenia is dose related and is associated with high levels of accumulated 6-TG nucleotides in bone-marrow cells. Measurement of TPMT activity is possible and can be used to identify patients who are at risk of accumulating high 6-TG levels with resultant bone-marrow toxicity and in whom azathioprine/6-MP therapy is more risky. This test is increasingly being used as a guide to the starting dose. Xanthine oxidase is also involved in 6-MP degradation to inactive metabolites and care should, therefore, be taken with patients who are co-prescribed allopurinol, which is an inhibitor of this enzyme.

Methotrexate

Methotrexate is a dihydrofolate reductase inhibitor. Folate-dependent metabolic pathways are inhibited with a resultant immunosuppressant effect due to reduced DNA synthesis, leukocyte proliferation and proinflammatory cytokine synthesis.

Indications

Methotrexate is used in chronically active CD that is corticosteroid resistant or dependent. Remission rates of 40% may be achieved after 16 weeks therapy and methotrexate may have a faster onset of action than azathioprine/6-MP. The drug may be continued as maintenance therapy, with 65% of patients remaining in remission at 40 weeks. Methotrexate has been used less widely than azathioprine/6-mp, and tends to be used in suitable patients where these agents have failed or have not been tolerated due to side effects. Methotrexate is not effective in UC.

Dosage and use

Methotrexate is given intramuscularly at a dose of 25 mg once weekly for 16 weeks and during this period the corticosteroid dose weaned down. If the patient tolerates the treatment and responds then maintenance therapy at a lower dose of 15 mg intramuscularly once weekly has been shown to be effective for at least 40 weeks. Oral maintenance therapy has not been shown to be effective.

Adverse effects

Nausea, abdominal pain, diarrhoea and mucositis may occur in up to 10%. Daily folic acid supplementation and weekly dosing are recommended to reduce the risk of such side effects. Concurrent therapy with other drugs that inhibit folate metabolism (e.g. sulphonamides, trimethoprim) should be avoided. Bone-marrow suppression and leukopenia is important, but is rarer (1%) than that seen with azathioprine/6-MP. Full blood count should be monitored weekly for the first month and monthly thereafter. Dose reduction or treatment withdrawal may be necessary if there is evidence of bone-marrow suppression. There are concerns over methotrexate-induced hepatic toxicity and liver fibrosis or cirrhosis may develop with long-term use. Available evidence in IBD patients suggests that hepatotoxicity due to methotrexate is not seen as frequently as it is in psoriasis patients. Methotrexate treatment should probably be avoided in patients with underlying liver disease or in those at risk of liver disease (e.g. alcohol excess, diabetes, obesity). Treatment should be stopped if symptoms or signs of liver disease develop. Abnormal liver chemistries are seen in 6% of patients at some stage during therapy and may be transient. Monitoring blood tests should be performed on a monthly basis and if the transaminases are markedly raised on one occasion (e.g. >120) or persistently raised over 3 months then treatment should be withdrawn and a liver biopsy considered. Since liver fibrosis/cirrhosis may be present in the presence of normal liver chemistries, some authorities recommend a screening liver biopsy after each cumulative 1.5 g of methotrexate given or after 2 years' treatment. Hypersensitivity pneumonitis occurs in up to 2% and should be suspected if cough and dyspnoea develop.

Ciclosporin

Ciclosporin is a peptide that inhibits nuclear transcription factor of activated T cells and prevents transcription of interleukin 2 as well as other pro-inflammatory cytokines. This results in diminished T-cell proliferation and an immunosuppressant effect.

Indications

Ciclosporin is used in severe acute UC that is not responding to intravenous corticosteroid therapy (see p. 132). It is rapidly acting and response rates of 60–80% are usually seen within 5 days. Ciclosporin is associated with serious adverse effects and it is not used as a long-term maintenance treatment. In acute severe UC ciclosporin therapy aims to avoid emergency colectomy, whilst enabling an alternative immunomodulatory such as azathioprine to be commenced for maintaining disease remission. Evidence suggests that 50% of such patients who respond to this approach will require a colectomy within 3–5 years because of recurrent disease. Ciclosporin has occasionally been used with success in severe CD, including fistulating disease.

Dosage and use

Ciclosporin is used at a dose of 2 mg/kg/day as an intravenous infusion. Concurrent corticosteroid therapy is usually continued, but may not be necessary. If there is no response to this treatment after 5–7 days, then surgical referral for a colectomy should be made. Those who do respond are converted to oral ciclosporin at a dose of 5 mg/kg/day in a divided dose (microemulsion formulation; Neoral®), which is continued for about 3 months whilst corticosteroids are weaned and stopped and azathioprine is started. Ciclosporin levels should be monitored to avoid drug toxicity. During intravenous therapy, a level of 250–400 ng/ml (monitor once or twice weekly) should be sought and during oral therapy the trough level should be 95–205 ng/ml; dosage will need to be adjusted accordingly.

Adverse effects

Ciclosporin has several potentially serious side effects. Headache, nausea, gingival hyperplasia, hypertrichosis, paraesthesias and tremors all occur commonly. Development of hypertension, electrolyte abnormalities (usually hyperkalaemia), renal impairment and abnormal liver chemistries occur in about 10% of patients and necessitate careful clinical and laboratory monitoring. These effects usually resolve on dose reduction or drug withdrawal. Seizures can occur and patients with hypocholesterolaemia (cholesterol <3.1 mmol/l) and hypomagnesaemia are at particular risk. Serum cholesterol and magnesium should be checked prior to treatment and if low (not uncommon amongst patients with severe UC), then ciclosporin should not be started. Patients receiving ciclosporin, corticosteroid and perhaps azathioprine therapy in combination are profoundly immunosuppressed and at risk of opportunistic infection. Some authorities recommend that such patients should receive *Pneumocystis carinii* antibiotic prophylaxis (as co-trimoxazole 960 mg on alternate days).

Infliximab

Infliximab is a chimeric (human IgG1 constant region and murine antigen-binding variable region) monoclonal antibody directed against tumour necrosis factor-alpha (TNF-α) and represents an important recent therapeutic advance in the treatment of CD. Infliximab acts by the neutralization of soluble and membrane-bound TNF-α and thus inhibits amplification of the inflammatory cascade seen in IBD. It may also result in destruction of TNF-α producing cells by complement fixation, antibody-dependent cytotoxicity and induction of apoptosis.

Indications

Infliximab is used in severe active CD that is refractory to treatment with corticosteroids and immunomodulatory agents such as azathioprine/6-MP and methotrexate or in patients who are intolerant of these agents. About two-thirds of patients have a good clinical response to a single-treatment infusion, usually within 2 weeks. One-third of patients may still be in remission 12 weeks after treatment. Infliximab is also useful for the treatment of CD patients with enterocutaneous and perianal fistulae and complete healing of fistulae for at least 4 weeks may be seen following a course of three infusions. The use of infliximab in UC has not been evaluated adequately so far and remains experimental. In those who respond satisfactorily to a single dose of infliximab, but then relapse, maintenance of remission may be achieved for up to 1 year if repeat infusions are given approximately every 8 weeks (actual timing determined by symptomatic relapse).

Dosage and use

For induction of disease remission in suitable patients, infliximab is given as a single intravenous infusion at a dose of 5 mg/kg. If maintenance treatment is required, a dose of 5–10 mg/kg is given at 8-weekly intervals. When used to treat fistulating CD, infliximab has been given as three 5 mg/kg infusions at weeks 0, 2 and 6.

Adverse effects

The limited data available suggest that infliximab treatment is relatively safe. Infusion reactions with urticaria, dyspnoea and hypotension can occur and may be treated with anti-histamines and corticosteroids. Delayed hypersensitivity reactions with rash, fever, arthralgia, myalgia and facial swelling have been observed amongst patients who are re-treated several months after previous treatment and the manufacturers do not recommend treatment intervals of more than 15 weeks. Other common side effects include headache, flushing, pruritus, nausea, abdominal pain, diarrhoea and dyspnoea. Congestive heart failure is made worse by infliximab and is a contraindication to treatment. Serious infections have occurred in patients treated with infliximab, including reactivation of latent tuberculosis. It is prudent to screen for this prior to treatment with a chest radiograph and perhaps a tuberculin skin test.

The formation of anti-infliximab antibodies (human anti-chimeric antibodies) may occur in patients receiving infliximab, with resultant decreased efficacy of subsequent infusions. Concomitant treatment with azathioprine or methotrexate may reduce formation of these antibodies. About half of patients receiving infliximab develop anti-nuclear antibodies. The significance is not known.

Antibiotics and anti-tuberculous therapy

Bacteria are implicated in the initiation and perpetuation of inflammation in IBD and there is a rationale for antibiotic treatment of the condition. However, with the exception

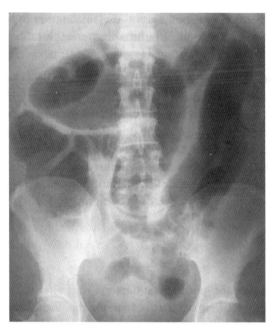

Fig. 5.6
Dilated colon in a patient with acute severe ulcerative colitis; such patients require combined management between medical and surgical teams and often require colectomy

Patients with severe colitis require hospital admission for intensive treatment and observation (see Fig. 1.2); both medical and surgical teams should participate. Regular clinical observations, including a daily stool chart, should be kept to assess the response to treatment. Daily full blood count, electrolytes, creatinine, albumin and CRP should be recorded. Stool cultures, *Clostridium difficile* toxin assay and parasite microscopy should be performed to exclude infective causes. Daily plain abdominal X-rays should be requested, looking for the development of megacolon (Fig. 5.6; colonic diameter >5.5 cm or caecal diameter >9 cm), until symptoms start to settle. Some centres advocate resting the bowel by keeping the patient nil by mouth until symptoms start to improve.

The mainstay of treatment is intravenous corticosteroids (hydrocortisone 100 mg qds). Antibiotic treatment is not required. Opiates, antidiarrhoeal agents and anticholinergics may precipitate development of toxic megacolon and should be avoided. 5-ASA drugs should not be commenced in patients not previously taking them, since they may rarely paradoxically exacerbate colitis.

Two-thirds of patients respond to this treatment, with resolution of pyrexia and tachycardia and reduction in bowel frequency to less than three stools per day without blood. Such patients can be switched to oral corticosteroids and discharged home for close out-patient follow-up. Patients who fail to respond adequately to 5–7 days of intravenous corticosteroid treatment should be considered for colectomy or intravenous ciclosporin treatment. More than eight stools per day, or a CRP of >45 in combination with more than three stools per day at day three of treatment have been shown to correlate with failure of medical therapy and requirement for a colectomy. On this basis ciclosporin therapy could be considered at this stage. Development of toxic megacolon that doesn't settle after 24 h, colonic perforation or severe colonic haemorrhage are also indications for colectomy.

Surgical treatment in ulcerative colitis

UC may be cured by surgery and about one-third of patients with UC will undergo surgical treatment, often within the first 10 years of diagnosis. Surgery may be performed on an emergency or elective basis.

Indications

Emergency surgery accounts for 20% of procedures performed in UC patients. It is usually performed for acute severe colitis that is either non-responsive to a reasonable trial of medical therapy or due to development of a complication such as toxic megacolon, perforation or massive haemorrhage.

About 70% of surgical procedures carried out in UC patients are performed on an elective basis. Elective surgery is usually for failure of medical therapy with persistent disabling symptoms. Sometimes surgical treatment is indicated if medical therapy is working, but resulting in unacceptable complications, e.g. corticosteroid-induced diabetes and drug-induced myelosuppression.

About 10% of procedures in UC patients are carried out for development of high-grade dysplasia or cancer in the diseased colon.

Surgical procedures

UC may be cured and long-term risk of malignancy eliminated by removal of the entire colon, i.e. panproctocolectomy. This may be achieved in a variety of ways and the operation selected depends upon the urgency of the situation, the patient's preoperative health and the patient's desire for anal continence.

Subtotal colectomy with end ileostomy is usually performed for acute severe colitis and its complications. The rectal stump is either directly closed or raised as a second stoma (mucous fistula). A restorative procedure may then be performed at a later date, when the patient has recovered from the acute illness. Some patients elect to keep a permanent end ileostomy, in which case the risk of development of malignancy in the remaining rectal stump must be considered.

For elective UC surgery, panproctocolectomy with permanent 'Brooke' end ileostomy is well established. However, over the last two decades restorative proctocolectomy, with creation of an ileal pouch, has become the surgical treatment of choice for UC. The colon and rectum are removed and the anal sphincters preserved. An ileal pouch is created using 2–4 limbs of distal ileum and this is anastomosed to the anal canal. By removal of the entire colon and rectum, the disease and future risk of malignancy are eliminated. The ileo-anal pouch preserves anal continence. In elective cases panproctocolectomy and creation of an ileo-anal pouch can be performed as a single-stage procedure. However, if

Table 5.7 Safety of inflammatory bowel disease medications in pregnancy and breast feeding

Medication	Pregnancy	Breast feeding
5-ASA	Safe	Safe
Corticosteroid	Safe	Safe
Azathiporine/6-MP	Probably safe	Not safe
Methotrexate	Contraindicated: abortifacient	Not safe
Ciclosporin	Probably safe	Not safe
Metronidazole	Avoid high doses	Avoid large single doses
Ciprofloxacin	Not safe	Not safe

Dysplasia is recognized as a premalignant mucosal lesion that predicts subsequent development of cancer. Early detection of dysplasia by surveillance colonoscopy in IBD patients, with subsequent colectomy in those in whom it is detected, may offer health benefits. However, as yet the reliability and benefits of colonoscopic surveillance programmes in IBD are unknown and their use in clinical practice is not routine. Current British Society of Gastroenterology guidelines recommend colonoscopic surveillance every 1–3 years from 10 years of disease duration in pancolitis and from 15 to 20 years' duration in left-sided colitis. Between two and four biopsies should be taken every 10 cm in order to be confident of detecting dysplasia. Colectomy should be recommended to the patient if high-grade dysplasia or a macroscopic dysplasia-associated lesion or mass (DALM) is detected. If low-grade dysplasia is detected, either an increase in the frequency of surveillance to 6 monthly or colectomy, should be recommended. Patients with PSC are at the greatest risk of colorectal cancer and they should have annual surveillance colonoscopy from the time of diagnosis.

Further Reading

Bebb JR, Scott BB. Systematic review: how effective are the usual treatments for ulcerative colitis? Aliment Pharmacol Ther 2004; 20:143–9.

Bebb JR, Scott BB. Systematic review: how effective are the usual treatments for Crohn's disease? Aliment Pharmacol Ther 2004; 20:151–9.

Cunliffe RN, Scott BB. Monitoring for drug side effects in inflammatory bowel disease. Aliment Pharmacol Ther 2002; 16: 647–62.

Evans JMM, McMahon AD, Murray FE, McDevitt DG, MacDonald TM. Non-steroidal anti-inflammatory drugs are associated with emergency admission to hospital for colitis due to inflammatory bowel disease. Gut 1997; 40: 619–22.

Eaden J. Review article: the data supporting a role for aminosalicylates in the chemoprevention of colorectal cancer in patients with inflammatory bowel disease. Aliment Pharmacol Ther 2003; 18 (Suppl 2): 15–21.

Forbes A, Britton TC, House IM, Gazzard BG. Safety and efficacy of acetarsol suppositories in unresponsive proctitis. Aliment Pharmacol Ther 1989; 3: 553–6.

Loftus CG, Loftus EV, Sandborn WJ. Cyclosporin for refractory ulcerative colitis. Gut 2003; 52: 172–3.

Papa A, Danese S, Gasbarrini A, Gasbarrini G. Review article: potential therapeutic actions and mechanisms of action of heparin in inflammatory bowel disease. Aliment Pharmacol Ther 2000; 14: 1403–9.

Podolsky DK. Inflammatory bowel disease. N Engl J Med 2002; 347: 417–29.

Rampton DS. Methotrexate in Crohn's disease. Gut 2001; 48: 790–1.

Rayner CK, McCormack G, Emmanuel AV, Kamm MA. Long-term results of low-dose intravenous ciclosporin for acute severe ulcerative colitis. Aliment Pharmacol Ther 2003; 18: 303–8.

Regueiro MD (ed.) Inflammatory bowel disease. Gastro Clin N Am 2002; 31.

Sandborn WJ. Nicotine therapy for ulcerative colitis: a review of rationale, mechanisms pharmacology and clinical results. Am J Gastroenterol 1999; 94: 1161–71.

Sandborn WJ, Hanauer SB. Infliximab in the treatment of Crohn's disease: a users guide for clinicians. Am J Gastroenterol 2002; 97: 2962–72.

Sandborn WJ, Targan SR. Biologic therapy of inflammatory bowel disease. Gastroenterology 2002; 122: 1592–608.

Sands BE. Therapy of inflammatory bowel disease. Gastroenterology 2000; 118: S68–82.

Watts DA, Satsangi J. The genetic jigsaw of inflammatory bowel disease. Gut 2002; 50 (Suppl III): iii31–6.

3. Treatment cannot be expected to cure functional disease, since there is no specific abnormality at which the treatment can be targeted. Therefore, a reasonable objective has to be negotiated with the patient prior to treatment.

4. Doctors often assume that a series of normal investigations reassures patients who are anxious about their symptoms. The opposite is actually true: in the case of endoscopy, the most anxious patients are the least reassured by a 'normal' result.

The commonest and only well-recognized functional disorders are IBS and FD; these will now be considered separately.

IRRITABLE BOWEL SYNDROME

What is irritable bowel syndrome?

IBS has no precise definition. It is generally accepted to be the combination of persistent abdominal pain or discomfort with disordered bowel habit in the absence of organic pathology. However, both more and less precise definitions are used in clinical practice. It is the diagnosis given to patients who have lower intestinal type symptoms (pain, bloating, diarrhoea, constipation) and who are found to have, or are anticipated to have, normal investigations. More precise symptom-based diagnostic criteria have been formulated beginning with Manning and colleagues who analyzed symptoms of patients with abdominal pain and disordered bowel habit who had no detectable organic disease and found six symptoms that were commoner in patients with IBS than those with organic disease (the Manning criteria) (see Box 6.1).

How common is irritable bowel syndrome?

The estimated prevalence of IBS depends on the definition used and, using three Manning criteria or the Rome criteria, population studies in the USA and UK have found a prevalence of between 3.6 and 15.5%. It is approximately twice as common in women with almost 50% having at least one IBS symptom.

What causes irritable bowel syndrome?

There does not appear to be a single cause for IBS. There is evidence that patients diagnosed in hospital with IBS have predisposing psychological factors. Symptoms appear to be precipitated by eating certain foods and there may be abnormal processing of sensory stimuli in the colon. More recent data suggest that patients with post-infective IBS and possibly others have microscopic changes in their colon (Table 6.1).

Food intolerance

Patients often report that certain foods exacerbate their symptoms. Whether this is a reaction to food content, form, smell or some other factor is very difficult to determine. Blinded challenge with blended foodstuffs passed down nasogastric tubes rarely

Table 6.1 Possible causes of irritable bowel syndrome

Cause	Evidence
Altered motility	Clustered contractions Response to smooth muscle relaxants
Altered sensation	Luminal distension thresholds Response to low-dose tricyclics
Microscopic inflammation	Mast cells in terminal ileum and colon Enteroendocrine cell hyperplasia Post-infective irritable bowel syndrome
Psychological	Life events Illness behaviour Mood disorder Response to psychological therapies
Diet	Patient complaints Response to exclusion/elimination diets Meal-induced 5-HT release

precipitates symptoms in patients who have reported intolerance. This suggests that the response is not an immunological or biochemical reaction to the constituents of the food. However, there is some consistency in the types of food that precipitate symptoms. Up to 66% of patients identify intolerances if foods are introduced sequentially following an exclusion diet. The most commonly reported food intolerances are listed in Box 6.2. The commonest, wheat, may be a response to colonic distension caused by fibre since many patients experience a worsening of symptoms with bran. Dairy product intolerance has been complicated by issues of lactose intolerance. The two are not synonymous and there is relatively poor correlation between lactase deficiency and symptoms; there is some evidence that lactase deficiency only produces symptoms when at least 250 ml of milk is

Box 6.2 Common food intolerances in irritable bowel syndrome

- Wheat
- Dairy products
- Coffee
- Potatoes
- Corn
- Onions
- Beef
- Oats
- White wine

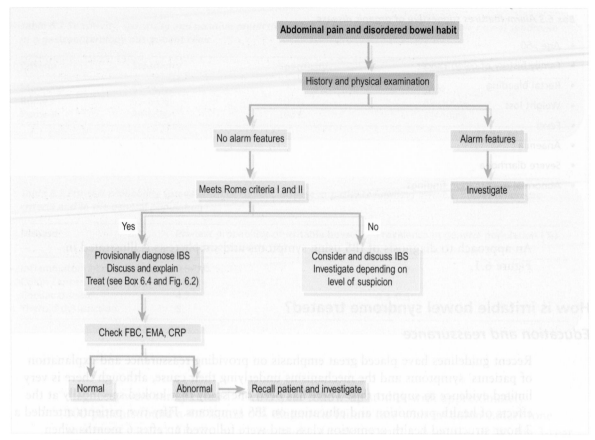

Fig. 6.1
Diagnosing irritable bowel syndrome

Box 6.4 General management of irritable bowel syndrome without specific treatment

- Give a functional explanation, avoiding the impression that it is imaginary, hysterical or psychosomatic
- Explain the facts about irritable bowel syndrome (IBS), e.g. common, distension hypersensitivity, food intolerance, precipitating life events, rarity of associated organic disease
- Consider no treatment
- Discuss simple symptomatic treatment
- Explain blood tests are to exclude rare diagnoses with similar symptoms
- Write to GP with normal results and offer to see again if alarm symptoms develop

---

symptoms in IBS (Box 6.2). If symptoms resolve, foods can be introduced one at a time to identify the precipitant. Even more restricted elimination diets can also be used with a slightly higher prospect of success.

Skin-prick testing with food allergens is not recommended. It is a test for food allergy and the non-specific nature of the results may be very confusing.

Pharmacological intervention

Almost all treatments used for IBS have no substantial evidence base to support their use. Large well-designed studies have only been carried out for the new 5-HT receptor acting agents and guidelines for the use of other agents has to be based on a multitude of small studies with variable entry criteria, control treatments and outcome measures. The variety of outcome measures, particularly for global symptom improvement, makes individual trials difficult to compare and individual drugs difficult to select for patients. It is much simpler to identify the most troublesome symptoms and attempt to treat these.

Smooth muscle relaxants

Meta-analysis of 26 double-blind trials found a significant benefit for this class of drugs over placebo, with improvement in 64% compared with 45% on placebo. Benefit was shown both for pain and global symptom score. Individual benefit could not be shown for all drugs and the best results were seen with those with an anticholinergic action, but this could have been a feature of the size and number of studies involved. Peppermint oil, which probably acts via relaxation of smooth muscle, has not consistently been shown to benefit patients with IBS.

Bulking agents

Simple advice on increasing fibre in the diet has not been specifically studied, even in patients with constipated IBS. Wheat fibre supplements do increase stool weight and decrease whole gut transit times, but drop-out rates in the trials were high and many patients experience worsening of their symptoms. Proprietary soluble fibre supplements, such as isphagula husk, increase stool frequency with less adverse events being reported.

Antidiarrhoeal therapy

Opioid receptor acting drugs have been studied in IBS. The peripherally acting agent loperamide reduced stool frequency and urgency in two trials at doses of between 4 and 12 mg daily. Codeine had a similar effect in a single study.

Tricyclic antidepressant drugs

Tricyclic antidepressant drugs and the newer 5-HT reuptake inhibitors both have effects on gut transit at doses that are below those used for depression. One large study with 50 mg trimipramine significantly reduced pain in IBS, but the power of the study was reduced by multiple treatment arms with different dosing intervals. Nocturnal dosing had the best results. Other studies with 50–150 mg have reported benefit with desipramine and amitryptiline. Constipation is the commonest side effect. A starting dose of 50 mg at night possibly increasing to 150 mg is appropriate. Drugs with significant antimuscarinic effects such as amitryptiline should be avoided in constipated patients, but perhaps specifically selected in those with diarrhoea.

Bile salt sequestering agents

IBS with normal bile salt retention does not have a significant response to colestyramine. Patients diagnosed with IBS who are found to have severe bile salt malabsorption do

147

respond, but, arguably, they do not have IBS and some turn out to have inflammatory bowel disease. Colestyramine is unpalatable to some patients and many prefer using other anti-diarrhoeal agents even when bile salt malabsorption is well documented.

5HT-receptor acting drugs

An important study showed that alosetron, a 5-HT 3 antagonist improved faecal urgency, diarrhoea and abdominal pain in women with diarrhoea-predominant IBS. The effect was small, but lasted throughout the treatment phase with symptoms recurring on withdrawal of the drug. Unfortunately, upon general release of the drug in the USA, several patients developed severe constipation and ischaemic colitis and a number died. This may have been because the indications for use of the drug when it was generally released were much broader than the strict entry criteria in the relevant studies. The drug has now been reintroduced at low dose (1 mg daily) on a limited-use programme for women with refractory symptoms. Similar studies with 5-HT 4 agonists have shown benefits in patients with constipation-predominant IBS. Tegaserod, a partial 5-HT 4 agonist, accelerated orocaecal transit times in IBS and several studies have shown an improvement in constipation, abdominal pain and bloating in women with IBS. Again the effect is small but significant.

It is impossible to know whether these sophisticated drugs are achieving results because of careful targeting of receptors important in the pathogenesis of IBS or they are acting simply as anti-diarrhoeal agents or laxatives in appropriately chosen patients. No comparison has been made with conventional anti-diarrhoeal drugs or laxatives and the question remains unanswered.

Psychological therapies

These can really only be considered in a small minority of patients, since they require considerable use of resources from specialized services across more than one specialty. However, there are a number of trials showing benefit for many forms of psychological therapies. The main criticism of trial design is always the adequacy of the control treatment. It is very difficult to control for psychological therapies without both unblinding the study and using a degree of less specific psychological treatment in the control group.

The most interesting findings are with hypnotherapy. Both individual and group hypnotherapy have been shown to have significant benefit for patients with IBS compared with patients receiving similar amounts of physician contact without hypnosis. In the largest study to date, 71% of patients initially responded to therapy. Of these, 81% maintained their improvement during the 6-year study period with the majority of the remaining only having a slight deterioration of symptoms. It appears to have long-lasting effects and be more successful with younger patients and those without serious psychopathology. There is recent evidence that this might be mediated through normalization of rectal distension pain thresholds.

Small studies have also shown benefit with relaxation therapy, biofeedback, cognitive behavioural therapy and dynamic psychotherapy, but their lack of adequate control groups and the tiny numbers involved make interpreting the results very difficult.

Probiotics

General interest in probiotics, increased prevalence of *Clostridium difficile* infections and the findings of evidence of abnormal colonic fermentation in patients with IBS has precipitated interest and a few small trials with probiotics. One study of 12 patients found no benefit with Lactobacillus plantarum 299v. Another slightly larger study found significant reduction of abdominal pain with 4 weeks treatment. A randomized-controlled trial with 60 patients using Lactobacillus plantarum (DSM 9843) for 4 weeks reduced abdominal pain and flatulence at 1 year.

Other treatments

Chinese herbal remedies used in one well-designed study showed benefit for patients with IBS compared with placebo. Benefit was only maintained in those with an individualized therapy and the results have not been repeated since. Care was taken to monitor liver enzymes and no adverse events were detected over the 8-week treatment period.

Summary

IBS is a common disorder that can be diagnosed without the use of extensive investigation in young patients without alarm symptoms. Explanation of diagnosis and likely precipitants with simple advice about diet may be the only treatment required. Pharmacological therapy is of limited efficacy, but can be targeted at specific symptoms. New 5-HT receptor acting drugs have a significant benefit over placebo for women with IBS, but whether the effect is any greater than with older therapies is unproven. A summary of management is shown in Figure 6.2.

FUNCTIONAL DYSPEPSIA

What is functional dyspepsia?

Peptic ulcers, particularly duodenal, are becoming less common whereas other acid-related disorders such as gastro-oesophageal reflux are becoming more common. Most patients with symptoms suggestive of these classic peptic disorders have no demonstrable organic disease. To be more positive about this increasingly common disorder and to relate it to other similar disorders, the term FD was created. Dyspepsia accounts for 3–4% of consultations in general practice and is largely responsible for the 19 million prescriptions per annum for acid-lowering drugs in England.

In recognition of the similarity of symptoms with those associated with organic disease, attempts have been made to sub-classify FD. Patients with predominant heartburn are said to have reflux-like dyspepsia, predominant epigastric pain ulcer-like dyspepsia and predominant bloating and early satiety dysmotility-like dyspepsia. There is some evidence that such classifications are useful in predicting those that might respond to treatment.

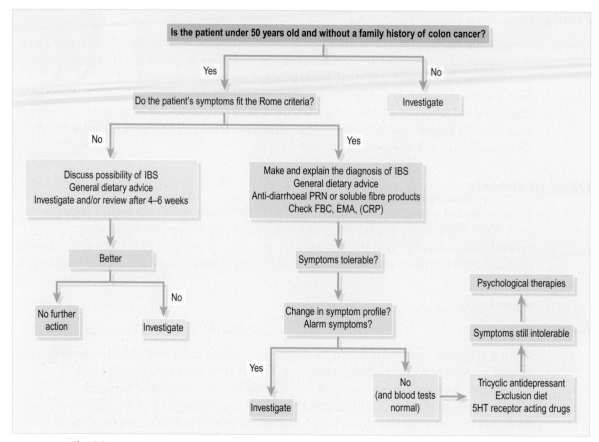

Fig. 6.2
Summary of management for irritable bowel syndrome

Two large trials with omeprazole showed benefit for proton pump inhibitors only in patients with reflux- and ulcer-like dyspepsia.

However, symptom profiles are not static and half of patients have symptoms that overlap more than one category and half change their symptom profile over a 1-year period.

How common is functional dyspepsia?

Population surveys in the UK suggest a prevalence of all dyspepsia of 38–40%, one in four patients consulting their GP and one in five of those consulting having an endoscopy or barium study. A similar USA study found 26% with dyspepsia plus 41.6% with oesophageal symptoms. A Scandinavian survey suggested that within 1 year, 34 people out of 1000 would seek medical advice in general practice with a new episode of dyspepsia and four of them would have alarm symptoms. However, most of them, 55% in one survey, would have FD.

What causes functional dyspepsia?

Psychological influences

Like other functional disorders, there is a higher incidence of psychological morbidity in patients with FD compared with asymptomatic controls and a higher incidence of adverse life events preceding symptoms. There is evidence for centrally mediated motor and sensory effects. Central inhibition of vagal tone causes impaired fundal relaxation and antral motility, altered gastroduodenal motility and gastric stasis in some patients, whereas anxiety enhances visceral sensitivity.

Evidence for these effects comes from studies carried out with hospital out patients who actually have the same levels of psychological disturbance as patients with organic disease, suggesting that psychological morbidity is a feature of hospital consultation rather than FD itself. Whole-population studies have suggested that it is the reporting of and consultation for symptoms that is driven by psychological factors rather than the symptoms themselves.

Disordered motility

Early research on the causes of FD focused on motility because of the huge interest in possible motility disturbances in IBS. Up to 50% of patients with non-ulcer dyspepsia (NUD) were found to have delayed gastric emptying, but this correlated poorly with symptoms and rectification with drugs did not necessarily improve symptoms. More sophisticated scintigraphic studies suggested that there was a gastric accommodation disorder with the fundus failing to relax to accommodate a meal, thus causing the antrum to become abnormally distended. Further studies suggested that this was due to a failure of reflex relaxation of the fundus in response to duodenal distension. This anomaly could potentially be enhanced by acid entering the duodenum and impairing its emptying. Abnormal duodenal emptying might exacerbate duodeno-gastric reflux, which is associated with many dyspeptic conditions, including gastric ulceration, alcoholic gastritis and gallstones. Bile acids disrupt the gastric mucosal barrier exposing it to luminal acid.

Distension hypersensitivity

The last 20 years has seen a change in emphasis from disordered motility to disordered sensitivity. Studying visceral sensitivity in functional GI disorders relies on using a reliable stimulus that can distinguish between normal sensation and hypersensitivity. Early experiments used luminal distension as a stimulus. This was partly because luminal distension was easy to perform, but also because organic disorders and experimental interventions associated with distension such as obstruction were known to be painful.

The first studies were carried out in the colon over 25 years ago and have been adapted to study upper gastrointestinal sensation. Most showed lowered pain/discomfort thresholds, lack of site specificity for visceral hypersensitivity, poor localization of symptoms and poor sensory discrimination.

151

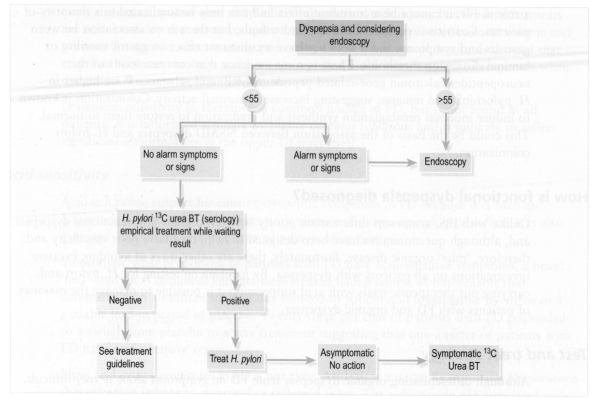

Fig. 6.3
Test and treat strategy for managing dyspepsia. Adapted with permission from British Society of Gastroenterology guidelines

functional disorders. Those trials with H2 antagonists found placebo responses varying from 25% to 62%. Most of these showed a small benefit for H2 antagonists over placebo, but many showed no benefit. Two comparator trials with proton pump inhibitors suggested superiority over H2 antagonists for uninvestigated dyspepsia and a subsequent trial in FD suggested benefit for lansoprazole over ranitidine. A small study with omeprazole showed a modest benefit over placebo (32% vs 14%).

Recently two large trials with omeprazole at doses of 20 and 10 mg found small benefits over placebo (38.2% and 36% versus 28.2%). Use of the Rome sub-classifications found the greatest benefit for patients with reflux-like dyspepsia, 54% with 20 mg ($P = 0.05$) and 45% with 10 mg ($P = 0.05$) compared with 23% with placebo. Patients with ulcer-like dyspepsia also benefited, 40% with 20 mg ($P = 0.05$) and 35% with 10 mg ($P = 0.08$) compared with 27% with placebo. Those with dysmotility-like dyspepsia did not benefit.

Helicobacter pylori *eradication*

If *H. pylori* causes some FD the most pertinent issue is whether *H. pylori* eradication improves symptoms. This assumes that any effect of *H. pylori* is reversible, which may not be the case given the chronicity of infection prior to detection and eradication. Many studies of *H. pylori* eradication have been published. Most were criticized for being too small, with insufficient follow-up using insensitive outcome measures until two studies were published in the same issue of *The New England Journal of Medicine*. They were much larger than previous studies, with 1 year's follow-up using previously validated scoring systems to assess outcome.

Both groups studied hospital patients only. McColl's group used relatively lax entry criteria accepting most patients presenting with symptoms referable to the upper GI tract. Using the strict primary outcome of complete resolution of symptoms, they found significant benefit for eradication therapy. Despite this, the average symptom score did not fall significantly more than with placebo. This may have been because the study was not powerful enough to show a significant difference or that only a subgroup responded. In particular, it is possible that the study group was enriched with 'missed' ulcer patients, since there was a high prevalence of peptic ulceration in symptomatic placebo patients who were subsequently re-endoscoped (four of six), which would tend to exaggerate the benefits of eradication. More recent data showing that 12.6% of *H. pylori* infected FD patients develop ulcers over a 2-year period support this interpretation.

Blum et al. had stricter entry criteria, recruiting only those with upper abdominal pain and discomfort. Despite this, they showed no significant benefit compared to placebo, either using the strict primary-outcome measure of complete resolution of symptoms, or reduction in average symptom score. They were more rigorous in excluding peptic ulceration (which was found in 3%) by re-endoscoping all patients at 3 and 12 months.

One explanation of the difference in outcome of the two studies was the poor placebo response in McColl's study (7%). This was uncharacteristically low for studies of functional disease, but may be explained by the longer follow-up or the more exacting definition of treatment success. Alternatively, blinding may have been compromised by the use of metronidazole, which frequently causes side effects.

McColl's study supported the hypothesis that some patients with FD achieve long-term benefit from *H. pylori* eradication, although these patients may have actually been 'ulcer' patients with no, minimal or simply missed findings at initial endoscopy. Both studies showed that most patients did not benefit and indeed some may have deteriorated.

The contradictory results of these studies may partly have reflected the difference in study populations and to overcome this problem two meta-analyses have been carried out. Again, the results are contradictory. The first found a small benefit over placebo in contrast to the second, which found none. Laines's analysis, which found no benefit, omitted four studies used in the previous analysis and included five not previously included. In particular, it excluded the largest study to date. This study had only been published in abstract form at the time, but was probably excluded through failing to provide an adequate definition of treatment success. However, it strongly influenced the outcome of the earlier meta-analysis and explains the main difference in outcome.

With no uniformly agreed disease definition, outcome measure, nor trial duration and with innumerable possible treatment regimens, it is not surprising that different meta-

McColl K, Murray L, El-Omar E et al. Symptomatic benefit from eradicating Helicobacter pylori infection in patients with nonulcer dyspepsia. N Engl J Med 1998; 339: 1869–74.

Moayyedi P, Soo S, Deeks J, et al. Systematic review and economic evaluation of Helicobacter pylori eradication treatment for non-ulcer dyspepsia. Dyspepsia Review Group. BMJ 2000; 321: 659–64.

Talley NJ, Silverstein MD, Agréus L, Nyrén O, Sonnenberg A, Holtmann G. AGA technical review: evaluation of dyspepsia. Gastroenterology 1998; 114(3): 582–95.

Thompson WG, Longstreth GF, Drossman DA, Heaton KW, Irvine EJ, Muller-Lissner SA. Functional bowel disorders and functional abdominal pain. Gut 1999; 45(Suppl 2): II43–7.

Gastrointestinal bleeding: acute and chronic

7

INTRODUCTION

Gastrointestinal (GI) bleeding accounts for about 8–10% of acute hospital admissions and is the commonest emergency managed by gastroenterologists in the UK. The majority of these admissions are due to acute upper-GI bleeding. The incidence varies from 50 to 150 per 100 000 population with an average of about 100 per 100 000 population per year, the incidence being highest in low socio-economic groups. Thus, an average-sized district general hospital serving a population of 300 000 can expect about 300 admissions per year related to GI bleeding. A UK audit published in 1995 reported 11% mortality in patients admitted to hospital because of bleeding and 33% mortality in those who developed GI bleeding while hospitalized for other reasons. However, in the absence of malignancy or organ failure, the National Audit reports a mortality in those aged less than 60 years of only 1.3%. This is because most deaths occur in elderly patients with other significant co-morbidities. The steep increase in mortality with advancing age and co-morbidity is compounded by the ingestion of non-steroidal anti-inflammatory drugs (NSAIDs) and the use of aspirin for cardiovascular co-morbidities. It is likely that one-third of all patients over the age of 60 years admitted with GI bleeding will have taken one of these preparations. Furthermore, it is recognized that the prevalence of *H. pylori* infection, which is now a well-recognized cause of peptic ulcer disease, increases with age. Aspirin doubles the risk of bleeding, even at doses as low as 75 mg daily. The use of NSAIDs increases the risk of ulcer complications by a factor of four. A history of upper GI bleeding is a significant risk factor for recurrent bleeding in those taking aspirin or other NSAIDs.

ACUTE GASTROINTESTINAL BLEEDING

Initial evaluation

Patients admitted with acute GI bleeding should ideally be the responsibility of a medical and a surgical gastroenterologist with joint care between the two teams. It is essential to admit these patients into a ward where adequately trained nurses and junior doctors are available 24 h. Some hospitals have set up special 'GI Bleed Units' to facilitate this process. It is essential to categorize patients at the time of admission into high or low risk of death. Rockall and colleagues defined independent risk factors (Table 7.1) that were subsequently shown to accurately predict death. This scoring system can be completed only after endoscopic findings are included, hence an early endoscopy (within 24–48 h) is essential. A pre-endoscopy Rockall score can be calculated, although its utility is not well established. In practice the definition of mild, moderate and severe risk, remains a matter of clinical judgement taking into account: age, co-morbidity and the severity of the bleeding episode. Blood samples should be taken and sent to the laboratory immediately for urgent measurement of full blood count, urea, creatinine, electrolytes, clotting profile, blood group and cross match. External examination, particularly to look for signs of chronic liver disease, is essential and will help in the overall management of the patient. The initial evaluation should focus on haemodynamic status.

Once the patient is reasonably stable a good history should be taken including previous admissions with GI bleed, abdominal surgery, alcohol use, bleeding disorders, liver disease and warfarin, NSAID or aspirin use.

Resuscitation

Intravenous access should be obtained with a wide bore (18G green; or even the wider bore 16G grey) cannula inserted in a forearm vein. In cases of haemodynamic compromise, volume replacement with normal saline should be started while awaiting blood transfusion. Given the lack of evidence in favour of colloids, crystalloids such as 0.9% sodium chloride (normal saline) are the convenient and inexpensive choice for fluid resuscitation. If the haemoglobin concentration is less than 10 g/dl in a haemodynamically compromised patient, it is sensible to start blood transfusion, as the haemoglobin will continue to drop with fluid resuscitation. The requirements for blood transfusion should be guided by the severity of blood loss and haemodynamic status.

Table 7.1 Rockall scoring system for risk of re-bleeding and death after admission to hospital for acute gastrointestinal bleeding

Variable	Score			
	0	1	2	3
Age (years)	<60	60–79	>80	
Systolic blood pressure (mm Hg)	>100	>100	<100	
Pulse (beats/min)	<100	>100		
Comorbidity	Nil major		Cardiac failure, IHD, other major comorbidity	Renal failure, liver failure, disseminated malignancy
Diagnosis	Mallory Weiss tear, no lesion, and no SRH	All other diagnoses		
Major SRH	None or dark spot			

Each variable is scored and the total score calculated by simple addition (maximum 11). SRH, stigmata of recent haemorrhage; IHD, ischaemic heart disease

Co-morbidity

Patients with known cardiac failure should be carefully monitored to avoid excessive fluid overload due to over-aggressive fluid resuscitation. Critically ill patients with cardiovascular, respiratory, renal and other co-morbidities will require central venous pressure and hourly urine output monitored and should be cared for in a high-dependency unit or, when intubation and respiratory support is needed, in the intensive care unit. Adequately resuscitated patients have a urine output of >30 ml/h and a central venous pressure of 5–10 cm H_2O with systolic pressure >100 mmHg.

Cirrhosis

Patients with cirrhosis are at high risk of infection following a GI bleed from any source and this may lead to septicaemia and spontaneous bacterial peritonitis. A broad-spectrum antibiotic such as ciprofloxacin (500 mg bd orally; or 200–400 mg bd by intravenous infusion over 30 min only if unable to take orally) should be given. This has been shown to increase survival and reduce infection.

Clotting abnormalities

Clotting abnormalities, especially in liver disease patients, should be treated with vitamin K1, 10 mg given slowly intravenously. Fresh frozen plasma (15 ml/kg body weight) should be considered if the prothrombin time is very prolonged (e.g. >7 s; INR >1.5).

Patients on warfarin

For patients on warfarin, it is important to determine the indication for anticoagulation. In patients with high risk of thromboembolism (e.g. those with mechanical prosthetic valve, recurrent thromboembolic events and atrial fibrillation with valvular heart disease) it is preferable to treat clotting abnormalities with fresh frozen plasma and/or a small dose of intravenous vitamin K1 (e.g. 0.5 mg). The aim is to normalize clotting temporarily pending endoscopic intervention and until the bleeding stops. The minimal anticoagulation required, weighing the risks and benefits of withholding anticoagulation, must also be considered. It is difficult to re-anticoagulate these patients when gastrointestinal bleeding stops if high doses of vitamin K1 are used.

In all other patients, warfarin can be withheld safely and clotting abnormality corrected with vitamin K1, 5 mg given slowly intravenously (and fresh frozen plasma if necessary). It is also important to review the need for long-term anticoagulation in these patients.

For patients over anticoagulated with warfarin (e.g. INR > 4) with major bleeding, administration of vitamin K1 is inadequate because its full effect is not seen for 12–24 h. The volume of fresh frozen plasma needed may be too large to be given safely. In this situation prothrombin-complex concentrates are indicated and should be discussed with the haematologist.

ACUTE UPPER GASTROINTESTINAL BLEEDING

This is arbitrarily defined as GI bleeding from a source proximal to the duodeno-jejunal junction. The presentation may be with haematemesis and/or melaena. The blood urea nitrogen is usually elevated (within 24 h) due to a sudden increase in the haemoglobin degradation and increased protein load to the gut. This may be normal in cirrhotic patients who may have subnormal urea levels to start with.

The causes are shown in Box 7.1. Peptic ulceration remains the single most common cause of upper GI bleeding in the UK and in the majority of countries in the world. It accounts for up to 60% of all episodes of upper GI bleeding. Most peptic ulcers are caused by *H. pylori* infection or NSAIDs. Variceal haemorrhage occurs in patients with portal hypertension, usually secondary to cirrhosis. A rise in the portal venous pressure of >12 mmHg results in the development of oesophageal and, less commonly, gastric varices, as well as in the other sites of portal systemic anastomoses. The two most important factors that determine the risk of variceal haemorrhage in cirrhotic patients are the severity of liver disease and the size of varices. Approximately 80% of patients with upper GI bleeding will stop bleeding spontaneously. In the remaining 20%, endoscopic intervention plays a pivotal role in stopping the bleed and also in preventing re-bleeds.

Role of endoscopy

Upper GI endoscopy is useful to:

- define the cause of bleeding, e.g. it is important to identify patients with varices, bleeding peptic ulcers, vascular lesions, cancer and other rarer causes

---

Box 7.1 Causes of upper gastrointestinal bleeding

- Peptic ulcer disease
- Oesophageal/gastric/duodenal varices
- Haemorrhagic gastritis
- Oesophagitis
- Mallory Weiss tear
- Upper gastrointestinal tumours
- Portal hypertensive gastropathy
- Gastric Antral Vascular Ectasia (GAVE or water melon stomach)
- Cameron ulcer within hiatus hernia
- Dieulafoy's lesion
- Corrosive ingestion, e.g. suicidal attempt with bleach ingestion
- Iatrogenic – post-endoscopic retrograde cholangiopancreatography sphincterotomy
- Haemobilia.

- assess risk of further bleeding. Endoscopic findings are crucial in assessing the risk of further haemorrhage and in the triage of the patients either for high-dependency care or for early discharge
- administer endoscopic treatment in the select group of patients who will benefit from endoscopic haemostasis.

Management of non-variceal upper gastrointestinal bleed

When an upper GI bleeding source is suspected, the test of choice for identifying and treating the bleeding lesion is endoscopy. There is no role for barium studies in the evaluation of acute upper GI bleeding. The timing of endoscopy remains a subject of debate, particularly for the patient who responds rapidly to volume resuscitation and has no further evidence of bleeding. While it may seem obvious that endoscopy would improve care, randomized trials indicate that diagnostic endoscopy does not improve mortality, re-bleeding rates, the need for surgery or length of hospital stay. The majority of patients (75–80%) stop bleeding spontaneously, limiting the impact of early diagnosis. Based on these data, patients are often initially admitted to hospital and have endoscopy performed electively within 24–48 h. The remaining 20–25% of patients with continuing or recurrent bleeding will benefit from urgent endoscopy after being adequately resuscitated. In this situation endoscopy can improve mortality and morbidity. Endoscopic therapy (with thermal coagulation and/or adrenaline injection of the lesion) is effective in the setting of actively bleeding ulcers and ulcers with a visible vessel in the base. Bleeding can be controlled in 85–90% of patients, with less than a 3% complication rate and significant decrease in re-bleeding and need for surgery. Mortality is decreased by about one-third. Endoscopic appearance of the ulcer is the best predictor of re-bleeding in peptic ulcer disease. The modified Forrest criteria, originally devised in Edinburgh, is widely used (Box 7.2). Laine and Peterson have reviewed the literature and have summarized the risk of re-bleeding and mortality according to endoscopic criteria (Table 7.2).

Bleeding ulcers

When an ulcer is found on endoscopy, it is essential to document its exact location, size and stigmata of recent bleeding (Box 7.2). Patients with major stigmata (i.e. active

---

Box 7.2 Modified Forrest classification for peptic ulcer haemorrhage

Class I: Actively bleeding ulcer
- I a spurting
- I b oozing

Class II: Non-actively bleeding ulcer
- II a non-bleeding visible vessel
- II b ulcer with surface clot
- II c ulcer with red or dark blue spots

Class III: Ulcer with clean base

Table 7.2 Risk of re-bleeding and mortality by endoscopic appearance of ulcer

Endoscopic finding (Forrest class)	Risk of re-bleeding	Mortality
Active bleeding (I a,b)	55%	11%
Visible vessel (II a)	43%	11%
Adherent clot (II b)	22%	7%
Flat spot (II c)	10%	3%
Clean base (III)	5%	2%

bleeding whether it be spurting or oozing blood from the ulcer, a non-bleeding visible vessel, or an adherent blood clot) should receive endoscopic therapy. In the case of an adherent blood clot, vigorous washing may dislodge it to reveal a vessel, which can then be treated.

Endoscopic therapies

Endoscopic therapies for ulcer bleeding are outlined below.

Injection   Adrenaline 1:10 000 injected with a disposable needle (variceal injection needle) produces blanching within a few seconds and stops bleeding in up to 95% of acutely bleeding ulcers (Fig. 7.1). About 5–15 ml is injected around the ulcer and then into the bleeding vessel. The volume depends on the ulcer size. Too little may not produce haemostasis (<5 ml) and too much (>15 ml) can get systemically absorbed and cause haemodynamic disturbance. Injection of sclerosants and alcohol does not produce any added benefit and can, in fact, cause complications such as necrosis and perforation. Other agents which stimulate clot formation (e.g. fibrin glue and thrombin) have been shown to achieve haemostasis. However, they are more expensive and not readily available.

Coagulation   Heater Probe (HP; Olympus, Japan) and Bipolar Coagulation Probe (BICAP; Gold Probe, Boston Scientific, Natick, MA, USA) produce thermal haemostasis

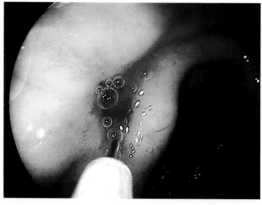

Fig. 7.1
Injection of adrenaline to control bleeding from a duodenal ulcer

as well as tamponade and mechanical compression (coaptive coagulation) of the bleeding vessel. The HP is applied as 5–6 s pulses of 30 joules each per tamponade station and acts as a heated coil of metal while the BICAP, with long pulses (7–10 s) at low power settings, 15–20 Watts, acts as a monopolar diathermy. In addition, HP has a water jet facility useful to wash the ulcer for better visibility and also aids in removing the clot. Argon plasma coagulation (APC) has been recently introduced as another mode of thermal haemostasis. It is delivered through a catheter probe inserted via the instrument channel of the endoscope and placed close to the mucosa (about 2–3 mm). When activated with a foot pedal it produces a flow of ionized argon gas, which coagulates the bleeding vessel and surrounding oozing tissue. It is a non-touch technique and care should be taken not to touch the mucosa wherein it can act like a monopolar diathermy and cause perforation. The disadvantages in using the APC are that mechanical compression of the bleeding vessel cannot be achieved and it may not be effective when there is a spurting vessel with plenty of blood, since the argon plasma is not really effectively formed in liquid medium. However, clinical studies using APC have shown results comparable to other thermal haemostasis modalities. It is best to use APC at power setting of 40–60 W, at 1-s pulses with gas flow rate of 0.8–1 l/min to coagulate the ulcer base and blood vessel after initial haemostasis is achieved with adrenaline injection (Fig. 7.2).

Mechanical closure   Endoclips have been introduced recently for endoscopic closure of minor perforations and also to clamp bleeding vessels during endoscopy (Fig. 7.3). They can be used to mechanically close the bleeding vessel and clinical trials have shown encouraging results. The original model was cumbersome to load the clip and deploy and hence was not popular. However, recently the disposable clips (QuickClip®, Olympus Japan) have been found easier to use. They are particularly useful when an active bleeding vessel or a non-bleeding visible vessel is seen. However, they may not be useful in chronic ulcers, which may have a fibrosed base, or with ulcers in awkward positions, which may be technically difficult to clip.

Combination therapy   The combination of adrenaline injection and thermal haemostasis has been shown to achieve better haemostasis and reduce re-bleeding rates quite significantly

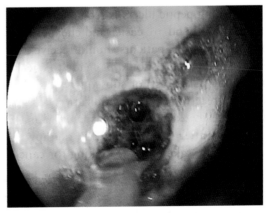

Fig. 7.2
Argon plasma coagulation applied to treat a duodenal ulcer following adrenaline injection

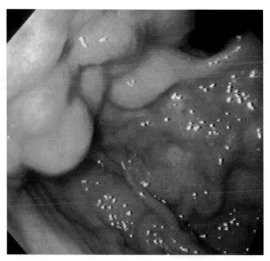

Fig. 7.7
Fundal gastric varices appearing like a bunch of grapes

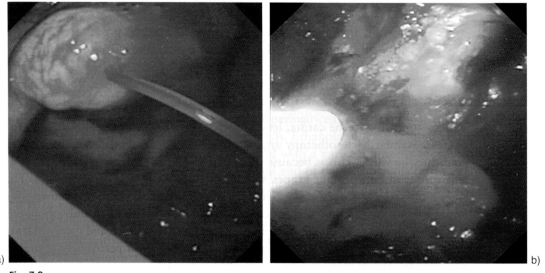

a)

b)

Fig. 7.8
Gastric varices, (a) actively bleeding, (b) histoacryl glue injection done with instantaneous haemostasis

but with less cardiovascular side effects, is as good as the combination of vasopressin and nitroglycerine and is the preferred drug therapy. It has been compared with somatostatin and balloon tamponade and found to be equally effective. Terlipressin is given in a dose of 1–2 mg intravenously, 6 hourly for 72 h during the acute episode. Somatostatin and its synthetic analogue octreotide, given intravenously cause selective splanchnic vasoconstriction with minimal side effects and reduce portal pressure and portal blood flow. The results of clinical trials have reported conflicting reports. It has not been consistently shown to be superior to vasopressin, terlipressin or balloon tamponade

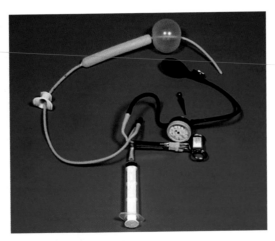

Fig. 7.9
Sengstaken tube. Courtesy of Dr David Patch

in reducing the failure to control bleeding. Although it is half as expensive as terlipressin, octreotide should probably only be used in patients with significant cardiovascular co-morbidity, which may preclude terlipressin use.

Balloon tamponade (Sengstaken tube) in acute variceal bleed

This form of treatment is highly effective and controls acute bleeding in up to 90% of patients, although about 50% re-bleed when the balloon is deflated. The Sengstaken tube has two balloons (gastric and oesophageal) with two aspiration ports oesophageal and gastric (Fig. 7.9). Inflating the gastric balloon alone with 200–300 ml air and with traction against the gastro-oesophageal junction will control the majority of the bleeds with minimal risk of oesophageal ulceration. However, in difficult cases with persistent oesophageal variceal bleed the oesophageal balloon needs to be inflated as well, to a pressure of 20–30 mmHg to control bleeding. The oesophageal balloon should be deflated and reinflated every 12 h to prevent oesophageal necrosis. The Sengstaken tube is associated with serious complications such as oesophageal necrosis, ulceration and aspiration pneumonia in up to 15–20% of patients. It is best to protect the airway by tracheal intubation and manage the patient in an intensive therapy unit. It may be life saving treatment in cases of uncontrolled bleeding, pending other forms of treatment or transfer to a specialist liver unit.

Transjugular intrahepatic porto-systemic shunt

This radiological intervention creates an intrahepatic shunt by placing a stent connecting the hepatic and portal veins (Fig. 7.10). Transjugular intrahepatic porto-systemic shunt (TIPS) is now widely used as rescue therapy in patients unresponsive to endoscopic management especially from bleeding gastric varices. Failure of endoscopic therapy has been defined as 'further variceal bleeding after two endoscopic treatments during a single hospital admission for an acute bleeding episode'. Used in this situation TIPS leads to immediate cessation of bleeding in up to 90% of cases.

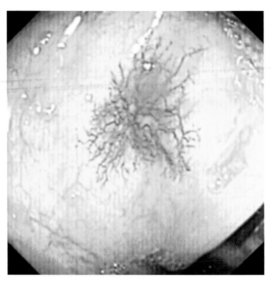

Fig. 7.15
Angiodysplasia of the caecum. Reproduced from GastroHep.com, courtesy of Blackwell's

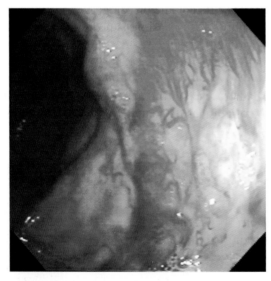

Fig. 7.16
Portal colopathy in a patient with idiopathic portal vein thrombosis

bowel. It is important to be extremely cautious, especially when treating lesions in the right colon with thermal coagulation, since the bowel wall is only about 2–3 mm thick and can very easily perforate. In general, the power settings for thermal coagulation methods should be approximately 50% lower than normal. Colonic tumours rarely present with severe bleeding. Endoscopic therapy with any of the above-mentioned thermal modalities or laser can control the bleeding.

Patients with massive rectal bleeding may require emergency mesenteric angiography to localize and control the bleeding site by coil embolization or gel foam embolization. Laparotomy, with or without on-table colonoscopy, would be the last choice if the patient continues to bleed without an identifiable source. There should be a low threshold to perform an upper GI endoscopy in patients presenting with acute rectal bleeding, especially when the proctoscopy or rigid sigmoidoscopy does not reveal any anorectal cause. Twenty five per cent of the patients will have an upper GI cause that can be easily identified and treated by an upper GI endoscopy.

CHRONIC GASTROINTESTINAL BLEEDING

Iron-deficiency anaemia

Iron-deficiency anaemia (IDA) is the most common presenting feature of chronic occult GI blood loss. It occurs in 2–5% of adult men and post-menopausal women in the developed world. While menstrual blood loss is the commonest cause in pre-menopausal women, blood loss from the gut is the commonest cause in adult men and post-menopausal women. IDA can also result from malabsorption secondary to coeliac disease, previous partial or total gastrectomy, bacterial overgrowth, Whipple's disease, lymphangiectasia and other rare malabsorptive conditions.

Definition

The diagnostic criteria for anaemia in IDA have varied in clinical studies ranging from Hb <10 to 11.5 g/dl for women and <12.5 to 13.8 g/dl for men. The lower limit of the normal range of haemoglobin concentration for the laboratory performing the test should, therefore, probably be used to define anaemia. Microcytosis (mean corpuscular volume (MCV) lower than the normal range) is characteristic of iron deficiency, but it may also occur in less common conditions such as thalassaemia, other haemoglobinopathies and in anaemia of chronic disease. Microcytosis may be absent in combined deficiency (e.g. iron and folate/B12 deficiency) that may be recognized by a raised red-cell distribution width (RDW). Serum ferritin concentration is the most powerful test to detect iron deficiency. A serum ferritin concentration of <12 mg/l is diagnostic of iron deficiency. In doubtful cases (e.g. anaemia of chronic disease) bone-marrow examination will confirm the diagnosis.

Evaluation and investigations

The diagnostic algorithm in these patients is debatable and often more challenging than in the acute bleed. History taking should include diet, menstruation and drug history including anticoagulation, aspirin and NSAIDs. Family history of haematological disorders (e.g. thalassaemia, sideroblastic anaemia), telangiectasia and bleeding disorders should be sought. Careful clinical examination to look for cutaneous signs (e.g. Osler–Weber–Rendu and Peutz–Jeghers syndromes) is important in addition to an abdominal and rectal examination. Whether to start with upper GI investigation or lower

GI investigation is a matter of clinical judgement and can be aided by patient's symptoms of dyspepsia or altered bowel habit. However, in elderly patients with more than one symptom this is not always true and can be misleading. The British Society of Gastroenterology has published guidelines that suggest running both upper and lower gastrointestinal investigations concurrently, or sequentially should the first prove normal. Upper gastrointestinal endoscopy reveals a cause in 30–50% of cases of IDA, although in the elderly lower gastrointestinal investigations are more likely to be diagnostically productive. Small-bowel biopsies from the second or third part of duodenum should be taken when performing endoscopy (unless the patient has a negative EMA test) as 4–6% of patients presenting with IDA have coeliac disease. With the exception of those diagnosed with gastric carcinoma or coeliac disease at upper endoscopy, all should go on to have a colonoscopy or double contrast barium enema (DCBE), since dual pathology occurs in 10–15% of patients. Flexible sigmoidoscopy is often done in addition to DCBE since small lesions may be missed in the sigmoid colon especially in the presence of diverticular disease and/or overlapping sigmoid loops. Omission of flexible sigmoidoscopy appears safe if digital examination is negative in the absence of rectal bleeding or change in bowel habit. If the IDA is transfusion dependent, small-bowel investigations including capsule endoscopy, enteroscopy and mesenteric angiography should be considered. Red-cell scanning is not useful in chronic occult bleeding. Diagnostic laparotomy and on-table enteroscopy may be considered in cases that have defied all other investigations and continue to require blood transfusions. Vascular lesions are the most common cause of occult small-bowel bleeding in the elderly and neoplasms account for the majority in younger patients. Small-bowel barium study is rarely of help unless abdominal symptoms are present. When the patient presents with abdominal pain, diarrhoea or intestinal obstruction, barium small bowel follow through will be useful to look for structural abnormalities (jejunal diverticulosis, neoplasm, Crohn's disease, intestinal tuberculosis etc.) in the small bowel. Meckel's diverticulum sometimes presents with occult blood loss and IDA. Diagnostic laparotomy is the most sensitive test whilst a technetium isotope scan may help in the diagnosis pre-operatively.

Management

If gastroscopy, small-bowel biopsy and colonoscopy are normal, iron replacement is recommended, with 3-monthly follow-up haemoglobin monitoring for 1 year and again at 2 years; additional replacement should be given as necessary if the mean corpuscular volume or haemoglobin falls below normal. Reassuringly, IDA does not return in most patients treated this way. Treatment of an underlying cause should prevent further iron loss, but all patients should have iron supplementation both to correct and replenish body iron stores. This is achieved simply with oral iron such as ferrous sulphate at a dose of 200 mg twice daily. Ascorbic acid enhances iron absorption and can be co-prescribed when response is poor. Parenteral iron should only be used when there is intolerance to oral preparations or in case of non-compliance. The haemoglobin concentration should rise by 2 g/dl after 3–4 weeks' treatment. Failure to do so is usually due to poor compliance, continued blood loss, malabsorption or misdiagnosis. Iron supplementation should be continued for 3 months after correction of anaemia to replenish iron stores.

Further Reading

American Gastroenterological Association Medical Position Statement: Evaluation and management of occult and obscure gastrointestinal bleeding. Gastroenterology 2000; 118: 197–201.

American Society for Gastrointestinal Endoscopy. Guideline on the management of anticoagulation and antiplatelet therapy for endoscopic procedures. Gastrointest Endosc 1998; 48: 672–6.

Bernard B, Grange JD, Khac EN et al. Antibiotic prophylaxis for the prevention of bacterial infection in cirrhotic patients with gastrointestinal bleeding: a meta-analysis. Hepatology 1999; 29: 1655–61.

Forrest JAH, Finlayson NDC, Shearman DJC. Endoscopy in gastrointestinal bleeding. Lancet 1974; 2: 394–7.

Goddard AF, McIntyre AS, Scott BB. Guidelines for the management of iron deficiency anaemia. Gut 2000; 46(Suppl IV): iv1–5.

Jalan R, Hayes PC. UK guidelines on the management of variceal haemorrhage in cirrhotic patients. Gut 2000; 46(Suppl 3-4): 1–15.

Jensen DM. Endoscopic diagnosis and treatment of severe hematochezia. Techniques in Gastrointest Endosc 2001; 3: 177–84.

Laine L, Peterson WL. Bleeding peptic ulcer. N Engl J Med 1994; 331: 717–27.

Lewis B. Enteroscopy Gastrointest Endosc Clin N Am 2000; 1: 101–16.

Palmer KR. Non-variceal upper gastrointestinal haemorrhage: guidelines. Gut 2002; 51(Suppl IV): iv1–iv6.

Rockall TA, Logan RFA, Devlin HB et al. Incidence of and mortality from acute upper gastrointestinal haemorrhage in the United Kingdom. BMJ 1995; 311: 222–6.

Rockall TA, Logan RFA, Devlin HB et al. Risk assessment following acute gastrointestinal haemorrhage. Gut 1996; 38: 316–21.

Schulman S. Care of patients receiving long-term anticoagulation therapy. N Engl J Med 2003; 349: 675–83.

Seewald S, Sriram PVJ, Naga M et al. Cyanoacrylate glue in gastric variceal bleeding. Endoscopy 2002; 34: 926–32.

Swain P. Wireless capsule endoscopy. Gut 2003; 52(Suppl 4): IV48–50.

Waye JD. How I use the Argon Plasma Coagulator. Clinical Perspectives in Gastroenterology 1999; 2: 249–54.

Yamamoto H, Sugano K. A new method of enteroscopy: the double-balloon method. Am J Gastroenterol 2003; 17: 273–4.

Liver disease

8

INTRODUCTION

The term liver disease encompasses a wide spectrum of both acute liver injury as well as chronic conditions, which over a period lead to cirrhosis. Liver disease is one of the ten leading causes of death. Chronic liver disease is a growing problem in the UK. In contrast with decreasing mortality due to most other digestive diseases, the mortality from liver diseases shows a striking upward trend (Fig. 8.1). There has been a threefold increase in deaths from liver disease in England and Wales over the last three decades. Of particular concern is the fact that more than two-thirds of deaths in 2000 occurred in those under the age of 65. Although there is undoubtedly a rising incidence of liver disease related to obesity, most of the rise in mortality is due to alcoholic liver disease and its complications. In the West Midlands 1993–2000, there was a threefold rise in death from alcohol-related liver disease. Diseases of the liver and pancreas account for almost 75% of all in-patient care episodes in gastroenterology. Therefore, understanding the basic mechanisms, clinical presentation, immediate and long-term management of liver disease is an essential part of training in gastroenterology.

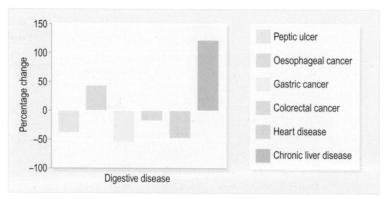

Fig. 8.1
Trends in mortality in the UK 1981–2000 (Data from Office of National Statistics)

INVESTIGATION OF PATIENTS WITH PRESUMED HEPATOBILIARY DISEASE

The assessment of patients with jaundice

The commonest presentations of liver disease are either decompensated liver disease or abnormal liver enzyme levels. Decompensated liver disease is most commonly manifest by the presence of jaundice and, in order of decreasing frequency, ascites, variceal bleeding and encephalopathy. Assessing the jaundiced patient involves the following key steps:

- Are there risk factors for liver disease in the history?
- Are stigmata of chronic liver disease present?
- What information is gained from the liver function tests?
- What critical information is required from further tests?

Risk factors for liver disease are alcohol excess, ethnicity (hyperendemic areas for viral liver disease), residence in an endemic area for viral hepatitis, blood-product exposure and intravenous drug use. Family history of liver disease or autoimmune disorders and a drug history are also important.

Stigmata of chronic liver disease rarely occur in the absence of cirrhosis and are palmar erythema, Dupuytren's contracture, clubbing, spider naevi, pigmentation, white nails and splenomegaly. Hepatomegaly is common in patients with alcoholic liver disease and primary biliary cirrhosis, but rare in other liver diseases.

The liver enzyme levels in the presence of jaundice mean relatively little. Alcoholic hepatitis is characteristically associated with minimal or no elevation of liver enzymes, in particular the alanine aminotransferase is never significantly elevated (>300 iu/ml) and hence other causes should be sought in this context. The traditional teaching that elevated transaminases are a pointer to hepatitic versus obstructive jaundice is wrong. A mixed picture of liver enzymes is almost universal in biliary obstruction due to stones, where there is presumably a significant cholangitic element. All patients require urgent ultrasound scanning to rule out biliary obstruction. A common catch is early biliary obstruction where the ducts have not yet dilated; this can occur in the first week of detectable jaundice, but is rare when the bilirubin exceeds 100 μmol/l. If the clinical suspicion of biliary obstruction is high, magnetic resonance cholangiography (MRC), endoscopic ultrasound, or repeating the ultrasound after 48 h may show biliary pathology.

The investigative pathway for patients with jaundice in whom biliary obstruction is excluded by ultrasound scanning is simple, with all patients requiring a drug and alcohol history and a full serological screen. It should be noted that jaundice with a very high transaminase level (AST >400) in hospital patients is most commonly due to ischaemic hepatitis (68%). Biliary disease and, more rarely, paracetamol overdose, acute viral hepatitis and autoimmune hepatitis should also be considered. There are very few other illnesses which present in this way.

Systemic diseases can frequently cause abnormal liver enzymes, but are unusual causes of jaundice. Haemolysis can present with jaundice and can co-exist in some patients with alcoholic liver disease. Other infective illnesses which may present with jaundice are leptospirosis, cytomegalovirus and Epstein–Barr virus infection.

Assessment of abnormal liver tests

Measurement of biochemical tests of liver function is now routine in the investigation of a wide range of symptoms and, indeed, as part of routine health checks. This has the potential to discover much significant liver and systemic disease at an early stage when specific symptoms of liver disease are not yet present, but also produces abnormal results in apparently healthy individuals. This is particularly so in the 'statin prescribing' era, when cardiovascular risk is calculated for a significant part of the population and interventions planned. As these drugs can and do cause significant liver injury, biochemical screening has increased.

Liver function tests

The usual liver-function tests include two separate types of test. Serum albumin and bilirubin provide a true measure of hepatic function, although both can be abnormal for a number of non-hepatic causes. The remaining tests are liver enzyme levels, usually alanine aminotransferase (ALT) or aspartate transaminase (AST) in combination with gamma glutamyl transpeptidase (GGT) and alkaline phosphatase (ALP). AST or ALT are sensitive markers of hepatocyte injury, but are also found in decreasing concentration in cardiac muscle, skeletal muscle, the kidney, brain, pancreas, lung and blood cells. As transaminases are present in highest concentrations in liver, significant elevation is usually due to hepatocyte injury.

GGT is found both in hepatocytes and in biliary epithelial cells. Its main utility is in the diagnosis of biliary tract disease, in combination with ALP. It is widely and incorrectly regarded as a sensitive and specific marker of alcohol misuse. Studies have shown that the sensitivity of elevated GGT for alcohol varies between 52 and 94%.

ALP is present in two major sites in the body, liver and bone. There are certain situations where a raised ALP is normal. In childhood, when bone growth is rapid, levels twice the adult normal are usual. In late pregnancy, placental alkaline phosphatase usually produces higher blood levels. An isolated raised ALP with a normal GGT is almost always bony in origin.

History

An asymptomatic individual found to have abnormal liver enzymes should have a history taken for specific factors that may predispose to liver disease or suggest another cause. Alcohol consumption, prior medical interventions, such as surgery or transfusion, intravenous drug use or tattooing should be included as should a detailed drug history, including non-prescribed or herbal remedies.

Physical examination

Physical examination aims to detect stigmata of chronic liver disease, including spider naevi, clubbing, hepatomegaly or splenomegaly. If present, these suggest significant liver disease as these signs are rarely present in the absence of hepatic cirrhosis. The history and examination should also aim to exclude non-hepatic causes for liver enzyme elevation. The commonest causes that may be difficult to diagnose clinically are right-sided heart failure or constrictive pericarditis, which can produce significant hepatomegaly and abnormal liver tests with relatively modest symptoms, and endocrine disorders, diabetes and thyroid dysfunction. The presence of obesity should be documented by body mass index:

weight [kg] divided by height [metres] squared

and, ideally, waist to hip ratio should also be recorded as the fatty liver variants now account for a significant proportion of elevated liver enzymes.

Further investigations

Further investigation is required if abnormal liver enzymes are found in the presence of stigmata of chronic liver disease or, in their absence, if the abnormality persists on a repeat sample after an interval of 2–3 months. Initial tests required are shown in Table 8.1. In young patients (<40 years) serum caeruloplasmin should be added to the list. Wilson's disease can be very difficult to diagnose, but a low caeruloplasmin is suggestive and should be followed by 24-h urinary copper levels, slit-lamp examination and, in some cases, penicillamine challenge and liver biopsy copper weight.

The purpose of initial serological screening is to establish a cause for liver enzyme elevation wherever possible. The serology is cheap and effective at producing a diagnosis. The route of investigation (ultrasound or blood tests) is generally directed by the pattern

Table 8.1 Investigations required in asymptomatic patients with elevated liver enzyme levels

Test	Abnormality	Interpretation
Full blood count	Macrocytosis	Specific for alcohol excess only if GGT elevated
	Thrombocytopenia	Suggests hypersplenism (portal hypertension)
	AMA positive, IgM raised	Diagnostic of primary biliary cirrhosis (PBC)
Autoantibodies and immunoglobulins	ASM/ANA positive, IgG Raised	Strongly suggestive of autoimmune hepatitis
Ferritin	Elevated	Suggests haemochromatosis, HFE mutations can confirm in 90%
Hepatitis B surface antigen	Positive	Implies chronic infection
Hepatitis C antibody	Positive	Suggests chronic infection
Anti-endomysial antibodies	Positive	Suggests coeliac disease
Alpha-1-antitrypsin level	Low	Suggests deficiency. Phenotype required. (PiZZ or PiM implicated)
Ultrasound of liver	Mass/dilated ducts	Tumour/stones

of enzyme abnormality. Elevated ALP and GGT should primarily be investigated by ultrasound followed by serology and the reverse for predominantly raised transaminases.

Results of initial investigation

This screening process will identify a variable proportion of diagnoses depending on the population studied. In a study of 19 877 Air Force recruits, 0.5% had abnormal transaminases, but a cause was found in only 12 (mainly viral hepatitis). In blood donors found to have a raised ALT, 48% had the abnormality attributed to alcohol, 22% to fatty liver and 17% to hepatitis C virus (HCV), although many patients did not have liver biopsy proof of diagnosis. There is evidence that even basic screening tests are not undertaken rigorously in either primary or secondary care settings. A primary care study of abnormal liver enzymes twice the upper limit of normal showed that, of 157 patients with no obvious cause, 58% had had no further test to elucidate the cause and no patient had the complete set outlined in Table 8.1. Sixty-two per cent on further investigation had a diagnosis requiring further management in secondary care and 20% had significant hepatic fibrosis.

Assessment of abnormal liver function tests in patients with normal screening blood tests

For the majority of patients with abnormal liver enzyme levels, the pattern is non-specific – commonly a raised ALT and GGT. The only investigation likely to produce a diagnosis in the absence of diagnostic serology in this situation is liver biopsy. The effects of alcohol, drugs and the non-alcoholic fatty liver variants can only be diagnosed on liver biopsy. Percutaneous liver biopsy does, however, involve a finite risk, primarily of haemorrhage, and hence the decision to offer liver biopsy has to be a balance of potential benefits of a diagnosis in the prevention of progressive hepatic fibrosis versus the risk. The presence of transaminase levels twice normal is associated with a histologically normal liver in only around 6%; hence there is usually a diagnosis to be made. The commonest diagnosis made on liver biopsy in this setting is fatty liver or non-alcoholic steatohepatitis (Table 8.2). This diagnostic group accounts for two-thirds of unexplained elevation of liver enzymes. Other important diagnoses were conditions such as anti-mitochondrial antibody negative primary biliary cirrhosis and autoimmune hepatitis. The presence of significant hepatic fibrosis varies in series using liver biopsy to investigate unexplained liver enzyme elevations between 12 and 50%; between 3 and 6% had cirrhosis.

A further important issue in the balance between risk and benefit of liver biopsy is the potential to alter the outcome for patients with chronic liver injury, by stopping the progress of hepatic fibrosis. This benefit is clear in conditions such as autoimmune hepatitis but less so in conditions such as alcoholic liver injury. Conditions with a specific treatment that can change the natural history of the liver injury are found in between 7 and 18% of patients undergoing biopsy for abnormal liver enzymes.

Non-alcoholic fatty liver disease (NAFLD) (i.e. fatty liver or non-alcoholic steatohepatitis) accounts for two-thirds of the patients having liver biopsy for abnormal LFTs. In those with simple steatosis, the condition is considered to have a benign course. In those with

Table 8.2 Findings on liver biopsy for unexplained abnormal liver-enzyme elevation in 354 patients

Final diagnosis	No (%)
Non-alcoholic steatohepatitis	120 (34)
Fatty liver	115 (32)
Cryptogenic hepatitis	32 (9)
Drug-related damage	27 (7.6)
Normal liver	21 (5.9)
Alcohol	10 (2.8)
Autoimmune hepatitis	7 (1.9)
Granuloma/sarcoid	6 (1.7)
Primary biliary cirrhosis	5 (1.4)
Primary sclerosing cholangitis	4 (1.1)
Haemochromatosis	3 (0.9)
Secondary biliary cirrhosis	2 (0.6)
Amyloid	1 (0.3)
Glycogen storage disease	1 (0.3)

significant inflammation, particularly with fibrosis on index biopsy (i.e. non-alcoholic steatohepatitis or NASH), about 10% progress to cirrhosis after 10 years. There is, as yet, no specific medical therapy for NASH. At present, in patients with suspected NASH, risk factors such as hypertriglyceridaemia and diabetes should be addressed and a programme of exercise and weight reduction tried before liver biopsy is offered. If these manoeuvres fail, biopsy will confirm the diagnosis and allow identification of those at significant risk of progression. These are suitable for clinical trials of new therapy. The algorithm in Figure 8.2 outlines the approach.

For the relatively small proportion of patients with cholestatic liver enzymes (raised ALP and GGT with normal ALT) and a normal abdominal ultrasound, more detailed biliary imaging with either magnetic resonance scanning or endoscopic retrograde cholangiopancreatography (ERCP) may be appropriate rather than liver biopsy, particularly if sclerosing cholangitis is suspected clinically.

ACUTE HEPATIC FAILURE

The term acute liver failure has been used to describe a potentially reversible condition, the consequence of severe liver injury, with an onset of encephalopathy within 12 weeks of the appearance of the first symptoms and in the absence of pre-existing liver disease. As the rapidity of onset of encephalopathy influences survival, it has been suggested that the terms hyperacute, acute and subacute should be used to define the sub-groups (Table 8.3) and the term 'fulminant' hepatic failure should be avoided. Acute hepatic failure is an uncommon, yet potentially fatal, condition with up to 66% mortality without liver transplantation.

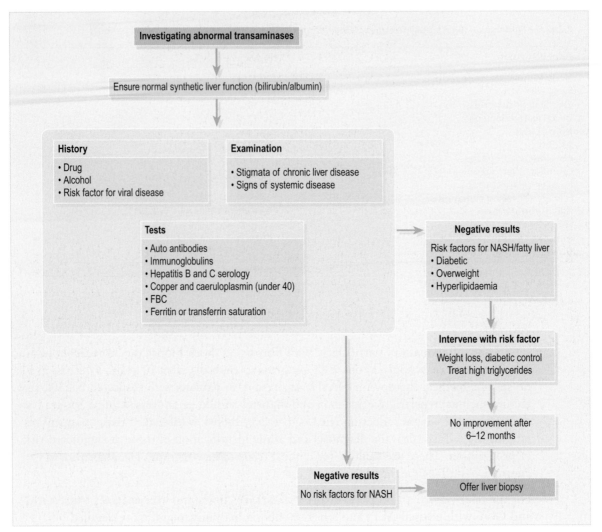

Fig. 8.2
Investigating abnormal transaminases

In most cases, massive hepatocellular necrosis occurs. In drug-induced liver injury it affects the centrilobular region in particular (Fig. 8.3). However, hepatic failure without necrosis occurs in acute fatty liver, complicating pregnancy or drug-induced mitochondrial toxicity characterized by accumulation of microvesicular fat in intact cells. Viral hepatitis and drug-induced liver injury account for most cases of acute liver failure (Table 8.4), although there is wide variation in the frequency of these in different countries. Paracetamol overdose accounts for over 70% of cases of acute hepatic failure in the UK, while viral hepatitis caused one-third of cases in India. Idiosyncratic hepatotoxicity is the cause of hepatic failure in 2–15% of cases.

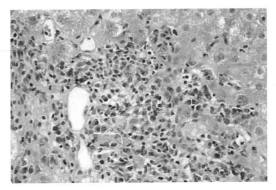

Fig. 8.3
Confluent necrosis around the central vein secondary to idiosyncratic hepatotoxicity

Table 8.3 Features of clinical syndromes under the umbrella term of 'acute hepatic failure'

Clinical Syndrome	Hyperacute	Acute	Subacute
Encephalopathy	++	++	++
Jaundice	≤7 days	1–4 weeks	5–12 weeks
Cerebral oedema	++	++	±
Coagulopathy	++	++	+
Bilirubin	+	++	++
Survival without transplantation (5)*	36%	7%	14%

*King's College Hospital, London 1972–1985 (prior to transplantation programme)

Table 8.4 Important causes of acute hepatic failure

Viral hepatitis	**Vascular events**
Hepatitis A, B, D and E	Ischaemic hepatitis
Herpes simplex	Veno-occlusive disease
Drug and toxins	**Others**
Paracetamol	Malignant infiltration
Idiosyncratic hepatotoxicity	Wilson's disease
Mitochondrial toxicity (nucleoside analogues)	Auto-immune hepatitis
Amanita phalloides (mushroom poisoning)	Acute fatty liver

Management

Identification of underlying aetiology is important as it guides both the medical management as well as predicting the outcome and hence, listing for liver transplantation (Table 8.5). Liver injury in paracetamol overdose is due to depletion of glutathione and, therefore, sulfhydryl donors such as N-acetyl cysteine, which replenish glutathione, limit the liver damage. Paracetamol toxicity is dose-dependent, but its effect is enhanced by induction of cytochrome p-450 by alcohol and antiepileptics, hence, the threshold for treatment should be reduced under such circumstances. Although patients receiving

191

Table 8.5 Indications to list for transplantation in acute hepatic failure

Paracetamol overdose
Arterial pH <7.3 (arterial lactate >3.5 mmol/l at 4 h*)

Or all three of:
Grade 3 or 4 encephalopathy
PT >100 s
Creatinine >300 µmol/l

Non-paracetamol acute hepatic failure
PT >100 s

Or any three of:
Age <10 years or >40 years
Aetiology: seronegative hepatitis, idiosyncratic drug hepatotoxicity
Jaundice to encephalopathy >7 days
PT >50 s
Creatinine >300 µmol/l

*Wendon J et al. Lancet 2002; 359(9306): 558

N-acetyl cysteine within 24 h of overdose have the best prognosis, benefit has been demonstrated even when the treatment is given after 36 h of ingestion of paracetamol. Early recognition of idiosyncratic drug-hepatotoxicity as a cause of acute hepatic failure is important as the withdrawal of the causative agent could reverse the liver injury.

Recognizing uncommon causes of acute failure could still influence the management. In patients with autoimmune hepatitis, steroid therapy is indicated and, in herpes hepatitis, early treatment with acyclovir improves outcome. Diagnosis of Wilson's disease is an indication for early transplantation as these patients deteriorate rapidly. Transjugular liver biopsy may occasionally be indicated to exclude malignancy in patients presenting with acute liver failure and hepatomegaly.

The onset of encephalopathy is often abrupt and may precede the appearance of jaundice. Cerebral oedema occurs in the majority of those with encephalopathy and is the leading cause of death. Raised intracranial pressure manifests with systemic hypertension, bradycardia, decerebrate rigidity progressing to pupillary changes and altered respiratory pattern. These patients should be managed by multidisciplinary teams at intensive care units with facilities to monitor intracranial pressure. Therefore, specialist liver units must be involved early in the management of acute liver failure with adverse risk factors (Table 8.5), especially when patients are potential candidates for liver transplantation. It is safer to transfer patients before grade III or IV encephalopathy develops.

Coagulopathy is typical of acute liver failure and is used as an indicator of prognosis. Abnormal coagulation may be compounded by thrombocytopenia. No attempt should be made to correct the abnormal clotting profile with fresh frozen plasma or cryoprecipitate before a decision regarding liver transplantation is made. Intravenous vitamin K can be used to correct any dietary deficiency in those with a history of alcohol abuse and is not contraindicated as it does not interfere with assessment of liver dysfunction. Up to 80%

cases of acute liver failure are complicated by systemic bacterial and fungal infection. Hence, regular microbial surveillance and aggressive treatment of presumed infection are essential. The benefits of prophylactic antibiotics to reduce infective episodes should be weighed against the risk of emergence of super-infections. The circulatory changes in acute liver failure resemble that of septic shock with effective hypovolaemia, but fluid replacement should be carefully monitored to avoid fluid overload and cerebral oedema. Oliguric renal failure develops in half of the patients, with acute failure worsening the prognosis. Renal support is essential to correct acid–base and electrolyte imbalances. Blood glucose should be monitored as hypoglycaemia is common.

CIRRHOSIS AND ITS COMPLICATIONS

In response to liver injury, cytokines released by the inflammatory cells and damaged hepatocytes activate hepatic stellate cells, which are the central mediators of wound healing. Activated stellate cells proliferate and secrete fibrillar collagen, resulting in excess fibrotic matrix. Extracellular matrix helps to contain the injurious agent. The injury response reaches a successful conclusion with the dismantling of repair apparatus. The extracellular matrix scaffold is taken down by matrix proteinases and activated stellate cells undergo apoptosis. Normal tissue structure is restored. When the injury is recurrent or chronic, the balance between fibrogenesis and fibrolysis tips in favour of fibrogenesis. Location of hepatic fibrosis (periportal, bridging, sinusoidal or pericentral) is characteristic for some types of injury. Over time, liver fibrosis progresses to cirrhosis, defined anatomically by the presence of nodules of hepatocytes separated by fibrous septae (Fig. 8.4). These fibrous septae in cirrhosis disrupt the architecture of the liver and impair liver function.

In patients with compensated cirrhosis, median 1-year and 10-year survival rates are 95% and 60%. Development and manifestations of portal hypertension have a major impact on prognosis in cirrhosis (Table 8.6). In those with compensated cirrhosis at diagnosis, the probability per year of developing major complication is 12% for ascites, 8% for gastrointestinal bleeding, 4% hepatic encephalopathy and 2% for hepatocellular carcinoma.

Portal hypertension

Portal hypertension occurs as a consequence of structural changes within the liver in cirrhosis, in combination with increased splanchnic blood flow (Fig. 8.5). Progressive collagen deposition and formation of nodules alter the normal vascular architecture of the liver and increase resistance to portal flow. Sinusoids may become less distensible with the formation of collagen within the space of Disse. Recent studies have suggested that activated hepatic stellate cells may dynamically regulate sinusoidal tone and thus portal pressure. Activated hepatic stellate cells become sensitive to the vasoactive substance endothelin, the concentration of which increases with fibrosis. In addition, liver injury results in a reduction in vasodilatory nitric oxide (NO) derived from hepatic endothelial cells. As a result of this imbalance, stellate cell contraction is promoted with consequent increase in sinusoidal resistance.

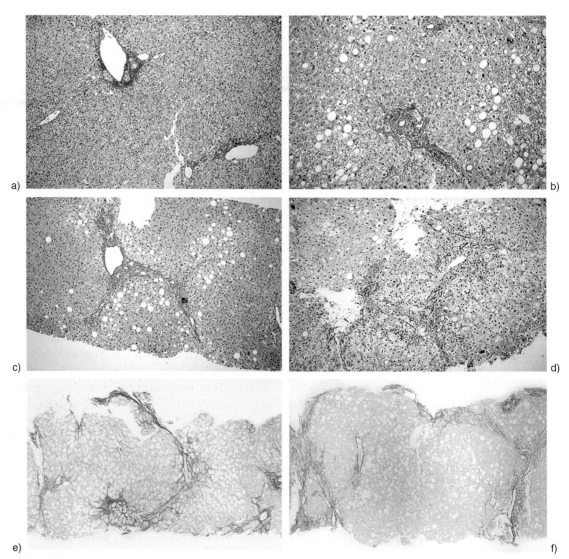

Fig. 8.4
Progression of liver fibrosis – serial liver biopsies demonstrating normal liver histology (a), through stages of increasing fibrosis (b, c), portal-central and portal-portal bridging (d), incomplete (e), to complete cirrhosis (f)

Table 8.6 Prognosis in different stages of cirrhosis

Stages	Mortality rate/year
No varices, no ascites	1%
Varices present, no ascites	3.4%
Varices present, ascites present	20%
Variceal bleeding, ascites present	57%

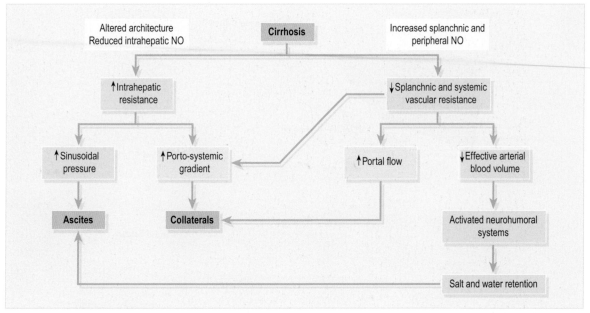

Fig. 8.5
Pathogenesis of portal hypertension

Splanchnic vasodilation with increased blood flow through the portal venous system is a major contributing factor in aggravating and maintaining portal hypertension. Peripheral vasodilation results in a reduction of systemic vascular resistance and mean arterial blood, which in turn lead to plasma volume expansion and elevated splanchnic blood flow. Marked overproduction of NO in the splanchnic and systemic vasculature has been shown to be the key to these haemodynamic changes. Thus, abnormal NO production by endothelial nitric oxide synthase (eNOS) plays a central role in pathogenesis of portal hypertension manifested by a deficit in intrahepatic NO and an increase in splanchnic NO. Further elucidation of mechanisms involved in eNOS regulation would allow better understanding of portal hypertension and open a new avenue of treatment.

OESOPHAGEAL VARICES

Formation of varices

Varices are part of portal-systemic collaterals and develop from the dilatation of pre-existent embryonic channels. The left gastric vein is responsible for the development of oesophageal varices, and short gastric veins arising from the splenic vein are responsible for the formation of fundal varices. Perforating veins communicate with submucosal and paraoesophageal venous plexuses and the latter are tributaries of the azygos venous system (Figs 8.6 & 8.7). Varices are already present in about 40% of compensated cirrhotics and the frequency increases up to 90% on long-term follow-up. Varices appear at a rate of 6% per year, and in 12% of patients per year small varices evolve into large ones.

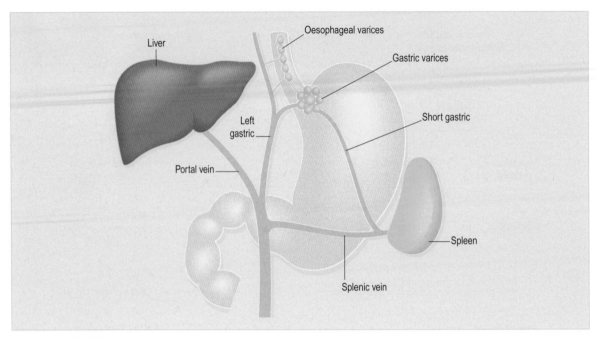

Fig. 8.6
Portal-systemic collaterals in portal hypertension

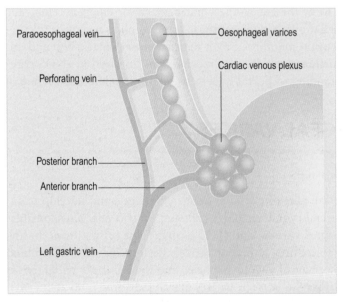

Fig. 8.7
Portal-systemic collaterals and oesophageal varices

Variceal rupture

According to 'explosion hypothesis', varices rupture because of increased variceal wall tension. Laplace's law explains how various factors interact to increase the wall tension, which is defined by the following equation:

$$\text{Tension} = \frac{(\text{variceal pressure} - \text{luminal pressure}) \times \text{radius of the varix}}{\text{thickness of the variceal wall}}$$

Accordingly, predictors of variceal haemorrhage are high wedged hepatic venous-portal gradient (WHVPG), size of the varix and the presence of red signs (cherry red spots and red wale markings). In addition, advanced Child–Pugh class (Table 8.7) would also predict variceal bleeding as a high score is likely to be associated with significant coagulopathy. A combination of these clinical features could be used to calculate a North-Italian Endoscopic Club (NIEC) index, which accurately estimates 1-year probability of variceal bleeding.

Investigations

Wedge venography

Measurement of wedged and free hepatic venous pressure (WHVPG) is a safe and reliable way of establishing the diagnosis of portal hypertension. Under fluoroscopic guidance, a catheter is 'wedged' into a hepatic vein (via the jugular or femoral vein). Pressure measurement when the catheter is wedged reflects the portal pressure. In extrahepatic portal hypertension (Table 8.8) WHVPG is normal. Wedged venography can also be used to image hepatic veins in Budd–Chiari syndrome. Injection of CO_2 when the catheter is wedged into the hepatic vein would result in a retrograde filling of the portal vein and demonstrate portal vein patency. CO_2 used as a negative contrast medium allows a quick and effective visualization of the portal vein.

In patients with cirrhosis, there is no risk of bleeding when the WHVPG is below 10 mm of Hg. The risk of variceal bleeding is markedly reduced when drug therapy reduces the WHVPG by 20% or below 12 mm of Hg. However, the timing of re-measurement of WHVPG and its clinical utility have not been firmly established.

Table 8.7 Child–Pugh classification

Feature	Points		
	1	2	3
Bilirubin (µmol/l)	<35	35–50	>50
Albumin (g/l)	>35	35–28	<28
Prothrombin time (prolongation in seconds)	1–3	4–6	>6
Ascites	None	Mild	Moderate
Encephalopathy	None	Grade 1–2	Grade 3–4

Grades:
A – 5–6 points, 0–5% mortality with shunt surgery
B – 7–9 points, 10–15% mortality with shunt surgery
C – 10–15 points, >25% mortality with shunt surgery

Table 8.8 Non-cirrhotic causes of portal hypertension

Conditions	Causes
Pre-hepatic	
Portal vein thrombosis	Intra-abdominal sepsis, upper abdominal surgery, Abdominal trauma
	Thrombophilic disorders
	Pancreatitis, pancreatic cancer
Banti syndrome	Occult/sub-clinical portal vein occlusion (from neonatal umbilical sepsis) presenting several years later
Hepatoportal sclerosis	Hypercoagulable states
(idiopathic portal hypertension)	Vasculotoxins, such as azathioprine, cyclophosphamide, methotrexate
Hepatic	
Sickle-cell disease	Sickled erythrocytes in sinusoids
Malignancy	Breast cancer, lymphoma, malignant melanoma
Amyloidosis	Amyloid in space of Disse
Post-hepatic	
Sinusoidal occlusion syndrome (veno-occlusive disease)	Post-bone-marrow transplantation (following cytotoxic induction therapy)
Budd–Chiari syndrome (hepatic vein thrombosis)	Myeloproliferative disorders, thrombophilic disorders, intra-abdominal cancers
Inferior vena cava thrombosis (obliterative hepatocavopathy)	Membranous web in IVC
Cardiac sclerosis	Congestive heart failure

Ultrasound scanning

Doppler ultrasound, power Doppler and harmonic resonance techniques allow detailed evaluation of portal system. Adequate examination with an ultrasound may often be limited due to technical factors.

Computerized tomography

Currently most scans performed are 'triple-phase' including an arterial, portal and a pre-contrast or delayed post-portal phase. Using multi-detector technology and fast gantry speeds, computerized tomography (CT) angiography has in many instances replaced conventional angiography.

Magnetic resonance imaging

Despite advances in CT technology some consider magnetic resonance imaging (MRI) to be more sensitive in the diagnosis of portal-vein thrombosis and the development of collaterals.

Management

Primary prophylaxis

According to Ohm's law, portal pressure is a function of portal venous flow and hepatic and portocollateral resistance. Non-selective beta blockers act both by decreasing cardiac output (beta 1 receptors) and by decreasing splanchnic arterial flow (beta 2 receptors) and thus reducing portal flow and the pressure. Treatment of patients with moderate and large varices with non-selective beta blockers halves the incidence of first variceal bleeding and six patients need to be treated to prevent one episode bleeding. If patients with small varices were included then the number needed to be treated increases to 10, but this strategy would eliminate the need to repeat endoscopic surveillance. Maximum tolerated dose of beta blocker is determined by incremental increases in dose to reach 25% reduction in resting heart rate or a decrease not below 55 beats per minute or the development of side effects. Using this method only 10% in a study group showed a reduction in WHVPG of >20% and 43% were considered non-responders. The addition of isosorbide mononitrate to reduce hepatic and portocollateral resistance does not increase the efficacy of primary prophylaxis and nitrate on its own may be detrimental. Patients who have contraindications to beta blockers or intolerance should be offered endoscopic banding as primary prophylaxis especially when the risk of bleeding is high (Child's C, large varices, red signs).

'Pre-primary prophylaxis' with beta blockers to prevent the appearance of gastro-oesophageal varices and hence to prevent first variceal bleeding, has not been shown to be effective. Therefore, patients with cirrhosis without varices at the time of diagnosis should undergo annual endoscopic surveillance. This may not be appropriate in patients who have a short life expectancy. For patients in Child's class A with no varices, repeat endoscopy may be warranted in 2 years' time.

Acute variceal bleeding

In the placebo-treated groups of randomized control trials, about 25% of those with gastro-oesophageal varices bleed with a 4% incidence of first bleeding per year. Variceal

Table 8.9 Key steps in the management of acute variceal bleeding

Do	Avoid
Adequate resuscitation: aim for Hb of 10 g/l, haematocrit of 30%, central venous pressure (CVP) of 5 mm of Hg	Overtransfusion: increases CVP and hence variceal pressure
Replace clotting factors: fresh frozen plasma for every 4 units of transfusion, platelets if <50 × 10⁹/l	Crystalloids
Early administration of vasoactive drugs (preferably terlipressin)	Nephrotoxic drugs, renal dose dopamine
Look for sepsis: diagnostic paracentesis, chest X-ray at admission; urine and blood cultures if indicated	
Prophylactic antibiotics (norfloxacin or ciprofloxacin orally), therapeutic antibiotics early if sepsis detected.	
Intravenous (iv) thiamine for those with alcohol excess	Withdrawal syndrome
Feeding via fine-bore nasogastric tube to start 24 h after bleeding has stopped. One dose of intravenous vitamin K 10 mg	High-sodium feeds
Therapeutic paracentesis if ascites is tense	Diuretics
Use Sengstaken-Blakemore tube when airway is protected	Keeping S-T tube with traction for >24 h

bleeding is one of the most serious medical emergencies with a mortality of 20–50% depending on the severity of the liver disease. Within the first 6 weeks, 30–40% re-bleed and the risk is the highest in the first 5 days. Therefore, goals in the management of acute variceal bleeding are to adequately resuscitate, to achieve haemostasis and to prevent re-bleeding. Key steps in the management are summarized in Table 8.9.

Drug therapy

Terlipressin is a synthetic triglycyl analogue of lysine vasopressin that is converted into vasopressin *in vivo* by enzymatic cleavage. It causes splanchnic vasoconstriction, thereby reducing portal flow and pressure. It has been used at doses of 1–2 mg intravenously every 4–6 h for up to 5 days. Terlipressin is effective in controlling bleeding and in reducing mortality. Unlike vasopressin it has a longer half-life, less systemic toxicity and it does not enhance fibrinolysis. Published data on the efficacy of terlipressin are homogenous and meta-analyses are concordant. When terlipressin was administered before admission to hospital, it reduced mortality in patients with advanced cirrhosis. In patients who received terlipressin before endoscopy, control of bleeding was achieved more frequently. Therefore, terlipressin should be administered as soon as possible in patients with upper gastrointestinal bleeding where there is a high index of suspicion that oesophagogastric varices are the source.

Octreotide is a cyclic synthetic somatostatin analogue with a long half life. Octreotide has been shown to improve the efficacy of endoscopic therapy. However, published data on octreotide are heterogeneous and meta-analyses are divergent. Hence, the efficacy of octreotide as first-line therapy is unclear.

Endoscopic therapy

Endoscopy is essential in the management of acute variceal bleeding. Diagnosis of variceal bleeding is established usually at first endoscopy and in about 25% of patients with cirrhosis a non-variceal cause of bleeding would be found. Endoscopic therapy could be performed at the time of first endoscopy.

Combination of vasoactive drugs with endoscopic techniques is better in controlling variceal haemorrhage than either treatment on its own. Endoscopic sclerotherapy and band ligation are the two techniques used in the management of oesophageal varices (see also p. 168). The studies comparing endoscopic ligation with sclerotherapy specifically in acute variceal bleeding have drawn conflicting conclusions. However, multiple trials comparing the two techniques in preventing re-bleeding have shown endoscopic ligation to be superior requiring fewer sessions for eradication of varices and to be associated with fewer treatment-related complications. Endoscopic band ligation is considered to be the preferred technique for prevention of re-bleeding.

Neither endoscopic ligation nor sclerotherapy has been a satisfactory treatment for fundal varices. In a recent randomized trial endoscopic injection of glue (n-butyl-2 cyanoacrylate) into fundal varices achieved initial haemostasis in 87% compared with 45% in those treated with band ligation, and was superior in preventing re-bleeding (31% vs. 54%). In this study, the group treated with glue injection received less transfusion and had lower mortality.

Antibiotic prophylaxis

Cirrhotic patients with gastrointestinal bleeding have a higher risk of developing bacterial infection during hospitalization compared with those admitted for other reasons. The frequency of infection increases with their Child's score. The spectrum of bacteria is similar to one described in patients with spontaneous bacterial peritonitis, hence similar pathogenetic mechanisms have been thought to be involved. Hypovolaemic shock associated with variceal bleeding has been shown to be associated with depressed reticuloendothelial system phagocytic activity and bacterial translocation. Endotoxins and cytokines related to sepsis induce platelet dysfunction and activation of the fibrinolytic system. Thus, infections predispose to recurrent variceal bleeding. Antibiotic prophylaxis in cirrhotics with gastrointestinal bleeding decreases the incidence of infections including spontaneous bacterial peritonitis (SBP), the frequency of re-bleeding and reduces the overall mortality by 10%. Norfloxacin (400 mg twice daily orally for 7 days), which is poorly absorbed, selectively decontaminates the intestine. Ciprofloxacin 500 mg twice daily is an effective alternative. In those where the drugs cannot be administered orally or by nasogastric tube, ciprofloxacin should be used intravenously.

Transjugular intrahepatic portosystemic shunt

TIPS is inserted by directing a needle under fluoroscopic guidance from the right hepatic vein to the right portal vein. The track is dilated to 8–12 mm and a metal stent is deployed to support the shunt wall. TIPS is effective in controlling acute variceal bleeding that is refractory to the combination of medical and endoscopic management. The latter combination controls bleeding in 80–90% of episodes and TIPS is used as 'salvage' therapy in those where a second endoscopic therapy fails to control bleeding. TIPS is effective in the control of bleeding from portal gastropathy.

TIPS is also more effective than endoscopic therapy in preventing re-bleeding, but this advantage is offset by increased frequency of encephalopathy and the need of continued shunt surveillance. TIPS does not improve survival.

Surgical management

Surgery has a limited role in the management of acute variceal bleeding complicating cirrhosis as TIPS offers a less invasive method of decompressing the varices than emergency portocaval shunts. Oesophageal transection and devascularization are now rarely performed. One randomized trial showed a partial (8 mm) portocaval shunt to be superior to TIPS in the reduction of re-bleeding rate. However, the re-intervention and mortality in the TIPS group in this study was higher than generally reported. Patient selection is the key in determining success from surgical portal systemic shunts. Liver transplantation offers improved survival in patients with Child's C cirrhosis, while shunt surgery has significant mortality (Table 8.7). In Child's A and B patients, benefits and risks of liver transplantation should be weighed against that for shunt surgery. The latter could be considered as an option in selected patients with non-cirrhotic portal hypertension.

Secondary prevention

Overall, about 70% of patients who have one variceal bleed, re-bleed. Non-selective beta blockers should be considered first-line treatment for the prevention of re-bleeding.

Patients who are non-compliant, intolerant or those with contraindications for beta blockers and those who are high risk (Child's C, large varices) should receive endoscopic ligation to eradicate the varices.

Other GI manifestations of portal hypertension

Ectopic varices

The portosystemic collaterals occurring at sites other than the cardio-oesophageal region are called ectopic varices. Duodenal varices are found in up to 40% of patients with portal hypertension undergoing angiography, while jejunoileal and colonic varices are frequent in those who have undergone abdominal surgery. Prevalence of rectal varices is 43% on endoscopy and 75% when endoscopic ultrasound is used.

Bleeding ectopic varices accounts for 1.5% of all variceal bleeds. Of ectopic variceal bleeds 35% occur in the small intestine, 25% from peristomal varices, 15% from colonic and 8% from rectal varices.

Portal hypertensive gastropathy

Diffuse macroscopic lesions seen in the gastric mucosa of patients with portal hypertension is referred to as portal hypertensive gastropathy (PHG). The lesions range from a 'mosaic-like pattern' in the mucosa (mild) to multiple 'red-point lesions', 'cherry-red spots' or 'black-brown spots' (severe). There is a wide variation in the reported prevalence of PHG, but the overall prevalence increases from 55% in those with recent diagnosis of cirrhosis to 90% in patients after sclerotherapy. Endoscopically confirmed acute bleeding occurs in about 2.5% from PHG during 18 months' follow-up and has 12.5% mortality. Chronic blood loss (2 g/dl drop in haemoglobin) occurs in 12% of patients with PHG during a 6-months' follow-up. Non-selective beta blockers reduce the risk of bleeding and chronic anaemia due to PHG.

Portal colopathy

Mucosal lesions resembling cherry-red spots or cutaneous spider telangiectasia have been described in 35–70% of patients with portal hypertension who were investigated for occult gastrointestinal bleeding. Their prevalence in consecutive candidates for liver transplantation is only up to 3%.

ASCITES

Ascites is a major complication of cirrhosis and occurs in 50% of patients during 10 years following the diagnosis. The development of ascites is an important landmark in the natural history of cirrhosis. The median 2-year survival is reduced from 90% for compensated cirrhosis to 50% in those with ascites. Therefore, occurrence of ascites indicates the need to consider liver transplantation as a therapeutic option. The majority (>75%) of patients who present with ascites have underlying cirrhosis, with the remainder being due to malignancy (10%), heart failure (3%), tuberculosis (2%), pancreatitis (1%) and other rare causes.

Pathogenesis of ascites

Portal (sinusoidal) hypertension is a pre-requisite for the development of ascites. Ascites rarely develops in those with a wedged hepatic venous-portal gradient (WHVPG) of <12 mm of Hg. However, patients with pre-sinusoidal portal hypertension (such as portal vein thrombosis) without cirrhosis rarely develop ascites. Portal hypertension increases the hydrostatic pressure within the hepatic sinusoids and favours the transudation of fluid into the peritoneal cavity. Initially, when excess interstitial fluid is produced across the sinusoidal vascular bed, it is drained by the lymphatics. However, soon the rate of lymph production exceeds that of removal and ascites begins to accumulate.

Sodium and water retention is critical in the pathogenesis of ascites. The classical 'underfill' or 'overfill' hypotheses of sodium and water retention are oversimplified as patients exhibit features of either expanded or contracted blood volume depending on posture and severity of liver disease. A unifying 'vasodilatation hypothesis' has been put forward to explain the known observations with regard to the development of salt-retaining states (Fig. 8.5). According to this, systemic vasodilatation in cirrhosis leads to a decrease in 'effective' blood volume and to activation of the renin–angiotensin–aldosterone system and sympathetic nervous system, leading to sodium and water retention. The mechanism that mediates arterial vasodilatation is unknown, but may involve increased endothelial synthesis of nitric oxide (NO), prostacyclin as well as changes in plasma concentrations of glucagon, substance P, or calcitonin gene-related peptide. The old concept that ascites is formed secondary to decreased oncotic pressure is false and plasma albumin concentrations have little influence on the rate of ascites formation.

Diagnosis

The underlying cause of ascites is frequently obvious from the history and physical examination. However, it is important to exclude other causes of ascites and, therefore, tests must be directed at diagnosing the cause of ascites. The essential investigations on admission include a diagnostic paracentesis and an abdominal ultrasound scan to evaluate the appearance of liver, pancreas, spleen and lymph nodes.

Abdominal paracentesis

Ascitic fluid is aspirated from a point about 5 cm medial and cephalad to the anterior superior iliac spine usually in the left lower abdominal quadrant. The inferior and superior epigastric arteries run just lateral to the umbilicus towards the mid-inguinal point and should be avoided. For diagnostic purposes, 20–30 ml of fluid should be withdrawn. Up to 1% of patients may develop abdominal haematomas due to paracentesis but serious complications such as haemoperitoneum or bowel perforation are rare (<1/1000 procedures).

Ascitic fluid investigations

An ascitic neutrophil count of >250 cells/mm^3 (0.25×10^9/l) or an ascitic total white-cell count >500 cells/mm^3 (0.5×10^9/l) is diagnostic of SBP in the absence of a known perforated viscus. About 15% of patients with ascites admitted to hospital have unsuspected

SBP and, therefore, all should have diagnostic paracentesis. Bloody ascitic fluid ($>50\,000$ cells/mm^3) occurs in about 2% of cirrhotics and, in one-third of these, there is an underlying hepatocellular carcinoma. However, in 50% of patients with bloody ascites, no cause can be found. Several studies have shown that direct inoculation of ascitic fluid into blood culture bottles will identify an organism in about 72–90% of cases, whereas only 40% are culture positive when ascitic fluid is sent in a sterile container to the laboratory.

Serum-ascites albumin gradient

Classification of ascites into exudates and transudates based on the ascitic protein concentration is outdated. Ascitic protein is >25 g/l in up to 30% of patients with uncomplicated cirrhosis, and patients with cirrhosis and tuberculous ascites may have a low ascitic protein. The serum-ascites albumin gradient (SAAG) is far superior in categorizing ascites with 97% accuracy. It is calculated as:

SAAG = Serum albumin concentration – ascitic fluid albumin concentration

SAAG of >11 g/l indicates a diagnosis of cirrhosis with portal hypertension (or cardiac failure, nephrotic syndrome), while SAAG of <11 g/l occurs in malignancy, pancreatitis and tuberculosis.

Other tests

Routine use of detailed analysis of ascites fluid has a low yield and is not cost effective. High ascitic amylase is diagnostic of pancreatic ascites and should be requested in patients with alcoholic liver disease. Gram-stain of ascitic fluid is rarely helpful. The sensitivity of smear for mycobacteria is very poor, while fluid culture for mycobacteria is 50% sensitive. Only 7% of ascites samples have malignant cells, yet, cytology is 60–90% accurate in the diagnosis of malignant ascites. Therefore, cytology should be performed when there is clinical suspicion of malignancy.

Treatment

Dietary salt restriction

A typical UK diet contains about 150 mmol of sodium per day, of which 15% is from added salt and 70% is from manufactured food. Severe salt restriction has been associated with lower diuretic requirement and faster resolution of ascites, but often leads to protein malnutrition. Dietary salt should be restricted to a no added salt diet of 90 mmol salt/day (5.2 g of salt/day).

Water restriction

There are no studies evaluating the role of water restriction on the resolution of ascites. However, water restriction for patients with severe hyponatraemia has become standard clinical practice. Specific vasopressin-2 receptor antagonists may be useful in the treatment of dilutional hyponatraemia.

Diuretics

Spironolactone is an aldosterone antagonist acting on the distal tubules and is the drug of choice (in a dose of 100–400 mg/day) in the initial treatment of ascites due to cirrhosis. Spironolactone achieves a better natriuresis and diuresis than a 'loop diuretic' such as frusemide. Most frequent side effects of spironolactone are those related to its antiandrogenic activity, such as decreased libido, impotence and gynaecomastia in men. Tamoxifen (20 mg twice daily) is useful in the management of gynaecomastia. Hyperkalaemia frequently limits the use of spironolactone on its own. Frusemide is a loop diuretic, which is used in a dose of 40–160 mg/day as an adjunct to spironolactone.

Generally, a 'stepped care' approach is used in the management of ascites. In patients with severe oedema, there is less need to be too restrictive about the rate of daily weight loss. Once the oedema has resolved but ascites persists, then the rate of weight loss should generally not exceed about 0.5 kg/day. Over-diuresis leads to hypovolaemia, renal impairment, hepatic encephalopathy and hyponatraemia.

Refractory ascites

This can be defined as ascites that cannot be mobilized or the early recurrence of which (i.e. after therapeutic paracentesis) cannot be satisfactorily prevented by medical therapy. This includes two different subgroups:

1. Diuretic-resistant ascites: ascites that is refractory to treatment with spironolactone 400 mg/day and frusemide 160 mg/day for at least 1 week and a salt-restricted diet of less than 90 mmol.
2. Diuretic-intractable ascites: ascites that is refractory to therapy due to the development of diuretic-induced complications that preclude the use of an effective diuretic dosage.

In patients who fail to respond, it is important to ensure that they are not consuming drugs that are rich in sodium or drugs that inhibit salt and water excretion such as NSAIDs. Compliance with dietary sodium restriction should be monitored by measurement of daily urinary sodium excretion. If urinary sodium exceeds the recommended sodium intake and the patient is failing to respond to treatment, then it can be assumed that the patient is non-compliant.

Therapeutic paracentesis

Several controlled clinical studies have demonstrated that large-volume paracentesis with colloid replacement is rapid, safe and effective. Large-volume paracentesis should be performed in a single session with volume expansion, preferably using 6–8 g of albumin/l of ascites removed. Serial paracentesis with and without albumin replacement have been evaluated in patients with tense ascites. There was a significantly higher rate of renal impairment, significant fall in serum sodium levels and a marked activation of renin–angiotensin–aldosterone system in those patients not treated with albumin. For a single paracentesis of <5 l, it has been shown that it is safe to omit volume expansion or to use non-albumin colloids.

Randomized controlled trials comparing Dextran-70 or Haemaccel with albumin suggest that these plasma expanders are clinically effective in the prevention of renal impairment. However, the use of artificial plasma expanders was associated with a significantly greater activation of renin–angiotensin–aldosterone. Analysis of data from all published studies also suggests that albumin is more effective in the prevention of hyponatraemia. With albumin, hyponatraemia occurs in only 8% compared with 17% for other plasma expanders.

Failure to give volume expansion can lead to 'post-paracentesis circulatory dysfunction' with impairment of renal function. Total paracentesis is associated with a marked reduction of intra-abdominal and inferior vena cava (IVC) pressure, leading to an immediate decrease in right atrial pressure (CVP). This is accompanied by an increase in cardiac output, a decrease in systemic vascular resistance, followed by a fall in pulmonary capillary wedge pressure and a decrease in the arterial blood pressure. The severity of post-paracentesis-circulatory dysfunction correlates inversely with patient survival.

Transjugular intrahepatic portosystemic shunt

Since elevated portal pressure is one of the main factors contributing to the pathogenesis of ascites, it is not surprising that TIPS is a highly effective treatment for refractory ascites. It functions as a side-to-side portocaval shunt. It is usually placed under local anaesthesia, and has largely replaced the use of surgically placed portocaval or mesocaval shunts. Numerous uncontrolled studies have been published assessing the effectiveness of TIPS in patients with refractory ascites. In most studies, technical success was achieved in 93–100% of cases, with control of ascites achieved in 50–92%. Prospective randomized trials have shown TIPS to be more effective in controlling ascites in up to 84% of patients compared with less than 45% in those treated with large volume paracentesis. Hepatic encephalopathy after TIPS insertion occurs in about 25% of patients and the risk is higher in those over the age of 60 years. TIPS is associated with a less favourable outcome in advanced Child–Pugh Class C patients. TIPS increases the cardiac preload and, hence, it may precipitate heart failure in those with pre-existing heart disease. TIPS insertion should be considered as a treatment option for patients who require frequent paracentesis (generally >3 a month). TIPS has also been shown to resolve hepatic hydrothorax in >70% of patients.

Spontaneous bacterial peritonitis

Spontaneous bacterial peritonitis (SBP) is the development of a mono-microbial infection of ascites in the absence of a contiguous source of infection. The prevalence of SBP in cirrhotic hospitalized patients with ascites ranges between 10% and 30%. When first described, its mortality exceeded 90%. However, in-hospital mortality can be reduced to around 20% with early diagnosis and prompt treatment.

Bacterial translocation, the phenomenon by which viable microorganisms from the intestinal lumen migrate to mesenteric lymph nodes and other extraintestinal sites, has been considered to be the main mechanism in the pathogenesis of SBP. In addition, activity of

Kupffer cells is reduced in cirrhosis. This is compounded by the fact that portosystemic shunts allow a proportion of circulating blood to escape the reticuloendothelial system, an important defensive system against bacteraemia. Fixation of complement to bacterial surfaces is a critical prerequisite for phagocytosis, and low serum concentrations of C3, C4 and haemolytic complement levels have been reported in patients with cirrhosis.

Diagnosis

Patients with SBP are frequently asymptomatic. However, a significant proportion has symptoms such as fever, abdominal pain or vomiting. Diagnosis should also be suspected in those who present with hepatic encephalopathy, impairment of renal function or peripheral leukocytosis without an obvious cause. A diagnostic paracentesis is mandatory in all patients with cirrhosis requiring hospitalization.

The diagnosis of SBP is confirmed when the ascitic neutrophil count is >250 cells/mm^3 (0.25×10^9/l) in the absence of an intra-abdominal and surgically treatable source of sepsis. Recent studies have demonstrated that using a reagent strip for leukocyte esterase designed for testing urine, the diagnosis of SBP can be made in 90% with a positive and negative predictive value of 98–99%.

Treatment

Escherichia coli, enterococci and Gram-positive cocci (mainly Streptococcus species) account for the majority of the episodes of SBP. Most published series have studied Cefotaxime as it covers 95% of the flora causing SBP and achieves high ascitic fluid concentrations. Other cephalosporins (ceftrioxone, ceftazidime) as well as coamoxiclav have been shown to be as effective in SBP. Although a large randomized study showed that albumin infusion (1.5 g/kg at diagnosis and 1 g/kg on day 3), in addition to antibiotic therapy, reduced the incidence of hepatorenal syndrome and improved survival, the conclusions of this study have been debated as the fluid support received by the control group has been considered inadequate.

Secondary prevention

Among patients who survive an episode of SBP, 70% develop a recurrence within 1 year. Oral norfloxacin (400 mg/day) reduces the probability of recurrence of SBP from 68 to 20%. In the UK, most centres use once daily ciprofloxacin 500 mg as prophylaxis against SBP.

Probability of survival at 1 year after an episode of SBP is 30–50%. Therefore, patients recovering from an episode of SBP should always be considered as a potential candidate for liver transplantation.

HEPATORENAL SYNDROME

Hepatorenal syndrome (HRS) is a functional renal failure that develops in patients with advanced cirrhosis (Table 8.10). There are two types of HRS. Type 2 HRS is a moderate

Table 8.10 International ascites club criteria for the diagnosis of hepatorenal syndrome

Major criteria
Decompensated liver disease with portal hypertension
Creatinine >1.5 mg/dl or glomerular filtration rate <40 ml/min
No hypovolaemia, ongoing bacterial infection or nephrotoxic drugs
No improvement on diuretic withdrawal and iv saline infusion (1500 ml)
Proteinuria <500 mg/day, normal renal ultrasound

Minor criteria
Urine volume <500 ml/day, sodium <10 meq/l, RBC <50/HPF, high-osmolality urine
Serum sodium <130 meq/l

renal failure that remains steady over long periods (months) and is associated with refractory ascites. Type 1 HRS is a rapidly progressive renal failure, usually developing in those with pre-existing type 2 HRS after a precipitating event such as severe bacterial infection. Splanchnic vasodilation associated with portal hypertension results in effective arterial hypovolaemia leading to activation of the sympathetic nervous system as well as the renin–angiotensin–aldosterone system, intense activation of which causes renal vasoconstriction. The kidney synthesizes vasodilatory prostaglandins and NO maintaining the homeostasis of renal perfusion. In association with a precipitating event, such as sepsis, there is a worsening of renal perfusion with activation of intrarenal vasoconstrictor mechanisms (angiotensin II, endothelin and adenosine) leading to type 1 HRS. A prolonged period of normalization of the circulatory volume over 3–4 days is needed for serum creatinine to fall.

Almost all patients with HRS Type 1 die within 2–3 weeks after the onset of renal failure. Numerous treatments have been tried for HRS over the years without any effect on prognosis. Recently, treatment with a combination of terlipressin and albumin infusion has been shown to be effective in reversing HRS. In a study involving 99 patients, renal function improved in 57% with a 25% 3-month survival and 13 patients underwent successful liver transplantation. The use of a molecular adsorbent recirculating system (MARS) in the management of HRS is currently being investigated.

HEPATIC ENCEPHALOPATHY

Hepatic encephalopathy complicates both acute and chronic liver diseases. In acute hepatic failure development of cerebral oedema can lead to cerebral herniation and death. In decompensated cirrhosis, chronic encephalopathy is a major clinical problem affecting the quality of patients' lives. The term sub-clinical encephalopathy has been replaced with 'minimal encephalopathy' as the latter is associated with impaired quality of life. Minimal encephalopathy is more likely in males with a higher Child's score and varices and with a positive response to five statements of Sickness Impact Profile.

Pathogenesis

Ammonia is still considered a key component in the pathogenesis of hepatic encephalopathy. The small bowel is quantitatively important in the generation of ammonia. A decrease in muscle mass in patients with cirrhosis reduces the ability of muscle to detoxify ammonia to glutamine. Glutamine, the product of ammonia detoxification, has been thought to lead to astrocyte swelling. Aquaporin-4, a specific water channel in the astrocyte, is a necessary route for water entry into the cells. Astrocytes in patients with chronic liver disease undergo osmotic adaptation by losing osmolytes, such as myo-inositol, taurine and glycerophosphocholine. The process of adaptation makes the brain vulnerable to a second osmotic challenge such as hyponatraemia. Many factors such as hypoxaemia, hypokalaemia and dehydration interact with ammonia. This explains the synergism observed in the development of encephalopathy. There is increasing evidence to show that functional alterations in the astrocytes result in impaired metabolic trafficking between neurons and astrocytes. Osmotic disturbances in the brain associated with cerebral oedema are seen in most patients with acute hepatic failure where there is less chance for astrocytic adaptation. Evidence from animal experiments suggests that glutamate synthesis by astrocytes triggers increased cerebral blood flow, which may contribute to the raised intracranial pressure.

Investigations

Diagnosis of hepatic encephalopathy should be based on sound clinical judgement (Table 8.11). Estimations of venous ammonia levels have been overused for the diagnosis of encephalopathy in patients with cirrhosis. To standardize neuropsychological testing in cirrhosis the 'Psychometric Hepatic Encephalopathy Score' has been proposed. This consists of six individual tests with a final score of between +6 and −18. A score lower than −4 is considered to be abnormal.

A hyper-resonant globus pallidus is a common finding in MRI of the brain of cirrhotics, but it is not an indicator of hepatic encephalopathy. Manganese accumulation is thought to be the cause of this abnormality.

Management

There has not been any major development in the treatment of hepatic encephalopathy in the last decade. Low protein diets are harmful for the hypercatabolic state in cirrhosis.

Table 8.11 Grading of hepatic encephalopathy

Grade 1	Subtle changes in sleep pattern and behaviour, best assessed by close relatives
Grade 2	Inappropriate behaviour, lethargy, slurred speech, asterexis
Grade 3	Stupor rousable by noxious stimuli
Grade 4	Coma

Nutritional recommendations include the provision of vegetable and dairy protein to meet increased metabolic needs.

Despite a lack of well-designed clinical trials, lactulose, a non-absorbable disaccharide, continues to be used, both orally and as an enema, as it inhibits ammonia producing bacteria in the gut as well as acting as a laxative. Antibiotics such as neomycin, metronidazole and non-absorbable rifaximin may be useful for short term (1–2 weeks) treatment. Zinc therapy has been considered to improve urea synthesis in malnourished patients. Sodium benzoate and phenylacetate, which are used in children with hyperammonaemia to facilitate elimination of nitrogen, have not been adequately tested in adults. A single dose of intravenous flumazanil (1 mg in 20 ml of 0.9% sodium chloride infused over 3–5 min) a central benzodiazepine receptor antagonist, results in transient improvement in a small sub-group of patients.

SPECIFIC LIVER DISORDERS

Gilbert's syndrome

Gilbert's syndrome is a common, benign, recessively-inherited condition in which the bilirubin level is higher than normal due to a deficiency of its glucuronidation by the liver. It affects 2–5% of the population. There is no associated increased morbidity. Those affected may notice jaundice at times of illness or fasting. In most cases it is discovered at routine testing of liver function. The likelihood of Gilbert's syndrome is so high when there is an isolated raised bilirubin found by chance, with normal red cell count and indices (thus excluding haemolysis as another cause), that further investigation is not indicated and the person can be reassured. Occasionally, it can cause confusion and in such cases genetic testing for an additional TA dinucleotide in the promoter region of the gene encoding for uridine diphosphate glucuronosyl transferase (UGT) on chromosome 2 can confirm the diagnosis.

Viral hepatitis

Viral hepatitis is much more common in the UK than is appreciated. Between 0.5 and 0.75% of the UK population is infected with hepatitis C virus (HCV) and 0.5% are hepatitis B surface antigen positive. Up to 2% of the UK population has evidence of prior hepatitis B virus (HBV) infection as evidenced by anti-core antibodies.

Hepatitis C

HCV is mainly spread by blood. The major mechanism of infection in the UK is intravenous drug use. This accounts for approximately 75% of cases. In the pre-HCV testing era (up to 1991), blood products also carried a risk of transmission. Blood products account for about 15% of HCV infection in the UK currently, although this proportion is declining, as new infections via this route are exceptionally rare. The haemophiliac population, prior to heat treatment of factor VIII concentrates in 1985, were particularly at risk with over 90% of patients with severe haemophilia being infected. The introduction of antibody screening of blood donors for antibodies to HCV has dramatically reduced the risk of infection by this route, with an estimated risk currently of 1 in 200 000 units. Worldwide, medical interventions or intra-familial transmission appear to be a major route of infection, but this is relatively rare in the UK. Sexual transmission does occur but is rare; most studies report only 1–4% positivity of partners in the absence of an alternative risk factor. Vertical transmission from mother to child can also occur. The risk of infection is between 1 and 6% and does not appear to be influenced by the mode of delivery or breast feeding.

In infected individuals, approximately 80% go on to become chronically viraemic. In this group who remain HCV RNA positive in serum, there is a risk of developing chronic liver disease, cirrhosis and hepatocellular carcinoma. In a number of different studies in different geographic areas the time from infection to the development of cirrhosis appears to be 20–30 years with hepatocellular carcinoma developing, on average, 10 years later. There are a number of factors that appear to either protect or enhance the risk of developing hepatic fibrosis. The outlook is worse in males, in patients infected at an older age and in those who drink excess alcohol. When all these risk factors are present, cirrhosis may develop in less than 10 years from infection. In low-risk groups, the time from infection to cirrhosis may exceed 50 years.

Assessing and treating hepatitis C

The key investigations in chronic HCV infection are shown below:

- Antibody to HCV
- Polymerase chain reaction (PCR) detection of HCV RNA in blood
- Viral genotype
- Viral load
- Activity of liver disease on biopsy
- Stage of liver fibrosis on biopsy.

About 80% of infected individuals will become chronically infected. The presence of antibody in the context of a patient with normal liver enzymes who is PCR-negative usually implies cleared infection and, if repeat testing confirms this, no follow-up is required.

Therapy for HCV evolved rapidly over the decade following its discovery in 1989. Current best therapy is pegylated interferon alpha and ribavirin. Overall cure rates, now with either the 12 kD or 40 kD pegylated interferons combined with ribavirin, are around 55% (Fig. 8.8). The National Institute for Clinical Effectiveness (NICE) has issued guidelines for the therapy of HCV that are based on the severity of liver injury and has approved pegylated interferon alpha and ribavirin as standard therapy for HCV. This implies that liver biopsy is still expected in the management of HCV infection, although the high success rates in genotype 2/3 infection make this somewhat controversial.

The major determinate of response to therapy is viral genotype. Genotypes 2 or 3 respond well to therapy with cure rates in excess of 75% with the use of 6 months treatment with

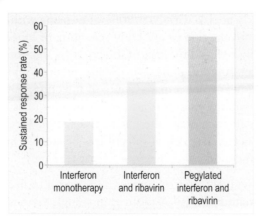

Fig. 8.8
Cure rates with evolving therapy for chronic hepatitis C

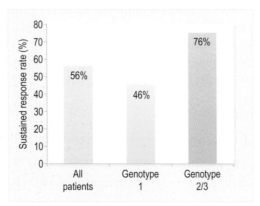

Fig. 8.9
Effect of viral genotypes on response rates to 40 kD pegylated interferon and ribavirin therapy

pegylated interferon and low-dose (800 mg per day) ribavirin. There is no benefit from longer or higher dose therapy. Genotype 1 is more resistant to therapy and requires 12 months' treatment with pegylated interferon and ribavirin at 1000–12 000 mg per day (based on body weight) with an overall sustained response rate of around 45% (Fig. 8.9). Genotype 4 behaves more like genotype 1. Other genotypes are rare in the UK and there are no data from trials about outcome or duration of therapy. The initial trials of standard interferon and ribavirin combination therapy established that there are other factors that influence response rates (Table 8.12). These factors also apply to pegylated therapy, which should be taken into account when planning dose and duration of treatment. Adherence to therapy is important to obtain maximum cure rates and the lower cure rates in patients with cirrhosis are primarily due to the fact that they can tolerate treatment less well. Many will start with thrombocytopenia or neutropenia, limiting the dose possible.

Early virological clearance from serum is strongly associated with cure. In genotype-1 infected patients who remain PCR positive at 12 weeks and fail to achieve a 2 log drop in

Table 8.12 Adverse response factors for pegylated interferon and ribavirin therapy

Factor	Significance of adverse factor
Genotype 1 or 4	Response rates fall from 75 to 45%
Viral load	$>2 \times 10^6$ copies per ml (high load) reduces response rate by approximately 10% in genotype 1 infection
Age >40	There is an 8% decrease in response rates for every decade increase in age
High body mass index	Patients over 90 kg have a 10% lower chance of cure
Severe hepatic fibrosis	Patients with cirrhosis tolerate therapy less well and have 10–15% lower chance of cure
Male gender	Males tend to be older and have more fibrotic liver disease, but even controlling for these factors have a 5–7% less chance of response
Afro-Caribbean ethnic group	Reduces response rates by 15%. The reason is unclear

Table 8.13 Significant side effects of interferon and ribavirin therapy

Side effect	% with side effect and impact on therapy
Flu-like syndrome	Occurs in 75%. Usually worst at initiation of therapy and rarely leads to discontinuation. Paracetamol helpful. Less severe with PEG interferons
Anaemia	A drop in Hb of about 3 g/dl is usual, caused by both haemolysis (ribavarin) and marrow depression (inteferon). Dose reduction and/or epoetin may be used if very symptomatic, especially for angina and heart failure. Drugs to be stopped if Hb <8.5
Neutropenia	A drop in WBC occurs in 80% of treated patients. Severe enough to cause discontinuation in 5% (Neutrophil count <0.5)
Thrombocytopenia	A fall occurs in 70%. Only usually significant in cirrhotics. Rare cause of discontinuation
Thyroid abnormalities	Occurs in 5%. Can be over or underactive. If under is usually permanent. Only common side effect to persist after stopping therapy
Depression	Mood altered in 50% or more. Clinical depression in 10%. Responds to usual therapy, but requires close monitoring

viral load, there is a 98% probability of non-response. This can be used clinically to discontinue therapy in patients who will not benefit from it.

Side effects of therapy are common and can be serious (Table 8.13). In reality, most contraindications to therapy are only relative and successful treatment can be provided even for patients with prior psychotic illnesses with good liaison with psychiatric colleagues. It is not possible for the 'amateur' to treat HCV successfully as it requires a significant amount of backup from nurse specialists, virology and histopathology to provide successful therapy. Response rates to treatment are very dependent on adherence to therapy and this can only be achieved with a high level of patient support. Up to 20% of hepatitis-C-infected patients are co-infected with HIV and all patients should be offered testing for this virus. Treating co-infected patients can be undertaken but it is complex and should be left to experts.

Table 8.14 Key tests in hepatitis B virus (HBV) infection and their implications (outside the setting of acute HBV)

Serological test/marker	Clinical implication
Hepatitis B surface antigen	Presence implies chronic infection
Hepatitis B e antigen	Presence implies replication of wild-type virus
Hepatitis B DNA	Direct measure of HBV replication
Anti-core antibodies	Presence implies cleared infection and immunity
Anti-surface antibodies	Vaccine-induced immunity

Acute HCV is relatively uncommonly identified as only about 2% of infections are icteric. It is, however, important to recognize it as treatment in the acute phase, even using interferon alpha monotherapy, has up to a 98% cure rate. Anyone presenting with an otherwise unexplained icteric illness who has a risk factor for HCV infection should be screened by PCR (antibodies will not develop for up to 3 months) and if detected should be offered treatment.

Hepatitis B

HBV is a common pathogen. Despite misinformation in most textbooks, it is relatively common in the UK (with a 0.5% prevalence of HbsAg positivity). Its major mode of spread is by vertical transmission with relatively small numbers of sexually transmitted/IVDU transmitted cases in the UK. It is, however, a disease predominantly of immigrants to the UK. The migrant populations from the Indian subcontinent, South East Asia and, more recently, Eastern Europe have a high rate of infection. Identification of an infected individual should prompt testing of other family members because of the mode of spread.

Hepatitis B serology and stages of infection

HBV has a highly unusual genetic structure, with a circular, partially double-stranded DNA genome. The HBV RNA template is encapsulated in hepatitis B core antigen (HBcAg) particles and reverse transcribed to produce negative-strand DNA. This is then used to synthesize an incomplete positive DNA strand and the virion is encapsulated with HBsAg before excretion from the cell. This complex process and the resulting virus components form the basis of serological tests essential in managing HBV (Table 8.14).

Liver-cell damage in both acute and chronic HBV infection is immunologically mediated. Cell-mediated and humoral immune responses occur in HBV infection and both are probably important in limiting and eliminating infection. There is invariably a humoral immune response directed against HBcAg and usually against HBsAg, but this response alone is not the cause of hepatitis as evidenced by liver disease in agammaglobulinaemic patients. The responses of HLA class I restricted cytotoxic T lymphocytes are thought to be the major mechanism of liver cell injury. The fact that patients with production of HBsAg alone in hepatocytes usually have little inflammatory liver disease suggests that the target of this attack is likely to be core antigen.

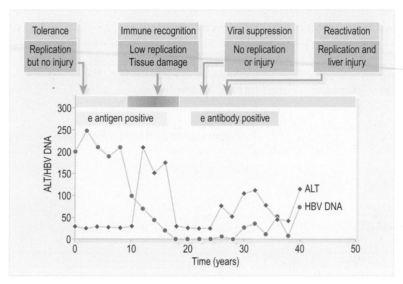

Fig. 8.10
The natural history of chronic hepatitis B infection

Chronic HBV infection occurs in phases, depending on the degree of immune response to the virus (Fig. 8.10). This is particularly true of patients infected in the first few weeks of life. If infected when the immune response is 'immature', there is initially little or no immune response to HBV. The levels of HBV DNA in serum are very high and the hepatocytes contain abundant HBsAg and HBcAg, but little or no ongoing hepatocyte death is seen on a liver biopsy because of the defective immune response. This state persists for a variable period of time; usually the degree of immune recognition increases over some years. When immune recognition starts to occur, the level of HBV DNA tends to fall and the liver biopsy shows increasing inflammatory liver disease. This inflammation and hepatocyte death produces hepatic fibrosis. Once this phase of infection is initiated there are two major possible outcomes: either the immune response is adequate, the virus being inactivated and then removed from the system, or the attempt at removal results in extensive fibrosis, distortion of the normal liver architecture and death from the complications of cirrhosis.

A third phase of HBV infection is now recognized (Fig. 8.10). This occurs late in the natural history of the immune response against HBV. In situations where the wild-type virus is inactivated but not eradicated, characterized by hepatitis B surface antigen positivity, e antigen negativity and undetectable levels of HBV DNA, there is still virus present in hepatocytes. This virus will be present in a number of forms, with viral mutants commonly produced. It is now well recognized that some of these mutant species can replicate in the presence of an adequate immune response against wild-type virus. This leads to re-emergence of HBV DNA in serum and can lead to progressive liver injury. These mutant strains may account for up to 60% of all replicating HBV infection in Europe. Recognition of this situation clinically is both important and relatively simple. It is important because reactivation of HBV replication carries a significant risk of the

Table 8.15 Basic management of hepatitis-B-infected patients

Clinical setting	Management
HBeAg positive HBV DNA high (>10^6/ml) Normal ALT	6-monthly ALT/HBV DNA No need for liver biopsy Therapy not indicated or effective
HBeAg positive HBV DNA low ALT elevated	Liver biopsy Treat with interferon if significant disease (lamivudine if cirrhosis)
HBeAg negative HBV DNA <10^4 + normal ALT	6-monthly ALT/HBV DNA
HBeAg negative HBV DNA >10^4 or Abnormal ALT	Liver biopsy Treat with lamivudine if significant disease

development of hepatic fibrosis and cirrhosis, and therapy is different from the usual 'wild type', e-antigen-producing HBV. It is simple to recognize as abnormal transaminases and significant levels of HBV DNA (>10^3 copies per ml) are present in the serum in patients who are HBsAg positive, but e antigen negative.

Diagnosing past HBV infection or establishing immunity to vaccine is easy serologically. If the virus is cleared after infection with HBV, antibodies to all viral antigens can be detected. The levels of most of these in blood, however, decline with time. This is particularly true of anti-HBsAg: after 1 year, most patients' levels of antibody have fallen below the level of detection in most commercially available assays. Despite this low level, immunity is still sufficient to prevent re-infection. Natural immunity is proven by the presence of IgG antibodies to HBcAg. These are a highly reliable marker of past infection and remain at detectable levels for a long period. Vaccine-induced immunity is directed purely against HBsAg epitopes and hence a vaccinated person will have detectable levels of anti-HBsAg, but no anti-HBcAg.

The key aim in any therapy for HBV is to inhibit viral replication. There is clear evidence that cessation of replication results in a reduction in inflammatory liver disease and improved outcome. Clearance of HBsAg as a result of therapy is uncommon. Hence, patients remain infected and there is a possibility of reactivation following therapy. The treatment used and its duration of therapy are substantially different in e antigen positive and negative patients with replicating HBV.

Management of e-antigen-positive patients (Table 8.15)

Interferon   Interferon-alpha was first shown to be effective for some patients who have e antigen positive HBV infection in the 1980s and it remains an effective therapy. Pegylated interferons are at least as effective and are more convenient for patients because of once rather than three times weekly administration. There are a number of factors that

Table 8.16 Factors affecting response to interferon therapy in e antigen-positive hepatitis-B infection

Factor	Effect on response
Elevated ALT/AST	Patients with normal ALT respond less well
Active interface hepatitis on biopsy	Patients with it respond better
Age	Younger patients respond better
HBV DNA level	Low levels (<10^6 copies/ml) respond better

can help predict the likelihood of response to treatment with interferon alpha and these help in the selection of patients who have the best chance of response to therapy (Table 8.16). Treatment of e antigen positive HBV requires 4 months' interferon therapy. If standard interferon is used it is in a higher dose than used for HCV infection (9 million units three times per week), but the same dose of pegylated interferons as for HCV. Increased duration of treatment does not significantly improve outcome. Overall, the probability of response to interferon therapy in chronic hepatitis B is between 25 and 40%.

Treatment of hepatitis B in patients who have significant fibrotic liver disease is rewarding because they have a relatively high probability of response and have most to gain from cessation of viral replication. Many patients have a substantial improvement in liver function if viral replication is stopped, but treatment in such patients does carry an increased risk. Interferon therapy produces viral clearance, at least in part, by inducing immune-mediated killing of infected hepatocytes and hence a transient hepatitis can cause severe decompensation requiring liver transplantation. In practice the risk of decompensation in Child's A patients is small, but lamivudine, which does not carry this risk, is the preferred therapy in patients with Child's B and C disease.

The most frequent pattern of response to interferon-alpha is shown in Figure 8.11. The HBV DNA level falls rapidly after initiation of interferon therapy. This is followed by a

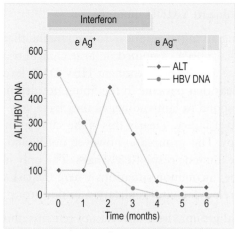

Fig. 8.11
Response to interferon therapy in e-antigen-positive hepatitis B infection

217

marked rise in transaminase values. This represents immune-mediated clearance of virus and HBV DNA levels quickly fall to undetectable levels. This is then followed within a few weeks by seroconversion to HBeAg-negative, HBeAb-positive status with complete normalization of transaminases. This type of response is seen in 25% of treated patients. Hepatitis B surface antigen usually remains positive, with a small proportion of patients clearing all markers of viral infection either during interferon therapy (2%) or many months after it (6%). A further proportion of patients show a late seroconversion some months after therapy.

Lamivudine   lamivudine, a nucleoside analogue, is a potent inhibitor of HBV DNA replication. Lamivudine has virtually no side effects, is given orally and has now been widely used in patients who have chronic HBV infection. Lamivudine has been shown to produce rapid inhibition of HBV DNA production and can result in e antigen/e antibody seroconversion and sustained inhibition of viral replication in approximately 30% of patients given 12 months' therapy. Its main limitation is the development of viral resistance. Emergence of lamivudine-resistant HBV is increasingly common with prolonged treatment. Genotypic resistance is detectable in 14–32% of patients after 1 year and increases to 38%, 49% and 66% after 2, 3 and 4 years, respectively. The resistance to lamivudine occurs because of mutations in the HBV polymerase gene (YMDD mutants), which allow the virus to replicate in the presence of lamivudine.

The emergence of lamivudine-resistant HBV is not necessarily associated with phenotypic resistance, i.e. loss of clinical benefit. If this occurs, the decision whether to continue with lamivudine or stop treatment depends on the clinical setting. There is no doubt that lamivudine resistance can be associated with severe histological liver damage, particularly in the post-transplant setting. It is, however, clear that YMDD mutants of HBV are generally less replication competent than wild-type HBV, with lower levels of HBV DNA present in serum. This means that therapeutic benefit can continue even if viral replication returns.

The optimal duration of lamivudine therapy remains uncertain. Approximately 35% of patients will have sero-converted to e antigen negative after 1 year of therapy and lamivudine can be stopped with continued monitoring. In patients who do not sero-convert, therapy is usually continued, but with an ever increasing risk of resumption of viral replication due to YMDD mutants.

Factors predicting an initial response to lamivudine therapy (removing HBV DNA from serum initially) have been examined in large clinical trials. The most important predictors of initial response are the pre-treatment HBV DNA level and the degree of inflammatory response. It is clear that patients in the 'immunotolerant' phase of their infection are those least likely to respond to lamivudine, as they have very high levels of HBV DNA and minimal or no liver injury. Clearly this is the same group who will not respond to interferon therapy. This group are, however, not ill and can be safely monitored without therapy until the immune response changes. The only indication to try lamivudine in this context would be uncommon situations where the risk of transmission to others was high. The chances of removing viral replication in this group are, however, low.

The other clinical group where uncertainty remains about lamivudine therapy is those with significant liver disease. There is no doubt that in patients with decompensated

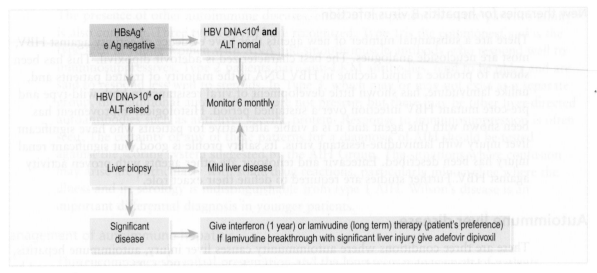

Fig. 8.12
Management of e-antigen-negative chronic hepatitis B infection

cirrhosis and ongoing viral replication, lamivudine is effective at suppressing viral activity and that liver function recovers. The only issue is the potential for long-term viral breakthrough in this group, which could preclude liver transplantation. This issue is likely to be resolved with the advent of alternative antiviral agents, which can be effective in the pre-transplant setting.

Treatment of e-antigen-negative chronic hepatitis B (Fig. 8.12)

In Europe, up to 60% of all replicating HBV infections now are in the late phase of infection, where initial inactivation of replication has occurred with later re-activation with so-called pre-core mutant viruses that can, presumably, avoid the immune response. It is well described that these mutants are generally much less responsive to therapy with interferon alpha. Patients may show a good rate of initial response to interferon with disappearance of HBV DNA from serum, but very frequently relapse after cessation of treatment. There is now evidence that giving interferon therapy for longer in such patients may improve the rate of loss of viral replication. A regimen of 6 million units three times a week for 24 months has been shown to produce a loss of viral replication in 30% of patients.

Lamivudine has been shown to be effective at removing HBV DNA from serum and normalizing transaminases. Unfortunately, this effect is not maintained in all patients, approximately 50% being HBV DNA-positive again in 18 months. This virological breakthrough is progressive in terms of the level of HBV DNA and accompanied by the return of biochemical and histological hepatitis in the majority over time. The management of pre-core mutant HBV, therefore, remains imperfect, but lamivudine clearly has a role in patients with significant liver injury.

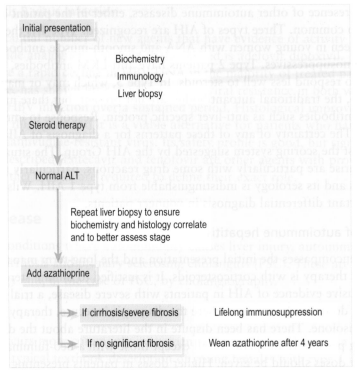

Fig. 8.13
Key steps in management of auto-immune hepatitis

diagnosis with the advent of widespread testing of liver enzymes and immunological profiles. M2 anti-mitochondrial antibodies are now diagnostic, less than 5% of patients with PBC do not have them, less if ELISA techniques are used to screen. Patients with M2 antimitochondrial antibodies and normal liver enzymes still have the disease and can be shown to have histological changes on liver biopsy and will develop deranged LFTs in follow-up.

Liver biopsy is not required to diagnose PBC. Its only role is in staging of disease and establishing prognosis where it still has utility for some patients. The sampling variability in PBC is greater than in conditions like HCV infection and this limits its usefulness.

Hepatomegaly is common in PBC and portal hypertension occurs early. Bone disease is possibly more frequent in patients with PBC, but not sufficiently severe to justify screening unless severely cholestatic and considering transplantation where osteoporosis will be accelerated and fractures are a significant cause of post-transplant morbidity. Cholesterol levels are almost always elevated in this biliary disease, but patients with PBC have a relatively low cardiovascular mortality and treatment is not usually required.

Management of PBC involves dealing with the symptoms not associated with severe liver disease (pruritus, Sjogren's syndrome and fatigue, Table 8.18) and an attempt to prevent

Table 8.18 Symptoms of primary biliary cirrhosis and treatment

Symptom	Therapy
Pruritus	Antihistamines at night Keep skin moisturized Colestyramine (start with low dose and build up) Rifampicin (cautious watch on LFTs) Naltrexone
Fatigue	No specific therapy Occasionally anti-depressants help
Sjogren's syndrome	Replacement tears and saliva

the development of severe liver disease by the use of ursodeoxycholic acid (UDCA). Although the data are far from convincing, it does appear that UDCA improves transplant-free survival in a number of large trials. The evidence is well summarized in a recent Cochrane review (Gluud & Christensen 2002) and most patients with PBC should be offered therapy. It has few significant side effects, but is expensive.

Primary sclerosing cholangitis

Primary sclerosing cholangitis (PSC) can affect bile ducts of any size. Unlike PBC it is more common in men and presents in young adult life (median age 45 years). Patients with ulcerative colitis are at markedly increased risk – about 1–3% of colitics will develop PSC and 70% of patients with PSC have colitis.

Diagnosis

Diagnosis of PSC is by cholangiography. Liver biopsy is less useful as the disease is characteristically patchy in distribution. It should be suspected in patients with cholestatic LFTs for which no other explanation is found. MRI cholangiography is now able to provide sufficiently detailed images of the biliary tree to make ERCP unnecessary in all patients, but it is still required in the majority. Other tests may point towards a diagnosis of PSC (ANCA positivity in 65%, ANA positivity in 55%) but none are helpful in isolation. There is a variant of PSC which affects only small intrahepatic bile ducts. This usually presents with cholestatic LFTs and the diagnosis is made on liver biopsy findings after an apparently normal cholangiogram. It has a generally better prognosis than PSC where duct changes are present at ERCP.

Management of primary sclerosing cholangitis

The management revolves around treatment of stricturing disease. This may present as recurrent cholangitis. The interventions possible are the use of UDCA, which is not proven to prevent progression of disease, although there is some suggestion that high doses may help, ERCP and stenting, rotating antibiotics and, if intractable, liver transplantation.

Alcohol-related liver disease

Alcohol excess is the commonest cause of end-stage liver disease in the UK and is part of a huge spectrum of illness caused by alcohol. The risk of developing liver disease in heavy drinkers is highly variable and dependent on a number of factors, the most important of which are, as yet, poorly defined genetic susceptibilities. If an individual is susceptible to alcohol-related injury then the risk of developing it is proportional to the level of alcohol intake. The pattern of drinking may play a role (binge drinking versus constant heavy intake), but this is controversial. Women are more susceptible than men (lower body weight, higher body fat and differing enzymatic degradation) and there has been a substantial rise in women presenting with severe liver disease due to alcohol over the last decade. In England in 2001, 21% of men had drunk more than eight units on at least 1 day in the preceding week and 9% of women more than six units. There is a worrying increase in the alcohol intake of children, with 24% of 11–15 year olds reporting that they had drunk alcohol in the previous week. The mean intake in those who did drink rose from five units in 1990 to 8.4 units in 2002. There are 5000 deaths per year from cirrhosis in the UK and the majority of these are alcohol related.

Liver disease due to alcohol can present acutely (alcoholic hepatitis) or with decompensated cirrhosis. The two often co-exist. Chronic liver disease due to alcohol is characterized by a number of histological processes (Fig. 8.1), key among which are accumulation of fat in hepatocytes together with evidence of liver cell damage (Mallory's hyaline, neutrophil infiltration). Very profound hepatocellular dysfunction is common.

Alcoholic hepatitis

Alcoholic hepatitis is, by definition, a histological diagnosis, but there is a recognizable clinical syndrome of alcoholic hepatitis requiring the following diagnostic features: jaundice, a history of alcohol excess, fever, leukocytosis and hepatomegaly. If present, the severity and mortality of alcoholic hepatitis is determined by the degree of hepatocellular dysfunction as described in the Maddrey discriminant function:

$$\frac{\text{plasma bilirubin } \mu\text{mol/l}}{17} + 2.4 \times [\text{patient's prothrombin time} - \text{control time in seconds}]$$

The 30-day mortality is 35–45% if the score exceeds 32. It should be noted that while Maddrey's original assessment of alcoholic hepatitis was only applied to patients with hepatic encephalopathy, many subsequent studies have used the discriminant function without encephalopathy being present.

It is key to the patient's long-term future that alcohol intake is minimized. A proportion of patients presented with a life-threatening illness will stop without significant interventions from the alcohol services, but many will not. Reduction in intake, but not abstinence, is a reasonable strategy in patients who do not have cirrhosis, but requires monitoring. Reduction in intake is important; even if abstinence is not achieved in patients with severe liver disease, reducing intake by 50% in patients with cirrhosis prolongs survival by 150%. Simply telling patients not to drink has an effect, but this is greatly enhanced by expert follow-up, at least in the short-term. Anti-craving drugs such as acamprosate have been widely used, but clearly have a limited role.

In the acute setting of alcoholic hepatitis, abstinence is taken for granted in this hospitalized population, although there is evidence that it is not achieved by a significant minority of patients, who continue to drink alcohol even though hospitalized. Careful supervision is important as is proper management of alcohol withdrawal and clear rules about abstaining from alcohol.

There are a number of medical therapies that have been used for acute alcoholic hepatitis. The longest standing of these is corticosteroids. A large number of studies have been performed, providing often opposing results. There is a general consensus that, if steroids have an effect, it is of relatively small magnitude and possibly greatest in females with active alcoholic hepatitis on biopsy where there may be a survival benefit at 30 days. No study has shown an improved survival at 1 year in steroid-treated groups compared to best supportive therapy, which includes nutritional support. If steroids are given, the accepted dose is 40 mg per day for 4 weeks. With such short-term therapy, there is no need to tail down the dose.

There is a single study showing survival benefit for patients treated for alcoholic hepatitis with pentoxifylline. This at least has the benefit of being a safe, oral therapy. It is important to recognize that the reduction in mortality seen in the trial of pentoxifylline was primarily due to a reduction in renal failure in the treated group. Further trials to confirm its effect are required.

Non-alcoholic fatty liver disease (NAFLD)

Non-alcoholic fatty liver disease includes a spectrum of clinicopathologic conditions characterized by lipid deposition in the hepatocytes in patients without a history of excess alcohol ingestion. The term NAFLD includes hepatic steatosis alone and non-alcoholic steatohepatitis (NASH), wherein there is lobular inflammation in addition to one of the following histological features:

1. Ballooning degeneration
2. Sinusoidal fibrosis
3. Mallory's hyaline.

The end-stage of NAFLD is thought to be cirrhosis (often labelled cryptogenic), wherein the typical histological changes of NAFLD may not be apparent.

Epidemiology

With the increasing incidence of obesity and type 2 diabetes, the incidence of NAFLD has also increased over the past decade. Although its true prevalence is unknown, NAFLD has been estimated to affect 10–25% of the general population. The prevalence of NASH is 1–5% in the general population, increasing to 20–33% in those with chronic elevation of liver enzymes. NAFLD occurs in about 2–3% of lean individuals compared with 20% in

Table 8.23 Indications for liver biopsy during the investigation of patients with haemochromatosis

Clinical signs of liver disease
Age >40 years especially with excess alcohol intake
Raised AST especially when other diagnosis are considered
Ferritin >1000 ng/ml
Platelets <200 x 10^9/l
Compound heterozygotes with raised iron indices/raised liver enzymes or clinical signs of liver disease
To calculate hepatic iron index in those who are neither C282Y homozygotes nor compound heterozygotes

Treatment

There is overwhelming evidence to show that regular phlebotomy before the development of cirrhosis or diabetes significantly reduces morbidity and mortality in patients with hereditary haemochromatosis. One phlebotomy removing 500 ml of blood (250 mg of iron) weekly or biweekly is appropriate in most patients. The haematocrit may be measured before each venesection, checking it is no lower than 20% below the starting value. Ferritin should be measured after 10 phlebotomies. The frequency of phlebotomy should be reduced when ferritin falls below 50 ng/ml. Most patients would then require at least 2–4 phlebotomies per year to maintain the ferritin below 50 ng/ml. Patients should be advised to consume red meat in moderation, although strict dietary restrictions are unnecessary. Excess alcohol and iron supplementation should be avoided. Large amounts of vitamin C has been reported to be associated with fatal arrhythmias in those with cardiomyopathy, presumably due to oxidative injury caused by rapid mobilization of stored iron. Therapy improves symptoms such as fatigue, and liver related abnormalities except cirrhosis resolve. Cardiomyopathy and arrhythmias also improve or resolve completely. Diabetes mellitus improves initially, although it does not usually disappear. Arthropathy and hypogonadotrophic hypogonadism due to haemochromatosis do not improve with phlebotomy.

Cirrhosis once established before phlebotomy has been thought to persist. Patients with decompensated cirrhosis may still need liver transplantation, although survival following liver transplantation has been lower than that in other indications for transplantation. The higher mortality is related to cardiac arrhythmias and infection. About 10–30% of patients with haemochromatosis die due to hepatocellular carcinoma and the risk of this is increased 200-fold in patients with cirrhosis. Elevation of serum alpha fetoprotein is seen in only one-third of the patients. Regular imaging with ultrasound scan is, therefore, the only realistic option for surveillance.

Wilson's disease

Copper is an essential trace element and is involved in diverse cellular functions such as mitochondrial respiration, antioxidant defence, melanin production, neurotransmitter (dopamine) metabolism, connective-tissue formation, iron homeostasis and peptide biosynthesis. Wilson's disease is an autosomal recessive inherited disorder of copper metabolism resulting in liver and/or neuropsychiatric disease. It occurs in all ethnic groups with a worldwide prevalence of 3 per 100 000 population. Wilson ATPase (ATP7B) is the product of the gene located on chromosome 13. Molecular genetic analysis of patients with Wilson's disease has revealed over 200 distinct mutations and most patients are compound heterozygotes. In hepatocytes, Wilson ATPase resides in the trans-Golgi network transporting copper into the secretory pathway leading to its incorporation into apocaeruloplasmin and excretion into bile. Biliary excretion is the only mechanism of copper elimination. Excessive accumulation of copper in the hepatocyte cytoplasm eventually results in cellular necrosis, leakage of copper into plasma and deposition in extrahepatic tissues.

Diagnosis

Patients with cirrhosis, neurologic manifestations and Kayser-Fleischer rings are easily diagnosed as having Wilson's disease. Increased awareness and systematic evaluation has enabled the diagnosis to be made earlier before the development of severe neurological complications and Kayser–Fleischer rings. The latter is present in about 50% of those without neurological symptoms and 10% of asymptomatic subjects. Most patients with Wilson's disease have some degree of liver disease even in the asymptomatic stage. Liver disease manifests itself usually between the ages of 8 and 18 years and the first presentation with liver disease is rare below the age of 5 years and over 40 years. Liver manifestations include asymptomatic hepatomegaly, raised enzymes, acute or chronic hepatitis, acute hepatic failure and cirrhosis. Other uncommon manifestations include hypercalciuria and nephrocalcinosis, chondrocalcinosis and osteoarthritis, sunflower cataracts and cardiac manifestations.

Acute hepatic failure due to Wilson's disease resembles that from other aetiologies and accounts for 6–12% of acute liver failures referred for transplantation. Acute hepatic failure is more common in women. A high index of suspicion is essential for the diagnosis since these patients require urgent liver transplantation to survive. A pattern indicative of Wilson's disease is Coombs-negative haemolytic anaemia, a relatively modest rise in serum transaminases (<500 units/l), normal or subnormal alkaline phosphatase and rapid progression to renal failure. An alkaline phosphate (unit/litre) to total bilirubin (µmol/l) ratio below 2 has been considered useful in the diagnosis, but this has not been confirmed in larger series.

The diagnosis of Wilson's disease in patients presenting with liver diseases is often difficult. None of the commonly used laboratory tests (listed in Table 8.24) alone allows a certain diagnosis and usually a combination of clinical presentation and laboratory tests is necessary to establish the diagnosis. Molecular genetic testing for diagnosis is cumbersome because of the number of mutations, each of which is rare and most patients are compound heterozygotes. Multiplex polymerase chain reaction should make mutational analysis for diagnosis feasible in the future. Currently it is only useful for screening the family of an index case with a known mutation.

Treatment

The mainstay of treatment for Wilson's disease remains life-long pharmacological treatment, but the choice of drug mostly depends on physician preference in the absence

Table 8.24 Laboratory tests for the diagnosis of Wilson's disease

Test	Typical findings	Limitations
Serum caeruloplasmin	<20 mg/dl	Low positive predictive value if used for screening Low in malabsorption, heterozygotes High with acute inflammation, pregnancy, contraceptive pills
Serum 'free' copper	>25 µg/dl	Dependent on the quality of assay High in chronic cholestasis, acute hepatic failure, poisoning
24-h urinary copper	>40 µg (0.6 µmol)/24 h	High in heterozygotes, chronic liver disease, autoimmune hepatitis, contamination
Urinary copper with D-penicillamine	>1600 µg (25 µmol)/24 h	Standardized only in children
Liver histology	Detection of copper by histochemical methods	Highly variable Present in chronic cholestasis Pathognomonic changes (focal copper stores by rhodanine stain) seen in about 10%
Hepatic copper	>75 g/g dry weight	96% sensitive, 90% specific

of comparative studies. Initial treatment for symptomatic patients should include chelating agents. Penicillamine mobilizes the copper and increases its urinary excretion and a daily dose of 1–1.5 g of penicillamine has been considered the 'gold standard' for therapy. To prevent deficiency induced by penicillamine, pyridoxine should be supplemented. About 20% of patients develop significant side effects on penicillamine. Trientine (750–1500 mg/day) is a copper chelator that is as effective with far fewer side effects. Zinc (zinc sulphate and zinc acetate) interferes with the uptake of copper from the gastrointestinal tract and also induces enterocyte metallothionein, which is an endogenous chelator of metals. Zinc has been used successfully as a first-line therapy as well as maintenance treatment in patients with symptomatic Wilson's disease. But in up to 15% of those who received zinc therapy as a first-line treatment, neurological symptoms worsened, requiring treatment with chelating agents.

Liver transplantation is the treatment of choice in patients with acute hepatic failure and decompensated cirrhosis. However, the role of transplantation in those with predominantly neurological symptoms is still uncertain.

Alpha-1-antitrypsin deficiency

Alpha-1-antitrypsin (AT) is a secretory glycoprotein predominantly derived from the liver that inhibits destructive neutrophil elastase. More than 75 variants of alpha-1-AT have been described, each inherited as autosomal codominant. Variants are defined by abnormal migration in serum phenotype analysis (by isoelectric focussing or agarose electrophoresis) and assigned a Pi (protease inhibitor) type. The most common normal variant is PiM found in over 95% of the population. The most common deficiency variant is PiZ and homozygosity (PiZZ) affects 1 in 1600–1800 live births. Liver disease affects 10–15% of PiZZ individuals. It is still unclear whether PiMZ state is associated with liver injury. Alpha-1-AT deficiency is associated with about 85–90% reduction in plasma levels. Injury to the lungs occurs by loss-of-function of alpha-1-AT while, in the liver, mutant protein is unable to traverse secretory pathways and hence is retained in the endoplasmic reticulum. The hepatotoxic effect is due to mitochondrial injury, caspase activation and release of free radicals.

Alpha-1-AT deficiency is the most common genetic cause of liver disease in children. It can present with neonatal hepatitis syndrome or with decompensated liver disease and portal hypertension in older children. In adults, it can present with raised liver enzymes, chronic hepatitis, cirrhosis, portal hypertension or hepatocellular carcinoma of unknown origin. Lung disease (emphysema) does not usually become manifest until the third or fourth decade. On liver biopsy, characteristic periodic acid Schiff positive, diastase resistant globules are seen in the hepatocytes. Liver disease is not always progressive and some affected children can lead normal lives for many years.

Avoidance of smoking will reduce the risk of emphysema by 1000-fold. Currently, there is no specific treatment for liver disease. Novel strategies of prevention and treatment with chemical chaperones (such as 4-phenylbutyric acid) that reverse the cellular misfolding of the mutant protein and immunosugar compounds (such as glucosidase and mannosidase inhibitors, which increase the secretion of alpha-1-AT) are currently being investigated. Patients with decompensated liver disease should be considered for liver transplantation.

Hepatocellular carcinoma

Hepatocellular carcinoma (HCC) is the fourth most common cause of death from cancer worldwide. It has been relatively uncommon in the Western world, but there is strong evidence from the USA that the incidence of HCC is rising, nine cancer registries reporting via the National Cancer Institute showed a 41% rise in mortality from primary liver cell cancer between 1980 and 1995 with a 70% rise in overall incidence (Fig. 8.14). HCC causes approximately 1500 deaths per year in the UK. HCC is unusual among

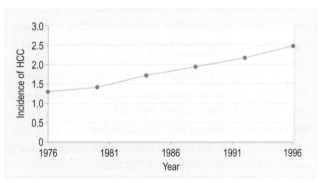

Fig. 8.14
Incidence (per 100 000 population) of hepatocellular carcinoma (HCC) in the USA

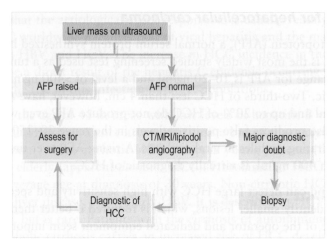

Fig. 8.15
Investigations required for a patient with known cirrhosis and a liver mass

In a patient not known to be cirrhotic who presents with a liver mass (Fig. 8.16), the initial investigation should be AFP. If raised, in the absence of a testicular primary, this confirms the diagnosis. If the lesion is potentially operable, then biopsy of the non-tumour liver may be required to determine the best treatment option. If the AFP is normal, a search for other causes (non-liver primary) and further radiological assessment of the mass are required. If investigations suggest HCC, then again biopsy of non-tumour liver will determine the surgical approach. Radiological imaging can exclude benign liver lesions with a high degree of sensitivity and specificity. Only in situations where considerable doubt exists will biopsy of the lesion be required.

Treatment of hepatocellular carcinoma (Table 8.26).

The only proven curative options are transplantation and resection, although ablative therapies may produce similar results. There are no randomized controlled trials comparing the outcome of surgical resection and liver transplantation for hepatocellular carcinoma. Both techniques are primarily suited to small volume unifocal disease and only a small proportion of patients with HCC in the UK will be suitable for either of these potentially curative treatments. The decision as to which therapy is appropriate will depend on availability of resources and individual tumour characteristics.

With transplantation, patients with single lesions of 5 cm diameter or up to three lesions of less than 3 cm, have an almost zero recurrence rate for the HCC. The prognosis after transplantation is the same as for a similar underlying liver disease without HCC.

Resection of HCC is a viable option, with short-term survival figures very similar to transplantation. Resection is only suitable for patients with excellent liver function (Child–Pugh A), because of the high risk of hepatic decompensation. The peri-operative mortality in experienced centres remains between 6 and 20% depending on the extent of the resection and the severity of pre-operative liver impairment. The residual liver after

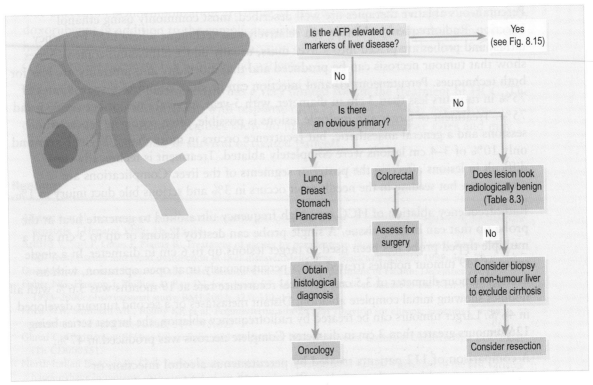

Fig. 8.16
Investigating a mass in the liver where the patient is not previously known to have cirrhosis

Table 8.26 Treatments for hepatocellular carcinoma (HCC)

Technique	Key factors in its use
Liver transplantation	Small volume disease, decompensated cirrhosis
Liver resection	Small volume disease, Child's A disease Treatment of choice for non-cirrhotic HCC
Chemoembolization	Inoperable, small volume HCC, good liver The only treatment for multifocal disease
Percutaneous alcohol injection	Less than 2 cm HCC ideal
Radiofrequency ablation	Up to 5 cm lesions treatable

resection continues to have a malignant potential. Recurrence rates of 50–60% after 5 years of follow-up after resection are usual.

Non-cirrhotic and fibrolamellar hepatocellular carcinoma should be treated by surgical resection where possible. The overall survival for fibrolamellar HCC at 5 years is 25–36% and, in non-cirrhotic non-fibrolamellar HCC, 5-year survival after surgical resection is approximately 25%.

237

Pancreatic disease

9

Diabetes mellitus is the most common medical condition resulting from a pancreatic abnormality. However, management of diabetes does not include any investigation or intervention directly related to the pancreas. Hence, it is not often mentioned under pancreatic diseases. Acute pancreatitis, chronic pancreatitis and pancreatic cancer are the major pancreatic conditions in which gastroenterologists are involved in the management.

ACUTE PANCREATITIS

Acute pancreatitis is an acute inflammatory process, with variable involvement of other regional tissues or remote organ systems. It is characterized clinically by the sudden onset of symptoms which usually resolve completely. Pathologically, the inflammatory process involves previously healthy gland which, on recovery, is expected to be morphologically and functionally normal. The reported incidence of acute pancreatitis in the UK ranges from 21 to 283 cases per million of the population and it accounts for about 3% of all admissions for abdominal pain.

Aetiopathogenesis

About 80% of acute pancreatitis is related either to stones in the common bile duct or alcohol excess (Table 9.1). About 10–15% of patients have no identifiable cause. It has been suggested that the majority of these have biliary sludge or microcrystals and that cholecystectomy could prevent further attacks. A proportion of idiopathic pancreatitis is attributed to sphincter of Oddi dysfunction and sphincterotomy has been proposed as a treatment. Activation of the zymogen trypsinogen to active trypsin is the critical step in the pathogenesis. Normally, the digestive enzyme zymogens, as well as lysosomal hydrolases, are synthesized on the endoplasmic reticulum. Both are then transported to the Golgi complex where zymogens are packaged in condensing vacuoles, carried towards the luminal surface and discharged in granular form, whereas lysosomal hydrolases are bound to receptors and transported to lysosomes. During the early stages of acute pancreatitis, the normal processes that result in the segregation of lysosomal hydrolases from zymogens appear to be disturbed. The mechanism underlying defective segregation varies according to the aetiology. In obstructive causes, ductal hypertension leads to

Table 9.1 Aetiology of acute pancreatitis

Obstructive causes
Common bile duct stone or sludge; obstructing tumours; parasites (e.g. ascariasis); duodenal Crohn's disease

Toxic causes
Alcohol abuse; scorpion sting

Drugs
Azathioprine; thiazides; furosemide; tetracycline; valproate; oestrogens

Infections
Mumps; mycoplasma; coxsackie;

Metabolic
Uraemia; hypertriglyceridaemia; hypercalcaemia

Other causes
Post-ERCP; trauma; ischaemia; systemic lupus erythematosis; necrotizing angiitis

endocytosis of zymogens from the acinar space and transportation to the lysosomal compartment. In other causes of pancreatitis, zymogen granules might fuse with lysosomes. Ethanol and drugs may cause direct toxic injury, while hyperlipidaemia in the microcirculation may lead to ischaemic insult or toxic injury secondary to excess free fatty acids. Once the autodigestion has been initiated, cytokines have a major role in amplifying the initial injury and leading to multiorgan failure.

Management

A history of abdominal pain and vomiting with epigastric or diffuse abdominal tenderness are common features in those with acute pancreatitis. It is important to exclude other causes of similar presentation such as visceral perforation, mesenteric ischaemia and leaking aortic aneurysm. The diagnosis is made when the serum amylase activity is >4 times above normal (or lipase activity twice the upper limit of normal) in an appropriate clinical setting. Lipase remains increased for longer than amylase and is more specific for the diagnosis. Plain X-rays of the chest and abdomen provide a base-line and help to exclude other causes of acute abdominal symptoms.

The initial prediction of the severity of the attack of acute pancreatitis has implications for management and prognosis. Clinical assessment alone has only 50% accuracy. Multifactor scoring systems such as Ranson (severe >2), Glasgow (severe >2), and APACHE II (severe >7) will improve the accuracy of severity assessment. The Glasgow scoring system has been validated in the UK population (Table 9.2). A peak C-reactive protein of >210 mg/l in the first 4 days or >120 mg/l at the end of a week is of independent prognostic value.

Imaging

Ultrasound is helpful in detecting gallstones, dilatation of the common bile duct and free peritoneal fluid, but the pancreas is visualized in only half of the cases. A computerized tomography (CT) scan is indicated when the diagnosis remains uncertain after the initial

Table 9.2 Glasgow Scoring System (score = no. criteria fulfilled)

Factors	Criteria of severity
Age	>55 years
White blood cell count	$>15 \times 10^9/l$
Glucose	>10 mmol/l
Urea	>16 mmol/l
PaO$_2$	<8 kPa
Calcium	<2 mmol/l
Albumin	<32 g/l
Lactate dehydrogenase	>600 units/l
Alanine transaminase	>100 units/l

investigations. CT scanning is also helpful in identifying the aetiology, especially in the elderly, to exclude a pancreatic tumour. All those predicted to have a severe attack should undergo dynamic CT scanning 3–10 days after the onset. This permits the assessment of the degree of pancreatic necrosis and predicts subsequent complications such as infected necrosis needing surgical intervention. Endoscopic ultrasound (EUS) can be used to identify the aetiology as well as to select patients for a therapeutic endoscopic retrograde cholangiopancreatography (ERCP).

Severe pancreatitis

About 20% of patients with acute pancreatitis have a severe attack and most of the deaths occur in this group. Patients who have cardiorespiratory compromise should be managed in high-dependency or intensive-care units for optimal support and management of metabolic complications. There is some evidence to support the use of prophylactic antibiotics (cefuroxime) in the prevention of septic complications. Prophylactic antibiotics are also indicated prior to invasive procedures such as ERCP.

Endoscopy

Early ERCP and endoscopic biliary sphincterotomy within 24–72 h of admission could significantly reduce morbidity (38–25%) and mortality (9–5%) in acute severe biliary pancreatitis. Early ERCP should be considered in acute biliary pancreatitis with jaundice, cholangitis, dilated common bile duct or a deteriorating course. ERCP guided pancreatic duct stenting could be useful in the management where there has been disruption of the main pancreatic duct leading to a pancreatic fistula or pseudocyst formation. Transgastric drainage of the pseudocyst can be performed safely using EUS guidance.

Surgery

Surgical debridement may be necessary when there is infected necrosis that does not respond to intravenous antibiotics. Local complications needing surgical management include a symptomatic pseudocyst not amenable to endoscopic drainage, involvement of

Table 9.3 Aetiology of chronic pancreatitis

Hereditary pancreatitis
- Point mutations in the cationic trypsinogen (PRSS1) gene
Cystic fibrosis
Tropical pancreatitis
- Serine protease inhibitor Kajal type 1 (SPINK 1) mutation
Congenital abnormalities
- Annular pancreas, pancreas divisum
Alcohol
Hyperparathyroidism

the splenic hilum by a pseudocyst, traumatic pancreatitis with rupture of the duct and pancreatic fistula with refractory ascites or pleural effusion. Pseudoaneurysms may form when inflammatory necrosis involves local vessels and lead to bleeding complications. These can be treated with angiographic transcatheter emobilization or by surgery.

CHRONIC PANCREATITIS

Chronic pancreatitis is a progressive inflammatory disease of the exocrine pancreas characterized by severe and recurrent episodes of abdominal pain associated with pancreatic inflammation, progressive loss of acinar tissue, and fibrosis. Each burst of inflammation leads to foci of interstitial or peripancreatic fat necrosis leading to pseudocyst formation and fibrosis. Ductal distortion and intraductal plugs of calcium carbonate can lead to pancreatic stones.

Epidemiology

The incidence of chronic pancreatitis varies from 1.6 to 23 per 100 000 per year throughout Europe, depending on the level of alcohol consumption. The incidence of chronic pancreatitis has been thought to be increasing. The causes of chronic pancreatitis are listed in Table 9.3. Alcohol accounts for 70–80% of cases of chronic pancreatitis. Mean consumption at the time of diagnosis varies from <50 g daily for 2 years to >150 g ethanol daily for 18 years.

Clinical manifestations

Pain is the predominant symptom in most patients with chronic pancreatitis, especially in the first 5–8 years of diagnosis. The pathophysiology of pain in chronic pancreatitis is poorly understood, but both pancreatic and extrapancreatic causes can account for the pain. Demonstration of a direct relationship between the degree of perineural inflammation and the clinical pain syndrome strongly supports the hypothesis of neuroimmune interaction as an important, if not predominant, factor in pain generation.

Increased pressure in the pancreatic duct and tissues can account for pain in a sub-group of patients. Raised intrapancreatic pressure might be related to secretion in the presence of an obstruction, and altering obstruction or secretion could modulate intensity and frequency of pain. Experimental evidence suggests that increased pancreatic and ductal pressure produce a compartment syndrome that could cause ischaemia, thus inducing pain. The ductal hypertension as an explanation for pain is supported by the fact that decompression of a dilated pancreatic duct by stenting or surgery relieves the pain. Pancreatic enzyme supplementation may also relieve pain in some patients because the proteases in the intestinal lumen regulate pancreatic secretion by cholecystokinin-mediated feedback. In those with pseudocysts, a well-recognized complication, drainage of the pseudocyst can give symptomatic relief.

Extra-pancreatic complications, such as common bile duct stricture and duodenal stenosis due to extensive fibrosis, can be the main cause of symptoms including pain. 'Groove pancreatitis', characterized by the formation of a scar plate between pancreatic head and the duodenum, was described in 20% of patients in a large series. Post-prandial pain in chronic pancreatitis could be due to compression of nerves and ganglia located in this groove.

Tests of pancreatic function

The exocrine pancreas produces 1 l of pancreatic juice daily, which consists of digestive enzymes secreted by acinar cells in inactive (zymogen) form and bicarbonate secreted by ductal cells. Once the pancreatic juice reaches the duodenum, the pro-enzyme trypsinogen is activated to trypsin by the brush border enzyme enterokinase. Trypsin in turn activates other proteases to their active forms.

Tests of pancreatic function are based on 'direct' measurement of pancreatic secretion or 'indirect' measurement of the effects of inadequate digestive enzymes. Direct tests are considered more sensitive, but there is no wide acceptance of a standard protocol regarding which secretagogue to use (secretin and/or cholecystokinin), which measurement to make (total volume or bicarbonate) and the normal ranges. Tests require collection tubes to be placed accurately. These are available in a few specialist centres each with individual modifications and standardization. Measurements of faecal elastase-1 and chymotrypsin are useful in demonstrating exocrine insufficiency in severe pancreatitis, but their sensitivity is low in mild pancreatitis. Quantitative faecal fat estimation is neither sensitive nor specific for pancreatic insufficiency and qualitative evidence of faecal fat with Sudan stain of stool does not prove malabsorption.

Ingested N-benzoyl-L-tyrosyl-paraaminobenzoic acid (NBT-PABA) is split by chymotrypsin to liberate PABA and the recovery of less than 50% of the ingested dose in a 6-h urine collection is considered abnormal. The fluorescein dilaurate (Pancreolauryl) test uses a similar principle with the measurement of the 10-h urinary excretion of fluorescein after hydrolysis of the ingested substrate by arylesterase. Both the indirect tests have >75% sensitivity in advanced disease, with much lower sensitivity in those patients with mild disease.

Imaging

A variety of imaging tests that delineate the structure of the pancreas can also be used to diagnose chronic pancreatitis. CT scanning is useful as the initial non-invasive test as it identifies structural changes in those with advanced disease. A CT scan does not consistently delineate minor branches of the pancreatic duct. Hence, a normal CT does not exclude the diagnosis. ERCP is the most widely used test to diagnose and classify chronic pancreatitis based on the changes in the pancreatic duct and the branches. ERCP allows decompression of the common bile duct or the pancreatic duct when indicated. However, ERCP is associated with a significant risk of complications, including acute pancreatitis. In at least 30% of cases, the minor ducts are inadequately opacified at ERCP making evaluation difficult. MRCP has the advantage of being non-invasive, but also is unable to define changes in the minor branches. Advances in technology could lead to standardization of 'functional MRCP' with an ability to quantitate stimulated pancreatic secretion, thus combining the advantages of imaging and exocrine function testing. EUS has an advantage over other techniques in that it can demonstrate structural changes in the pancreatic parenchyma as well as the duct. It is probably the most sensitive imaging modality in identifying mild chronic pancreatitis. The studies comparing EUS with ERCP and exocrine function tests are unable to assess the roles in the diagnosis of early pancreatitis. Long-term outcome in patients identified as early pancreatitis by EUS are awaited.

Treatment

Disabling pain is the main therapeutic challenge in chronic pancreatitis. The management of pain should be multidisciplinary as described later under pancreatic cancer. The Manchester 'oxidant stress' hypothesis implies that reactive xenobiotic metabolites and depletion of glutathione are critical for the development and maintenance of ongoing inflammation. Accordingly, antioxidants have been used in the treatment of painful chronic pancreatitis, although the data demonstrating their efficacy emerge only from a small, randomized placebo-controlled study and an audit. Endoscopic and surgical decompression, as well as resection, should be considered in those refractory to medical management, especially in those with obstructive complications of chronic pancreatitis.

Fat and protein malabsorption can be improved by oral pancreatic enzyme supplements. The activity of enzyme supplements is reduced in acidic pH in the duodenal lumen as may occur when bicarbonate secretion is reduced in chronic pancreatitis. Proton pump inhibitors, given with the enzyme supplements, can improve their efficacy.

Prognosis

The course of chronic pancreatitis is variable. About 50% continue to have episodes of significant pain even after 10 years from diagnosis, and up to 46% develop obstructive complications. Progressive fibrosis leads to loss of both endocrine and exocrine function of the pancreas. Diabetes develops in one-third of patients and exocrine insufficiency could manifest itself with diarrhoea, steatorrhoea and weight loss. Other complications include portal or splenic vein thrombosis and the development of pancreatic cancer. Overall, 21–35% of patients die over a period of 10 years, although the majority of mortality is not directly related to pancreatic disease.

PANCREATIC CANCER

Ductal adenocarcinoma accounts for over 90% of all exocrine pancreatic tumours and 80–90% of these occur in the head of the gland. Pancreatic cancer is the seventh leading cause of cancer mortality in the UK accounting for 6700 deaths per year. Age standardized annual incidence of pancreatic cancer in the West Midlands is 10 per 100 000 population and the difference in incidence between men and women is narrowing (annual incidence 12 and 10 per 100 000).

An association between pancreatic cancer and smoking has been consistently demonstrated. Of several other factors investigated, there is clear evidence that type 2 diabetes of less than 2 years' duration is associated with increased risk. There is a five- to fifteenfold increased risk of pancreatic cancer in association with chronic pancreatitis, while this risk is increased by fifty- to seventyfold in those with hereditary pancreatitis. In hereditary pancreatitis, age-accumulated risk begins to rise at 40 years of age and is 40% by the age of 75 years. Pancreatic cancer can also be associated with other cancer family syndromes. There is a high incidence of periampullary cancers (cancers within 1 cm of the papilla of Vater) in patients with familial adenomatous polyposis.

Clinical features and diagnosis

Three main symptoms of pancreatic cancer are pain, loss of weight and jaundice. Persistent back pain (indicating retroperitoneal infiltration) and severe, rapid weight loss have usually been associated with unresectability, although there are no specific symptoms that clearly identify patients with potentially curable pancreatic cancer. Periampullary tumours cause jaundice at a relatively early stage, which may account for their higher resectability. In contrast, jaundice in patients with cancer of the body or the tail of the pancreas usually is caused by hepatic or hilar metastasis and, therefore, indicates unresectability. The diagnosis of pancreatic cancer should be considered in older patients with type 2 diabetes of recent onset without a family history and in those with an unexplained attack of acute pancreatitis.

Apart from jaundice, there are usually no other signs. A small proportion of patients present with palpable gallbladder (Courvoisier sign). A palpable epigastric mass, ascites and an enlarged supraclavicular lymph node indicate unresectability.

Tumour detection

Laboratory liver tests cannot reliably distinguish between metastatic liver disease and an obstructed bile duct. Although the reported sensitivity of transabdominal ultrasound in the detection of pancreatic tumour is high, technical difficulties and inter-observer variation limit its use mainly to confirm bile-duct obstruction. EUS with an overall detection rate up to 97% is superior to helical CT, MRI and PET scanning in detecting small pancreatic tumours. With a provision for fine-needle aspiration and Trucut biopsy, EUS has an advantage over helical CT when alternative diagnoses are being considered. ERCP is important in the diagnosis of periampullary tumours by direct visualization and biopsy. When the clinical presentation is that of biliary obstruction, ERCP has the advantage of providing an opportunity to sample by brush cytology or histology (using biliary biopsy forceps) as well as to relieve jaundice and associated symptoms by biliary stenting.

Staging

The role of different techniques and imaging modalities in assessing resectability remains controversial. The assessment of local extension, vascular involvement, hepatic and nodal metastasis by helical CT correlates well with surgical findings in large tumours, while EUS is considered to be superior in staging small (<3.5 cm) tumours. The inclusion of EUS in the algorithm of preoperative assessment increases the clean Whipple's rate by 10%. Laparoscopy, including laparoscopic ultrasound, can detect occult hepatic and peritoneal metastasis not identified by other imaging modalities. Selective angiography is unreliable in predicting resectability and adds little information on arterial anatomy over that obtained by helical CT or MRI. It is, therefore, not routinely used in the management of pancreatic cancer.

Tissue diagnosis

Attempts should be made during the course of investigations to obtain tissue samples. Brush cytology at ERCP has a high specificity, but low sensitivity. Devices to obtain larger biliary biopsies are currently being tested. EUS-guided fine-needle aspiration (FNA) cytology offers a safe, sensitive and specific mode of obtaining a tissue diagnosis. The sensitivity of EUS-guided sampling can be increased further by Trucut biopsies when feasible (Figs 9.1a–c). The transperitoneal approach (CT guided or laparoscopic) has been associated with a risk of tumour cell seeding along the needle track or within the peritoneum and thus is not justified in those whose tumour is considered potentially resectable.

Treatment

Palliative drainage

Controlled trials of palliation of obstructive jaundice in patients with pancreatic cancer do not favour either stenting or surgical bypass. Median survivals after these treatments are similar. Stenting can be performed immediately with fewer early complications while surgical bypass has a better long-term stent patency. In most centres, palliative surgery is reserved for those with good performance status with longer life expectancy and for those where duodenal tumour invasion has resulted in gastric outlet obstruction.

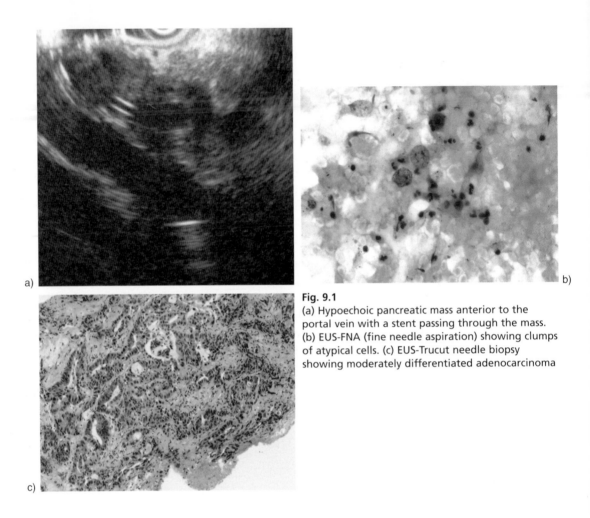

a)

b)

c)

Fig. 9.1
(a) Hypoechoic pancreatic mass anterior to the portal vein with a stent passing through the mass. (b) EUS-FNA (fine needle aspiration) showing clumps of atypical cells. (c) EUS-Trucut needle biopsy showing moderately differentiated adenocarcinoma

Endoscopic stent insertion at the time of ERCP has been associated with fewer procedure-related complications and lower mortality rates compared with the percutaneous transhepatic approach and, thus this is the method of choice. More than two-thirds of patients are successfully palliated by a single stent. The average patency of self-expanding metal stents is about twice that of plastic stents, which is about 4 months. Cost of a plastic stent is about 4% of that of a metal stent. Therefore, while patients with clearly unresectable pancreatic cancer with longer life expectancy are suitable for metal stenting, plastic stents may be appropriate in most patients awaiting staging, or those with short life expectancy. The percutaneous transhepatic approach is used in those where endoscopic approach is not feasible or has been unsuccessful.

The benefit of relieving jaundice before attempted resection of pancreatic cancer has not been consistently demonstrated. Therefore, routine stenting prior to surgery is not recommended. However, if definitive surgery is delayed more than 10 days, then it is common practice to perform endoscopic biliary drainage and defer surgery (for 3–6 weeks) until the jaundice settles.

Resection

There is a good correlation between post-operative mortality and both the caseload of the centre as well as the number of resections performed by the individual surgeon annually, indicating that pancreatic cancers should be managed at specialist centres. The rate of resectability is around 20%, while the 5-year survival after Whipple's pancreaticoduodenectomy is about 10%. Pancreaticoduodenectomy (with or without pylorus preservation) is the standard surgery for cancer of the head of the pancreas. Extended resections involving the portal vein and total pancreatectomy may be required in some cases, but resection in the presence of known portal-vein involvement is not justified. Lateral resection with splenectomy is indicated in localized cancer of the body and tail. The involvement of the splenic artery and vein is not a contraindication.

In a large trial adjuvant chemoradiotherapy showed no benefit, but there was a trend towards survival advantage with maintenance chemotherapy with 5-fluorouracil (5FU) and folinic acid (ESPAC). A further study comparing 5FU, gemcitabine and no adjuvant therapy is currently being conducted. At present, adjuvant therapy should be considered only in the context of a trial. In palliative chemotherapy for unresectable, metastatic or recurrent pancreatic cancer, gemcitabine should be the agent of choice, as it improves symptoms (pain control, performance status and weight gain) in 24% compared with 5% with 5FU.

Pain is a common symptom in patients with advanced pancreatic cancer. Management should include analgesics introduced according to the recommendations of the World Health Organization's progressive analgesic ladder. Coeliac plexus neurolysis is effective in pain control in 70% when performed early during the course of the illness. This could be performed at the time of palliative surgery or percutaneously. EUS-guided coeliac neurolysis is safe and cost effective in the management of these patients. Pancreatic duct decompression is rarely necessary.

Further Reading

Axon ATR, Classen M, Cotton PB et al. Pancreatography in chronic pancreatitis: international definitions. Gut 1984; 25: 1107–12.

Bramhall SR, Allum WH, Jones AG et al. Treatment and survival in 13560 patients with pancreatic cancer, and incidence of the disease, in the West Midlands an epidemiological study. Br J Surg 1995; 82: 111–15.

Forsmark CE, Chowdhury RS. Review article: pancreatic function testing. Aliment Pharmacol Ther 2003; 17: 733–50.

Gullo L, Pezzilli R, Morselli-Labate AM. Italian Pancreatic Cancer Study Group. Diabetes and the risk of pancreatic cancer. N Engl J Med 1994; 331: 81–4.

Kochman ML. EUS in pancreatic cancer. Gastrointest Endo 2002; 56(Suppl 4): S6–12.

Lowenfels AB, Maisonneuve P, Cavallini G et al. Pancreatitis and the risk of pancreatic cancer. N Engl J Med 1993; 328: 1433–7.

McClay R. Chronic pancreatitis at Manchester, UK. Focus on antioxidant therapy. Digestion 1998; 59(Suppl 4): 36–48.

Sahai AV. EUS in chronic pancreatitis. Gastrointest Endo 2002; 56(Suppl 4): S76–81.

Sebastiano PD, Mala FFD, Bockman DE, Friess H, Buchler MW. Chronic pancreatitis: the perspective of pain generation by neuroimmune interaction. Gut 2003; 52: 907–11.

Ulrich CD for the Consensus Committees for the European Registry of Hereditary Pancreatic Diseases, the Midwest Multi-Center Pancreatic Study Group and International Association of Pancreatology. Cancer in hereditary pancreatitis: consensus guidelines for prevention, screening and treatment. Pancreatology 2001; 1: 416–22.

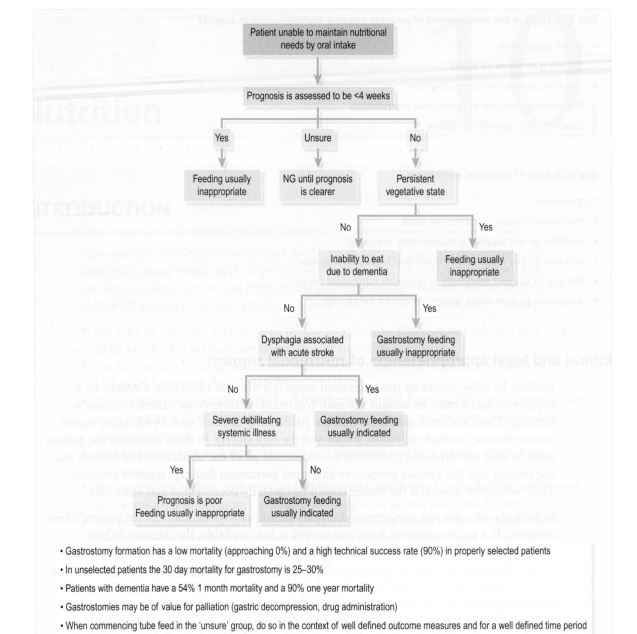

Fig. 10.1
Guide to determining the appropriateness of enteral feeding

The flowchart contains the following elements:

Patient unable to maintain nutritional needs by oral intake
↓
Prognosis is assessed to be <4 weeks
→ Yes → Feeding usually inappropriate
→ Unsure → NG until prognosis is clearer
→ No → Persistent vegetative state
  → No → Inability to eat due to dementia
  → Yes → Feeding usually inappropriate
    Inability to eat due to dementia
    → No → Dysphagia associated with acute stroke
    → Yes → Gastrostomy feeding usually inappropriate
      Dysphagia associated with acute stroke
      → No → Severe debilitating systemic illness
      → Yes → Gastrostomy feeding usually indicated
        Severe debilitating systemic illness
        → Yes → Prognosis is poor Feeding usually inappropriate
        → No → Gastrostomy feeding usually indicated

- Gastrostomy formation has a low mortality (approaching 0%) and a high technical success rate (90%) in properly selected patients
- In unselected patients the 30 day mortality for gastrostomy is 25–30%
- Patients with dementia have a 54% 1 month mortality and a 90% one year mortality
- Gastrostomies may be of value for palliation (gastric decompression, drug administration)
- When commencing tube feed in the 'unsure' group, do so in the context of well defined outcome measures and for a well defined time period
- In incompetent patients, the decision is that of the responsible physician but **communication** with all involved is essential

Table 10.1 Nutritional state assessment

Body composition (macro)	
Assessment of lean mass	Anthropometry, total body potassium, total body nitrogen, bioelectric impedance, urinary 3-methylhistidine, urinary urea:creatinine, aminoacid profiles, whole protein turnover (^{14}C leucine, ^{15}N glycine)
Assessment of fat mass	Anthropometry, bioelectric impedance, ultrasound, computerized tomography, essential fatty acid levels
Assessment of body water	Anthropometry, isotope dilution, bioelectric impedance, tissue hydration
Assessment of bone mass	Densitometry, radiogravimetry, bone biopsy, photon beam scanning, computerized tomography
Body composition (micro)	
Electrolytes and minerals	Sodium, potassium, copper, magnesium, calcium, phosphorus, iron, chromium, selenium, iodine, cobalt, zinc, manganese, molybdenum
Vitamins	Thiamine (red-cell transketolase)
	Riboflavin (red-cell glutathione reductase)
	Niacin (methylnicotinamide excretion)
	Pyridoxine (red-cell aminotransferase)
	Folic acid, B12, ascorbic acid, retinol, cholecalciferol, alpha-tocopherol, phylloquinone
Body function	
Hepatic secretory proteins	Albumin, pre-albumin, transferrin, haptoglobin, retinol binding protein, haptoglobin, orosomucoid, alpha-1-antitrypsin
Immune function	Total lymphocyte count, cell-mediated immunity, rosette-forming T cells, delayed cutaneous hypersensitivity, humoral immunity, complement C3
Muscle function	Maximum voluntary contraction, electrical stimulation

Current salt and water balance

In critical and high-dependency care, central venous pressure, in addition to clinical assessment and strict fluid balance charts, will help. In the general wards it may be necessary to depend on clinical assessment and then to promote strict fluid balance and precise daily weights for subsequent monitoring. It is worth asking bed-bound patients (or their relatives) for their height and weight if this is not recorded. It is good practice to estimate a patient's weight, before asking or looking at their records, so that, over time, the skill of reasonably accurate bedside assessment of weight and height can be developed. Allowance can be made for peripheral oedema or ascites by using Table 10.2.

Current state of micronutrients

Detailed mineral, vitamin and trace element function, serum and tissue levels and recommended daily requirements are available in most textbooks of nutrition. They should always be referred to when caring for severely malnourished patients, those who will require prolonged nutrition support and those with complex co-morbidity.

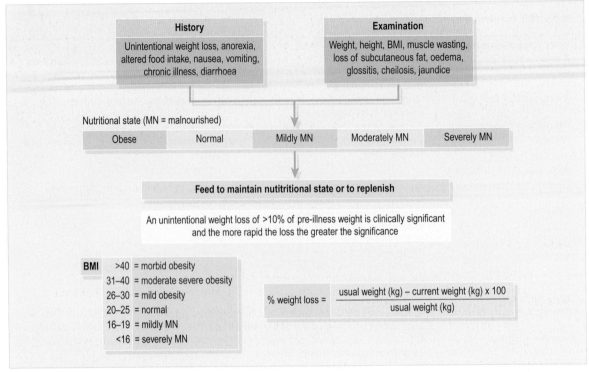

Fig. 10.2
Mini global nutrition assessment

Table 10.2 Estimation of fluid excess with oedema or ascites

Clinical finding	Estimated fluid excess
Oedema detectable only at ankle or sacrum	1 kg
Oedema to mid calf/lower back	5 kg
Oedema to mid thigh/scapulae	10 kg
Minimal, detectable ascites	2.2 kg
Moderate, evident ascites	6.0 kg
Severe tense ascites	14 kg

Impact of the clinical condition and of drug therapy

In this assessment consider:

1. Drugs – for example the frequent use of emesis-inducing drugs, or nebulized teratogenic drugs, which necessitate temporary but complete isolation of patients (e.g. ribavarin).
2. Therapies – for example the use of full face masks for assisted non-invasive ventilation, frequent trips to radiotherapy or theatre which interrupt feeding regimens, or the use of isolation due to immunosuppression.

Table 10.3 The estimated basal metabolic rate according to age, gender and weight (W) in kgs

Females kcal/24 h	Males kcal/24 h
15–18 years 13.3W + 690	15–18 years 17.6W + 656
18–30 years 14.8W + 485	18–30 years 15.0W + 690
30–60 years 8.1W + 842	30–60 years 11.4W + 870
>60 years 9.0W + 656	>60 years 11.7W + 585

3. Surgery – especially oropharyngeal or gastrointestinal surgery and the patient's nutritional state in the event of complications or delayed recovery.

Energy expenditure

Direct or indirect calorimetry is not always available and, most often, predictive equations, such as the Scholfield equation, are used combined with various corrective factors to take account of the clinical situation. Dietitians will normally calculate energy expenditure, but it is important to understand the calculations involved. The common steps involved are:

1. Determine basal metabolic rate (BMR) (Table 10.3).
2. Adjust for stress using Elia's nomogram. This is available in most dietetic and nutrition textbooks and allows correction of BMR for stress such as burns, severe sepsis or multiple trauma, infection and starvation.
3. Add corrective factor for activity and diet induced thermogenesis:

Bed-bound and immobile: + 10%
Bed-bound, mobile and sitting: + 15–20%
Mobile on ward: + 25%

Nitrogen losses

Measuring nitrogen balance is a dynamic measure of nitrogen loss and is useful in complicated and critical-care patients who are not in renal failure. It requires an accurate 24-h urine collection and its value is reduced if there are large non-renal losses such as burns, fistulae or severe diarrhoea. In the absence of accurate nitrogen balance studies, nitrogen requirements may be estimated as shown in Table 10.4.

Once the initial assessment is completed the outcome should be clearly documented in the patient's records and should include:

- an explanation of and evidence for the decision on whether or not to begin nutritional support. This is especially important when nutritional support is not being offered for ethical or legal reasons. If the decision cannot be made immediately, the plan for how it is to be achieved (MDT meeting, case conference, etc.) should be outlined. This helps to avoid unrest and anxiety for relatives and the ward team

Table 10.4 Nitrogen requirements according to the state of the patient

State of patient	Nitrogen g/kg/24 h
Normal	0.17 (0.14–0.20)
Hyper metabolic	
5–20%	
25–50%	
50%+	
Likely nitrogen depleted	0.2 (0.17–0.25)
	0.25 (0.2–0.3)
	0.3 (0.25–0.35)
	0.3 (0.2–0.4)

- the current nutritional state (height, weight, BMI) and fluid balance
- the nutritional requirements (fluid, calories, nitrogen, sodium, potassium, calcium and magnesium). This helps to avoid errors and confusion out of hours and at weekends
- the goals of treatment (e.g. target weight, maintenance until oral intake is possible)
- the plan for monitoring:
  - frequency and type of blood tests
  - details of required fluid balance
  - frequency of weighing
  - frequency of review.

DECIDING ON THE ROUTE OF ACCESS FOR ARTIFICIAL NUTRITION SUPPORT

The routes for artificial nutritional support are oral, enteral and parenteral (i.e. intravenous) in that order. None is mutually exclusive and it is important to use the most physiological route to its maximum capacity before moving on to the next route. For example, an elderly post-operative patient may not be able to manage enough nutrition with an oral fortified diet with supplements and may, in addition to this, be prescribed overnight tube feeding. Another exception is a patient with the short bowel syndrome who may continue oral feeding but require parenteral nutrition as well.

It is essential that the types of tubes for parenteral and enteral feeding be standardized across any individual hospital campus. New tubes and accessories should never be introduced until everyone potentially involved in their use has been trained. Simple changes, such as new connectors, different coloured appliances or tubes, can cause great difficulty on the wards. It should be remembered that patients on intensive-treatment units (ITU) and high-dependency units (HDU) will eventually move to a general ward, often at night or at the weekend, so that staff training in all areas is important.

In enteral feeding, if the patient requires artificial feeding for more than 4–6 weeks, stoma feeding is usually more appropriate. However, if feeding is for less than this, nasogastric

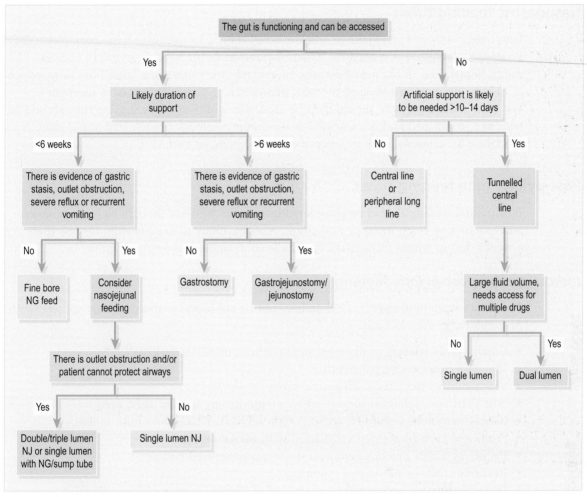

Fig. 10.3
Choosing the route of access

tube feeding should generally be used. There are exceptions, such as a patient with head and neck cancer who may need artificial feeding for less than 6 weeks, but may benefit from stoma feeding whilst receiving radiotherapy to the mouth or throat. Another exception is a patient with extensive burns who, though needing feeding for many months, may have to rely on nasogastric tube feeding because of difficulty with abdominal access.

In parenteral feeding, a patient needing support for less than 2 weeks may well manage with standard centrally or peripherally inserted central lines. A patient needing parenteral support for longer than this will usually need a tunnelled line.

An outline for choosing route of access is detailed in Figure 10.3.

Nasogastric feeding tubes

Fine-bore (5–8F) polyurethane or silicone tubes should be used and large-bore PVC tubes avoided, unless there is a need for gastric aspiration or the need to give very viscous drugs. Sometimes, in the post-operative or critical-care situation, a large-bore tube, which is already in place, will be used to 'trial' nasogastric feeding. If the trial is successful, however, a fine-bore tube should then be used. The position of the feeding tube should be reviewed, confirmed and documented at the commencement of each feed and if there is any cause for concern, such as an episode of coughing or vomiting.

Post-pyloric tube feeding tubes

Post-pyloric feeding should be considered in patients who are thought to have an intact and functioning small intestine and colon, who are likely to need feeding for less than 6 weeks, but in whom intragastric feeding is contraindicated or not possible.

Indications for post-pyloric feeding

Patients in whom intragastric feeding may not be appropriate and who may succeed with post-pyloric feeding include:

- Gastric stasis relating to diabetes, malnutrition, or pelvic surgery
- Uncomplicated severe pancreatitis
- >15% burns associated with gastric stasis
- Post gastro-oesophageal surgery when a jejunostomy has not been sited
- Multi-organ failure and ITU patients with high gastric residues but no ileus
- Prolonged (>72 h) assisted ventilation with BIPAP or CPAP
- Recurrent highly emetic chemotherapy in malnourished patients
- Recurrent therapy associated vomiting
- Bone-marrow transplantation
- Severe gastro-oesophageal reflux in patients who cannot protect their airways.

Types of post-pyloric feeding tubes

The available feeding tubes are:

- single lumen over the wire
- single lumen weighted
- single lumen memory coil (Benjmark®)
- single lumen balloon
- any of the above with an additional nasogastric or sump tube
- double lumen
- triple lumen.

Choice of post-pyloric tubes

Deciding which type of tube to use depends on the severity of gastric stasis and the risk of reflux and vomiting.

In patients with acute pancreatitis or severe gastric stasis, at risk of aspiration, the choice is between the following:

- A triple lumen tube
- A double lumen tube
- A single lumen post-pyloric tube and a standard nasogastric tube or sump tube.

The triple and double lumen tubes are larger and may be uncomfortable for alert patients so, if artificial feeding is likely to be needed after gastric emptying has improved, the third option is chosen.

In all other patients a single lumen post-pyloric tube is the tube of choice.

Positioning of post-pyloric tubes

These tubes can be positioned endoscopically, radiologically or during laparotomy. The broad outline for deciding on a method of insertion is:

- If gastric emptying is presently normal and there is no vomiting, consider bedside placement as for a nasogastric tube. Use a single lumen memory coil or balloon tube and confirm spontaneous passage either by X-ray or migration of tube 8–12 h later. Prokinetics may be used but are usually not necessary.
- If gastric emptying is not normal or the patient is vomiting, the preferred placement method is radiologic providing the patient is clinically well enough to go to the X-ray department or screening is available.
- If the patient cannot go to the X-ray department easily (e.g. being ventilated or the tube is to be positioned in theatre) and there is no screening facility available, endoscopic placement is preferred.

Methods of endoscopic placement of post-pyloric tubes

The two main methods of endoscopic placement are as follows:

1. 'Over the wire':
   a. the guide wire is passed through the biopsy channel of a gastroscope into the jejunum
   b. the scope is removed and the wire is re-routed through the nose using a short tube passed through the nose and out of the mouth
   c. the jejunal tube is passed over the nasojejunal guidewire
   d. position is confirmed by screening or X-ray
2. 'Differential friction'. This technique is mainly suitable for the single lumen Benjmark tubes:
   a. a suture is secured to the end of the tube
   b. the tube is passed into the oesophagus to 30 cm
   c. then the gastroscope is passed and the friction between the two at cricopharyngeus and gastro-oesophageal junction will carry the tube forward to pylorus
   d. if the tube coils in the fundus a forceps may be used to catch the thread and guide the tube down along greater curve to the antrum (this is rarely necessary)
   e. the scope is passed to the distal antrum only, as the feeding tube enters the duodenal cap

   f. As the tube is seen to enter the duodenal cap, digital pressure is placed on the tube against the pharynx and the scope is withdrawn to the gastro-oesophageal junction

   g. The digital pressure is then released and the scope is passed forward to the distal antrum/pylorus again

   h. e–g is repeated until the feeding tube is at about 115 cm at the nose without coiling in the stomach or mouth

   i. digital pressure is then applied to the tube against the pharynx again and the scope is removed

   j. ease of guidewire removal is a good indicator of satisfactory position, but this can be confirmed by X-ray.

This method is only suitable for intubated and ventilated patients and is not suitable using conscious sedation.

Securing feeding tubes and post-placement care

Securing feeding tubes and post-placement care is of the utmost importance. It is essential that nursing staff caring for the tubes understand:

- the difference between nasogastric and post-pyloric tubes
- which ports to use in multiport tubes (it is easy for unaware staff to feed through the gastric port and aspirate through the jejunal port of a triple lumen tube)
- which drugs are safe to instil down the tubes without the risk of blockage
- the importance of flushing
- the importance of documentation
- all tubes should be secured at two areas:
  - single lumen tubes should not usually be secured at the nose, but rather at the cheek, then over the ear and secure again at the neck
  - triple lumen tubes should be secured at the nose and again at the cheek
  - in patients where there is a high risk of displacement or the clinical condition makes repeat access difficult (multiple trauma, large burns, post upper GI surgery) then the tubes should be secured using a postnasal sling or bridle.

Particular problems with post-pyloric feeding tubes

- Position at the nose or X-ray are the only ways of confirming a stable position; aspiration and auscultation are inappropriate
- All flushes must be sterile
- Detection of absorption failure and ileus is difficult, especially with single lumen tubes
- There are few bio-availability data available on drugs given jejunally.

Gastrostomy, gastrojejunostomy and jejunostomy

The types of tubes available are shown in Box 10.3.

In deciding which stoma to recommend, remember that:

- gastrostomies are the stomas of choice as they allow bolus feeding and are easier to care for long term. The commonest indications are:

Box 10.3 Types of feeding tube

- Gastrostomy – semi rigid internal fixator
- Gastrostomy – balloon internal fixator (initial placement)
- Gastrostomy – balloon internal fixator for surgical placement (sutured in place)
- Gastrostomy – pigtail internal fixator
- Gastrostomy – balloon internal fixator (replacement for established stoma tracts)
- Gastrojejunostomy without gastric aspiration facility
- Gastrojejunostomy with gastric aspiration facility
- Jejunostomy – semi rigid internal fixator
- Jejunostomy – balloon internal fixator
- Surgical jejunostomy (sutured in place) – non-cuffed
- Surgical jejunostomy – cuffed
- Low-profile gastrostomy and jejunostomy buttons

- neurological disorders (stroke, motor neuron disease, Parkinson's disease, multiple sclerosis)
- oropharyngeal or oesophageal cancer
- long-term supplemental enteral feeding (cystic fibrosis, short bowel, Crohn's).
- gastrostomies should be used with caution, or not at all, in patients with severe gastro-oesophageal reflux, gastric outlet obstruction, ascites, gastric or peritoneal malignancy, hepatomegaly and gastric varices
- gastrostomies can be used in peritoneal dialysis, but haemodialysis or low-volume peritoneal dialysis may need to be used to allow the stoma to form and there is the risk of peritoneal infection and loss of the peritoneal route for dialysis
- jejunostomies can be used following upper GI surgery or in patients with long-term gastric dysmotility
- gastrojejunostomies may be used for the same indications as jejunostomies, but are more difficult to manage. However, they are particularly useful when gastric aspiration and distal feeding or drug administration may be required (e.g. in palliative care).

When deciding how to form stomas it needs to be remembered that:

- most gastrostomies and jejunostomies can be formed endoscopically, radiologically, with X-ray screening or ultrasound, or surgically
- it is important that skill in all three areas is available so that all patient groups can be catered for
- patients with head and neck cancers may manage radiologic placement better. Furthermore, there is a risk of tumour seeding if the feeding tube is pulled passed the tumour in endoscopic placement
- patients in whom good endoscopic transillumination cannot be achieved may need radiologic or surgical placement

- large hiatus hernias may need to be reduced before a gastrostomy is placed
- surgical placement will be more convenient in patients who are having upper GI surgery
- when the internal fixator is a balloon or a pigtail the stoma should be secured using Brown Muller® fixators to prevent free gastric perforation in the event of early, accidental displacement.

Parenteral nutrition access

The catheters available are shown in Box 10.4.

Often, in short-term nutrition in ITU or oncology, the catheter to be used will already be in place. If a catheter needs to be chosen for parenteral nutrition, the choice will depend on the length of time it is estimated the patient will need nutritional support and whether or not access is needed for drugs, other fluids and sampling. If multiple lumens are required for drugs or other fluids then it is appropriate to use multi-lumen lines. Most units dedicate one lumen for parenteral nutrition use. It is most important that all lumens are handled with strict aseptic technique during dressing, manipulation and sampling and drug administration to avoid infection.

Implantable devices are only used for long-term home parenteral nutrition.

DECIDING ON THE NUTRITIONAL REGIMEN: SOME SIMPLE RULES

- Prescription of parenteral nutrition and complex enteral feeding regimens should be multidisciplinary and always completed with the support of dietitians and pharmacists. Although long delay in starting nutritional support for a patient is harmful, it is rarely a matter of urgency to start feeding. In the acute, short-term situation, more harm can be done by overfeeding than underfeeding or not feeding.
- Energy intake should not exceed 40 kcal/kg/24 h. Glucose oxidation reaches maximum at 4–5 g/kg/24 h. At levels of greater than 6 g/kg/24 h the increase in glucose oxidation and, therefore, oxygen consumption can cause respiratory distress.
- Energy expenditure as fat is normally about 1–1.5 g/kg/24 h, but for critically ill patients it is about 0.8–1 g/kg/24 h.
- Nitrogen intake should not usually exceed 0.3 g/kg/24 h.

Box 10.4 Types of catheters used for parenteral nutrition

- Standard single and multi-lumen central catheters
- Peripherally inserted central catheters (PICC)
- Tunnelled single or double lumen catheters
- Implantable devices

- Fat has 9.4 kcal/g, carbohydrate about 3.75 kcal/g and amino acids have approximately 2.7 kcal/g nitrogen. The fat:carbohydrate ratio is approximately 40:60 in most regimens.
- Fluid requirements are usually 30–35 ml/kg/24 h. A more accurate estimation can be achieved using the formula: fluid requirement = 1500 ml × body surface area (m^2). In addition, 2–2.5 ml/kg/day will be needed for each °C if the temperature is >37°C and additional fluid losses (diarrhoea, fistulae, burns, etc.) must be added to the total.
- Sodium and chloride requirements are each 1–1.5 mmol/kg/24 h. If the serum sodium is low and the patient is estimated to be in fluid balance, then the additional sodium required can be estimated using the equation:

  0.2 × body weight in kg × (140 – measured serum sodium mmol/l)

- Potassium requirements are 1–1.5 mmol/kg/24 h. If the serum potassium is low the additional potassium required can be estimated using the equation:

  0.4 × body weight in kg × (4.0 – measured serum potassium mmol/l)

- Calcium requirements are 0.1–0.15 mmol/kg/24 h. To correct serum calcium for a low albumin use the formula:

  $$\text{Corrected calcium} = \text{measured calcium mmol/l} + \frac{(40 - \text{serum albumin g/l})}{40}$$

- Remember that in long-term critically ill patients, persistently elevated calcium may mean calcium loss from bone. Using a bisphosphonate may be appropriate.
- Magnesium requirements are 0.1–0.2 mmol/kg/24 h and phosphate requirements are 0.5–0.7 mmol/kg/24 h (see re-feeding syndrome).
- Most standard enteral and parenteral regimens will have adequate vitamin, mineral and trace elements when prescribed to meet the patient's nutritional needs.

Parenteral regimens

The components of parenteral regimens are outlined below.

Nitrogen

There are a large variety of standard amino acid solutions commercially available. Higher strength solutions with nitrogen contents of more than 18 g/l can be used when volume control is important. These solutions do not contain some amino acids, such as glutamine and cysteine, because of problems with stability. Dipeptide solutions such as glycyl-L-glutamine, glycyl-L-tyrosine and L-alanyl-L-glutamine are available as a source of these less-soluble, heat-labile amino acids. These solutions may be used in some hypermetabolic states, but caution is advised in renal and liver impairment.

Carbohydrate

This is usually supplied as a glucose solution. The solutions are usually in concentrations from 5 to 50% weight/volume and are available with or without electrolytes.

Lipid

Emulsions of lipid usually consist of soya bean long-chain triglycerides (LCT) emulsified with egg-derived phospholipids. They are available as 10, 20 and 30% weight for volume concentrations. Medium-chain triglyceride (MCT) mixtures are also available. Structured MCT/LCT, n-3-fatty acids and short-chain fatty acids are presently being investigated as substrates for parenteral nutrition.

Electrolytes, trace elements, vitamins and water

To compound a parenteral nutrition formulation, the most important requirement is an aseptic facility. This usually means a Class A aseptic room with a horizontal laminar flow cabinet where staff work in full aseptic clothing. When prescribing parenteral nutrition, consideration must always be given to the pharmacy implications. Prescribing complex regimens with numerous additions in the evening or at weekends make it difficult, if not impossible, for the pharmacy to meet the need. The parenteral formulations most often used are:

- 'big- bag' compounded *de novo*, where all components are compounded in a 2–5 l bag, which has appropriate addition ports
- 'standardized big bags' with minor additions. These can be two-in-one that do not contain fat, or all-in-one that do. These bags have a limited shelf life. The additions required are limited and usually involve electrolytes, minerals and vitamins only
- multilayered bags. In these bags the fat, glucose and nitrogen components are in separate chambers, which can be easily broken by external pressure when the bag is ready for use. These bags have a much longer shelf life, but again may involve the addition of electrolytes, minerals and vitamins.

Enteral regimens (i.e. oral or tube feeds)

There is a rapidly increasing list of enteral products available and a logical and efficient approach to choosing a product for a patient can best be achieved by considering three broad areas:

1. *Main categories*. These are shown in Box 10.5.
2. *Generic attributes*. The generic attributes to be considered for enteral prescriptions are shown in Table 10.5. Most feeds are lactose- and gluten-free.
3. *Classification*. The main types of enteral feed are shown in Table 10.6

MONITORING OUTCOME OF NUTRITIONAL INTERVENTION

The purpose of monitoring is to ensure adequacy of the nutritional regimen prescribed and to detect and minimize feeding-related complications at an early stage.

In the initial assessment the monitoring regimen will have been decided upon. This, in turn, will have depended on the clinical and nutritional condition of the patient and the type of feeding regimen employed. Most monitoring regimens will involve all or some of

Box 10.5 Diet

Fortified oral diets
Regular hospital diet can be fortified by adding a carbohydrate or fat module (see below) or simply adding butter, cream or extra sugar. The purpose is to make food energy-dense so that patients with poor appetites can get 'more for each bite'.

Oral supplement/sip feeds
Patients who cannot manage enough with fortified diet can add energy-dense liquid supplements that can be made up on the ward (Buildup®, Complan®) or are available in multiple flavours in tetra packs.

Sip feeds may also be used at the sole nutrition source (e.g. in the early phases of exclusion diet or in the management of Crohn's disease).

Tube feeds
These feeds may be given as the sole nutrition source or as a supplement to oral diet.

Table 10.5 Generic attributes to be considered for enteral prescriptions

Consideration	Presentation	Source and notes
Nitrogen	Whole protein, peptides and amino acids	e.g. whey, casein, soya
Carbohydrate	Malt dextrin, mono- and oligo-saccharides	e.g. corn, potato
Fat	LCT, MCT, free fatty acids	safflower, sunflower
Energy density and distribution	kcal/ml	e.g. amount from nitrogen, carbohydrate and fat
Fibre	g/l (usually about 15 g/l)	e.g. wheat bran, ispaghula husk, soy polysaccharide
Electrolyte composition	mmol	
Vitamin and mineral content	Expressed as volume required to meet RNI; % RDA/L	
Energy density	kcal/ml	usually 1–1.5 kcal/ml
Osmolarity	mmosm/l	the high osmolar elemental and peptide feeds may cause osmotic diarrhoea in patients with short bowel
Stabilizers		a rare, but 'hidden' source of dietary intolerance
Palatability and acceptance	Multiple flavours and consistencies	

RNI, recommended nutritional intake; RDA, recommended daily allowance

the following, at varying degrees of frequency depending on the clinical condition and the feeding regimen:

• Clinical and ethical appropriateness of current feeding regimen
• Nutritional adequacy of regimen
• Tube, stoma or catheter site (position, security, infection, accessories)

Table 10.6 The main types of enteral feed

Classification	Attributes	Use
Polymeric	Whole protein Maltodextrin and LCT (to a specified calorie density) ± fibre ± flavouring	Used as sip feeds, supplemental feeds and as tube feeds. May be used in addition to oral diet or as nutritionally complete feed
Semi elemental	Mono or oligo peptides Mono-oligosaccharides LCT/MCT ± flavouring	Sip or tube feeds May be used in pancreatic or intestinal malabsorptive states, but has high osmolar load
Elemental	Nitrogen as amino acids Carbohydrate as glucose Fat as free fatty acids ± flavouring	Sip or tube feeds May be used in pancreatic or intestinal malabsorptive states, but has high osmolar load
Modular	Nitrogen, carbohydrate, fat, electrolytes, vitamins and trace elements as individual powdered/liquid mixes	To individualize a patient's diet usually in conditions of possible complex food intolerance
Disease/organ specific/inborn errors of metabolism	Specific to disorder (e.g. renal failure or phenylketonuria)	
'Nutritional pharmacotherapy'/ novel substrates	Additional glutamine, arginine, nucleotides, etc.	Very little evidence base

- Has the patient actually got what was prescribed
- Food chart if appropriate
- Fluid balance charts
- Anthropometric measurements as appropriate (e.g. weight, skin fold thickness, hand dynamometry, bioelectric impedance)
- Clinical condition such as temperature, fluid balance, haemodynamic state, drug chart and change in disease management plan (e.g. surgery and chemotherapy)
- Biochemistry (sodium, potassium, phosphate, glucose, magnesium, calcium, LFT, albumin and trace elements).

DEALING WITH COMMON PROBLEMS

Generic problems

Communication

Working within an MDT that advises other teams is often difficult. Communication and clear definition of roles and responsibilities is essential. Remember that, although the patient's *primary* team has consulted you as a member of the NST, they may expect or

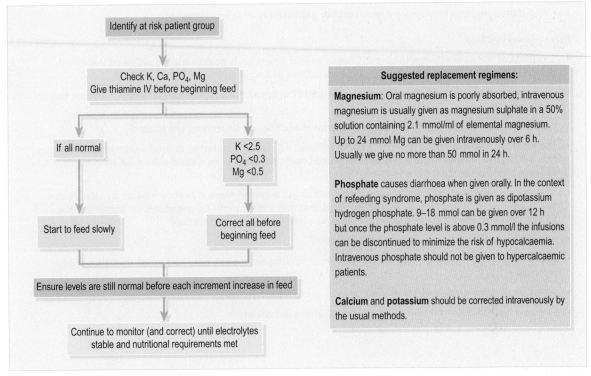

Fig. 10.4
Management of refeeding syndrome

The flowchart in Fig. 10.4 contains the following text:

Identify at risk patient group

Check K, Ca, PO₄, Mg
Give thiamine IV before beginning feed

If all normal

K <2.5
PO₄ <0.3
Mg <0.5

Start to feed slowly

Correct all before beginning feed

Ensure levels are still normal before each increment increase in feed

Continue to monitor (and correct) until electrolytes stable and nutritional requirements met

Suggested replacement regimens:

Magnesium: Oral magnesium is poorly absorbed, intravenous magnesium is usually given as magnesium sulphate in a 50% solution containing 2.1 mmol/ml of elemental magnesium. Up to 24 mmol Mg can be given intravenously over 6 h. Usually we give no more than 50 mmol in 24 h.

Phosphate causes diarrhoea when given orally. In the context of refeeding syndrome, phosphate is given as dipotassium hydrogen phosphate. 9–18 mmol can be given over 12 h but once the phosphate level is above 0.3 mmol/l the infusions can be discontinued to minimize the risk of hypocalcaemia. Intravenous phosphate should not be given to hypercalcaemic patients.

Calcium and **potassium** should be corrected intravenously by the usual methods.

presume support for a number of aspects of the patient's care, including gastroenterological problems, complex electrolyte problems and daily fluid balance.

Refeeding syndrome (Fig. 10.4)

During starvation or relative starvation there is a shift in the energy generating metabolic pathway from glucose metabolism to ketone metabolism. The former is highly dependent on phosphate and the latter is not. In conditions where predominant ketone metabolism is combined with low levels of body potassium, phosphate, magnesium and thiamine, the ability to revert from ketone metabolism to glucose metabolism is severely curtailed. Such conditions most frequently encountered in clinical practice include alcoholism, anorexia nervosa, chemotherapy, frail elderly (especially on diuretics), diabetes and small-bowel disease. In these situations a sudden glucose load will switch off ketone metabolism, switch on an unsustainable glucose metabolism and the result may be confusion owing to metabolic encephalopathy; pulmonary oedema owing to impaired myocardial contractility and arrhythmia; respiratory failure owing to impaired diaphragmatic and intercostal muscle contractility; proximal myopathy and, more rarely, dysphagia, ileus, rhabdomyolysis and haemolysis. Patients at risk should be identified during initial nutritional assessment. Potassium, magnesium, calcium and phosphate should be measured and corrected before the feed is commenced. In these situations it is advised to give additional thiamine.

Box 10.6 Procedure report following a non-surgical gastrostomy or jejunostomy

Report should include:

- condition of the patient's mouth care (this ensures that attention is paid to the condition of the mouth during the procedure but also encourages ward staff regarding mouth care)
- whether or not pre-procedure antibiotics were used (The British Society of Gastroenterology advises the use of antibiotics)
- how position of stoma was identified (transillumination, finger indentation, ultrasound)
- the absence of air aspiration (prior to gastric perforation) during instillation of local anaesthetic (recording this is a helpful reminder of the risk of interposed bowel, the procedure should always be abandoned if air is aspirated before the stomach is entered)
- how many percutaneous punctures were required to get access (if there is post-procedure peritonitis one puncture suggests that this is a controlled fistula and that a leak might be controlled by tightening the fixation devices; more than one puncture raises concern about free perforation)
- at what distance the tube was secured at skin level
- if additional securing devices (e.g. Brown-Muller or sutures) were used, how and when they should be removed
- where to find the guidelines for managing and caring for the stoma
- who and how to contact in the event of complications or concern

Safe duration without nutritional support

In general, nutritional support is needed when patients have been fasting for longer than 7 days, but this depends on the underlying nutrition state and current illness.

Tube problems

Blockage of tubes that have been difficult to site is the commonest problem. This is avoided by clear instruction to nursing staff on tube care. When tube blockage occurs, a 30–50 ml syringe should always be used to try to unblock it before using a smaller syringe. The pressure exerted by smaller syringes risks rupturing the tubes.

Stoma problems

Early problems

There are a number of frequently encountered early problems following stoma formation, but often a good procedure report (Box 10.6) will alleviate many of the problems associated with post-procedure care:

Some discomfort and erythema at the site is usual. Pain relief should be given and the patient monitored.

- Severe pain and peritonism suggest a leak, infection or free bowel perforation. Free air on plain film of abdomen occurs following the procedure in over 30% of patients and is not, by itself, an indication for intervention.

- A leak can be identified by X-ray tubogram and can usually be remedied by tightening the fixator devices. A major leak suggesting free perforation or tear may require surgical intervention.
- Direct injection into the peritoneal cavity on tubogram indicates both a displaced tube and a free viscus perforation (assuming that position in the bowel lumen was confirmed at initial insertion) and indicates the need for laparotomy if the patient is fit.
- If there is localized peritonism and there is not a free perforation, then the stoma should be put on free drainage and should not be used to feed or administer drugs; pain relief and intravenous fluids should be given and the patient kept under regular review until the situation settles.
- When there are early complications, the temptation to remove a gastrostomy tube (outside of a laparotomy situation) should be resisted, especially in the first 2 weeks, as this would result in a free perforation. It is easy to remove balloon and pigtail initial placement tubes at the bedside and inexperienced junior staff may consider doing this.
- Infection at the stoma site will need swabs and antibiotics.
- It is always difficult to confirm the position of a replacement jejunostomy and a tubogram is usually necessary.

Problems after discharge

When patients are discharged to the community with feeding stomas the most frequent problems include the following:

- The tube falls out. This is most common with balloon and pigtail tubes. These stoma tracts close very rapidly. It is important that a replacement balloon tube is placed as soon as possible. If replacement is easy and gastric contents are aspirated, then the tube can be used to feed. If replacement is difficult and/or there is no aspirate, confirmation of correct placement using a tubogram will be needed.
- The stoma becomes infected. Providing there is no evidence of abscess formation, swabs and antibiotics will be sufficient, but an abscess may need surgical intervention.
- The peristomal skin becomes excoriated. In this situation support from the stomatherapist should be sought.
- Failure to monitor the patient's condition. Patients with stroke disease or multiple sclerosis may have significant improvement in their swallowing. Unless there is regular reassessment this and the patient's ability to eat may be missed.

Removing a gastrostomy

When asked to remove a gastrostomy remember:

- there is a risk of free gastric perforation if tubes are removed within 6 weeks of placement
- if the internal fixator is a pigtail, then turning the 'lock' to undo the pigtail will allow withdrawal of the tube
- if the internal fixator is a balloon, then deflation of the balloon will allow removal

Table 10.7 Sodium content of some drug infusions

Drug	Approximate sodium content
Normal saline 1 l	150 mmol
Ciprofloxacin 400 mg iv	30 mmol
Fluconazole 200 mg	15 mmol
Flucytosine 2.5g	34 mmol
Foscarnet 6 g	93 mmol
Metronidazole 500 mg	13 mmol

- if the internal fixator is rigid and the patient has no adhesions, strictures or gut motility problems (scleroderma, etc.), then the tube can be cut at skin level and allowed to fall into the stomach, otherwise it will need to be removed endoscopically.

Parenteral feeding problems

Sepsis

The cause of sepsis is often due to the clinical condition and not the parenteral line, but with new fevers it is best to stop the feed, culture the line and the peripheral blood (and any other clinically relevant cultures). Most lines can be salvaged with the appropriate antibiotics, but sometimes, especially in unstable septic patients, the line may need to be changed. It is best to wait until the patient is afebrile before siting a new feeding line.

Drugs

Some drugs alter electrolyte balance (e.g. amphotericin, ciclosporin and diuretics). Another problem is the electrolyte content of the various drug regimens in use. Some drug infusions can contain large amounts of sodium as shown in Table 10.7.

Further Reading

Elia M. Enteral and Parenteral Nutrition in the Community. British Association for Parenteral and Enteral Nutrition, Maidenhead, 1994.

McAter CA. Current Perspectives on Enteral Nutrition in Adults. British Association for Parenteral and Enteral Nutrition, Maidenhead, 1999.

Lennard-Jones JE. Ethical and legal aspects of clinical hydration and nutritional support. British Association for Parenteral and Enteral Nutrition, Maidenhead, 1998.

Nightingale JMD. Intestinal Failure. GMM Press, London, 2001.

Payne J, Grimble G, Silk D. Artificial Nutrition Support in Clinical Practice. GMM Press, London, 2001.

Pennington CR. Current Perspectives on Parenteral Nutrition in Adults. British Association for Parenteral and Enteral Nutrition, Maidenhead, 1996.

Silk DBA. Organisation of Nutritional Support in Hospitals. British Association for Parenteral and Enteral Nutrition, Maidenhead, 1994.

Sizer T. Standards and Guidelines for Nutritional Support of patients in Hospitals. British Association for Parenteral and Enteral Nutrition, 1996.

Stratton RJ, Green CJ, Elia M. Disease related malnutrition: an evidence based approach to treatment. CABI Publishing, 2003.

Stroud M, Duncan H, Nightingale JMD, British Society of Gastroenterology. Guidelines for enteral feeding in adult hospital patients. Gut 2003; 52(Suppl vii): vii1–vii12.

Modern endoscopy

INTRODUCTION

The practice of safe and accurate endoscopy is one of the initial skills, if not the main one, that any gastroenterology trainee wants to master. It remains an essential part of any gastroenterologist's diagnostic and therapeutic armamentarium throughout their career, no matter which sub-specialist area they ultimately choose to develop. Even though other forms of investigation may supersede some aspects of diagnostic endoscopy, there remains the ever-increasing demand for endoscopy therapeutics.

This chapter will introduce important concepts and topics in endoscopy, both in terms of patient care and provision of a good endoscopy service. It also lists useful practical guidelines for managing the patient in the endoscopy room (such as antibiotic protocols, managing the diabetic patient, etc.). However, it is beyond the scope (sic) of this chapter to describe how to perform individual techniques.

A BRIEF HISTORY

Before the 19th century, even from ancient times, there were a handful of documented attempts to visualize the interior of the body using various forms of rigid tubing with candlelight. By the 1930s Rudolf Schindler was producing exquisite colour drawings of gastric pathology using a semi-rigid endoscope and a retrievable miniaturized 'gastrocamera' was manufactured in the 1950s to take photographs from within the stomach. At about this time advances in technology allowed the development of the coherent fibreoptic glass bundle and the use of a recognizable fibreoptic endoscope was reported by the late 1950s. Instrument development was taken on by the Japanese camera manufacturers, improving the flexibility, robustness and waterproofing while reducing the endoscope diameter and increasing the working channel size. Finally, microelectronic developments, particularly of the charged coupled device (CCD) and piezo-electric crystals, ushered in a new era of video and ultrasound endoscopy. This has allowed further evolution of not only endoscopic diagnosis, but also training and working (assistants and trainees can see as clearly as the operator). Electronics allow new ways of imaging the mucosa and submucosa outside of the visible spectrum to open more opportunities to improve patient management.

Thus, gastrointestinal (GI) endoscopy has changed rapidly over the last 40 years, from a somewhat limited procedure to one that has seen an explosion of utility, experience, complexity and, as a result, demand. Currently in the UK about 2% of the population undergoes one endoscopy per annum and this is likely to rise when colorectal cancer screening is introduced. How to manage endoscopy, with limited resources, as a service to patients, therefore, becomes an important part of any gastroenterologist's ability to care for the population.

ENDOSCOPY UNITS

Concomitant with the rise in use of endoscopy was the requirement for a safe environment in which to practise. Trainee endoscopists probably concentrate just on the ability to learn how to endoscope, but it is important to appreciate the setting that allows safe and efficient endoscopy. Early endoscopy rooms were often no more than side rooms on a general ward, using general nursing staff as endoscopy assistants. Modern endoscopy requires properly designed areas and dedicated endoscopy nursing staff. The minimum suggested elements are shown in Table 11.1 and design guidance can be found from

Table 11.1 Aspects of endoscopy unit design

Main user	Zones required	Notes
All	All	Environment must be easy to clean and aesthetically pleasing
Patients	Entrance and reception	Must include disabled access, toilets, children play area
	Administrative	Often much larger area required for notes storage
	Assessment and preparation	Must allow private, dignified clerking and preparation for patients. Ideally linked to nearby clinics and a separate waiting area away from the general waiting area
	Procedure rooms	Suggested size 5.5 × 5.0 m, one larger for X-ray equipment and anaesthetic trolley. Two rooms per 250 000 population
	Recovery areas	Must allow for monitoring of sedated and non-sedated patients, private changing, nursing desks, refreshments, trolley storage, private interview areas for results
	Quiet room	For post endoscopy interviews
	Toilet facilities	
Staff	Changing rooms	Including lockers and shower facilities
	Rest area	With kitchen area
	Offices	Ideally, on site for nurse manager, lead endoscopist, nurse practitioners
	Training and information	Seminar room with video links and library
Support	Decontamination	Large enough to comply with latest cleaning and safety standards. Dry storage for endoscopes
	Storage	Accessories, equipment transport cases, office consumables,
	Linen and waste utility	cleaner. Space for information hubs and video processing
	Water, oxygen, vacuum, electricity	Includes video link, computer data networks
	Security	Must be physically secure and alarmed

Department of Health NHS Estates Department, as 'building note 52', published in 1994. Nevertheless, many hospitals have had to cope with the evolutionary nature of endoscopy in a limited space, leading to wide variations in the quality of service, particularly from the patient's perception of privacy and dignity.

Most endoscopy units have had to fit into clinical area shapes designed for other purposes, such as ward space or clinic areas, quite often for activity levels based on the past rather than the future. The processes surrounding endoscopy are very complex, not just because of the variety of endoscopy procedures, but because of all of the administrative processes before and after. Once a patient has been booked on to a list there follows a succession of steps from reception, to nurse assessment, preparation, final consent, the procedure itself, recovery and discharge planning. A unit has to cope with in-patients and out-patients, ensure equipment is available, serviced and decontaminated, have the right skill mix of nursing and endoscopist staff for all that day's activities. Ideally, the flow of patients should follow a path that does not cross back on itself or other processes. There is no standard or best design of an endoscopy unit. Design considerations such as the size of various waiting zones, keeping clean areas from contaminated paths, and the number of trolleys each unit needs depends on the case mix handled in each unit.

The layout of the procedure room itself also has a significant impact on the efficiency of working. Three areas interact: the patient (trolley) space, the endoscopist space and the assistant area. Like the overall patient pathway, workflows within a room should not cross over each other. The patient trolley should be able to be turned through 180°. The endoscopist requires access to the nearby endoscope, drugs, gloves and aprons and a separate sub area with notes, radiographs and computer data entry. The nurse-assistant zone is much larger, requiring additional access to accessories, storage and separation of contaminated equipment and specimens from clean areas. The room should have dimmable lighting, piped oxygen and suction, have anti-static floor coatings and not be cluttered by cabling trailing over the floor.

Room design is also influenced by the type of procedure and the rationale of patient pathways. Early designs operated on the basis of not just performing the endoscopy, but also pre-assessment, clerking and consent, as well as some recovery time. This has the attractiveness of simplicity, but is inefficient for turnover. Modern rooms are generally run to maximize procedure time with other pre- and post-procedure tasks occurring elsewhere. Procedure rooms may be specialized for one type of endoscopy and hold particular storage areas, accessories and equipment, while others may need to cater for all procedures. This imposes a trade off between flexibility for scheduling patients and efficiency for running specialist lists.

Recovery zones need to be large enough to cope with the variations in numbers of patients electing to have sedation, with all bed spaces having piped oxygen, suction, oximetry and availability of blood-pressure monitoring, with sufficient staff to cope with this. Once recovered, patients require good information to plan management and help them understand the findings. Ideally, this should be done in areas separate from the patients arriving for assessment.

Endoscopy units, therefore, house a complex collection of processes that require compromise to allow flexibility. A good endoscopy-unit design augments the optimum patient pathway and does not restrict it.

MODERNIZING ENDOSCOPY – THE UK EXAMPLE

Development of endoscopy in the UK has been somewhat haphazard, whilst being a victim of its own success. Despite the overwhelming utility of endoscopy in diagnosis, for example of cancer where it has replaced upper GI barium studies, endoscopy has remained a somewhat Cinderella specialty as far as funding and profile is concerned. It has also suffered from variable clinical ownership, with endoscopy units around the country being under the wing of physicians, surgeons, radiologists and general practitioners (GPs). This has led to variations in the quality of clinical leadership and in the standard of training, staffing and patient care in the face of increasing demands. Endoscopists have many other conflicting demands on their time outside of the service. Information about incoming referrals both in quality and quantity are often absent, with multiple routes of referral and lengthy waiting times. Quite often this has led to reduction in morale and, ultimately, less than ideal patient care and hence complaints.

In parallel with the emergence of clinical governance in medical practice, endoscopists have been learning how to standardize the quality of care from various pilot projects around the country. This is now being promoted by the NHS Modernisation Agency. At the heart of every endoscopy service should be the patient experience. Each patient should expect a timely, safe and accurate endoscopy performed in pleasant surroundings by competent and caring staff. Every step of the 'journey' from referral to discharge has potential pitfalls, but key areas for a good endoscopy service are:

- good clinical leadership in the unit: nursing and medical
- assessing and reviewing processes (mapping processes, the 'patient pathway')
- knowing what patients need (patient feedback)
- knowing what the demand for the service is (the rate of referral)
- knowing how much work there is to be done (the numbers already waiting)
- planning and using the capacity of resources (equipment, rooms, endoscopists) effectively
- knowing the outcomes of the work done (quality and quantity)
- looking for new ways of coping or altering with demand.

Quite often the above information is either unavailable or inaccurate and, therefore, it is not surprising that endoscopy units struggle to cope with quality control. Detailed analysis of what actually happens during the average endoscopy list can be quite illuminating when it comes to measuring how much time is lost through delays. In an ideal world each list would start promptly, never be cancelled, each patient would arrive on time with no 'DNAs', time between cases would be minimized by rapid turnover, endoscopes would always be ready and plentiful, staff would not require breaks and there would be no other interruptions.

Of course, we all know the real endoscopy list is not like this. Analyzing each step does require much effort, but it is a rewarding exercise for planning the true capacity of each hospital. While the maximum achievable usage is probably about 80% of the total available time, most units who do this exercise find they are running at 40–50%! Estimating capacity is not just a case of multiplying how many of a certain type of endoscopy are done per week by an average reasonable procedure time. Actual times, obtained by observing every procedure, are required – there is quite a variation in times depending on the individual trained endoscopist, the type of endoscopy procedure and if trainees are present. Thus, endoscopy capacity is not just dependent on the number of endoscopists or the number of rooms.

Similarly, understanding the true demand on the service is fundamental to being able to plan that service. Demand is not simply a matter of the number of endoscopies referred and the potential time taken to perform that procedure, but must include all the ancillary activities before and after endoscopy itself.

When faced with increasing demands on the service and rising waiting lists, the most obvious solution is to try and obtain extra endoscopists or rooms, but this may not actually be necessary if unused capacity can be released.

So what can be done to improve efficiency and release unused capacity? Some measures to improve efficiency are easier than others. Ascertaining why some lists start late may allow better planning with the endoscopist concerned and enforcing a no late cancellations rule on endoscopists should prevent sudden rescheduling of lists. Trying to use replacement endoscopists to work on cancelled lists through annual leave sounds simple, but quite often trained endoscopists are already busy elsewhere. Implementing guidelines for referral or follow-up may cut out unnecessary endoscopies, for example a test and treat policy to reduce the need for diagnostic endoscopy in simple dyspepsia, increasing the interval between Barrett's follow-up surveillance or reducing the variability between endoscopist's opinions for follow-up of colonic polyps. These are outlined in the respective chapters. Enforcement of follow-up protocols reduces the variability and confusion seen where individual endoscopists (particularly early in their career) determine arbitrary follow-up intervals, often erring on the side of caution. This can be applied to new cases as well as to current cases (the 'backlog') by review of all case notes.

Reducing time lost through patients not attending (DNAs) is more difficult. Traditionally, a clinician would request an endoscopy and often the patient would just be sent an appointment time for that clinician's list. This led to multiple waiting lists within one unit and great complexity for scheduling. Setting up systems where patients can negotiate a time convenient to them requires more administrative time as well as the introduction of pooled waiting lists. This latter change can be quite challenging for some clinicians. One method is for a patient to take their request form to the endoscopy centre to book their own time, which could be on any suitable list (surgical, medical or nurse practitioner). They also obtain all the correct information booklets and consent forms at the same time. This booked admission system reduces DNA wastage and is a central part of NHS modernization and should be fully implemented by 2005.

More expensive solutions include funding extra endoscopists (nurse practitioners and clinical staff) to increase capacity, one-stop clinics to simplify patient pathways, obtaining extra endoscopes if turnover is a problem and introducing extra sessions (weekends or evenings). The latter may be temporary to cut through the backlog, but will only be effective if the other measures are in place to stop the backlog accumulating again.

The key to most of this is information. Calculation of true capacity as suggested above may show where the bottlenecks are and form the basis of business cases. A weekly check on waiting times allows the adjustment of lists to optimize any trends. Clearly this requires a robust information system. Keeping control of demand and waiting times does require effort from the entire team and identifying an enthusiastic lead clinician for endoscopy helps to focus the task.

The ultimate outcome of this sort of strategy is to improve the patient experience and where some or all of these measures have been introduced, patient feedback through questionnaires and interviews has been very favourable. Patient surveys in the past have identified the two main concerns of uncertainty and frustration of not knowing when an appointment will be and issues around lack of information. Endoscopy units employing these measures also notice reduced number of complaints from patients and referring medical staff.

INSTRUMENT DECONTAMINATION

Endoscopes are very expensive, complex and delicate instruments and will not withstand steam autoclaving, as used in the sterilization of surgical instruments, between cases. Instead, endoscopes must undergo 'high-level disinfection' before and after each use. It is important that all endoscopists know how to perform this task, especially when using instruments out of normal working hours. Endoscopy accessories can, however, be sterilized by standard theatre techniques, although there is a trend to use single-use disposable items. The best practice is to decontaminate all equipment to a standard suitable for all patients, whether immunocompromised or not.

There are two equally important phases – physical removal of debris from the endoscope internal and external surfaces, followed by chemical neutralization of microbiological agents. The first commences the moment the patient is extubated, where the endoscopist should initiate aspiration of warm soapy water up through the biopsy channel. This is followed by the dismantling of any removable items from the endoscope and thorough brushing of each channel with a clean brush at least three times, as well as the exterior of the instrument with a clean toothbrush. An endoscope has at least three channels to clean (positive pressure air/water supply and suction channels in the umbilical cord and the combined biopsy channels) using detergent/enzymatic cleaner. The instrument is tested for leaks and damage. The second phase uses an automatic washer disinfector. There are several on the market and it is important you know how to operate your machines.

In the UK, new regulations, known as 'HTM 2030', are tightening up decontamination machine issues. It is important to involve local microbiology and infection-control departments, as inspection panels will be appointed with the power to close units if standards are not met. Key points are:

- one endoscope per washing machine tub
- every irrigation channel to record cleaning fluid flow data
- all instruments and accessories to be traceable to each use, patient and cleaning cycle
- all staff to be properly trained, assessed and protected
- machines to be housed in purpose built rooms
- very frequent testing of disinfectant power and replacement
- regular microbiological assessment of machines and even deliberate challenge
- water supply decontamination standards.

Clearly these standards have implications for the turnover of endoscopes during a working list, as well as the overall cost of endoscopy.

In addition, all staff have to be trained in the health and safety regulations for the use of disinfectants to avoid injury to health and in wearing appropriate protective clothing. Two per cent glutaraldehyde was a commonly used agent until concerns around the immune sensitizing action prompted its withdrawal. Alternative agents are now used, listed in Table 11.2, although all are necessarily toxic. For the rare instance where a patient with suspected vCJD requires endoscopy, previously vCJD exposed endoscopes are available from the national CJD surveillance unit, as they cannot be reliably decontaminated.

Once decontaminated, endoscopes are stored and dried. At the end of the day they are stored in vertical hanging cupboards, ready for a further decontamination cycle before the next use. Ideally, only single-use accessories would be used and biopsy valves and covers used only once, but economic considerations may prevent adoption of this policy.

The only additional precautions required relate to patients known or suspected to host MRSA, which may contaminate the endoscopy room requiring extra cleaning after

Table 11.2 List of disinfectants used commonly in the UK

Agent	Suggested contact times	Comments
Ortho-phthalaldehyde (Cidex OPA)	5 min	Very poor at destroying spores
Succine dialdehyde ± formaldehyde (Gigasept, Gigsept FF)	5 min	Very poor at destroying spores
Peracetic acid (NuCidex, Perascope, Gigasept PA)	5 min, but 20 min for mycobacteria	Can penetrate biofilms Very labile, requires daily changes
Superoxised water (Sterilox, Suprox)	5 min 10 min for mycobacteria	Produced by electrolysis machine on site Careful monitoring of endoscope condition required
Chlorine dioxide (Tristel)	5 min 10 min for mycobacteria	Corrosive, requires very good ventilation, careful monitoring of endoscope condition
Alcohol	5 min	Damaging to endoscopes, for drying channels only, flammable

serving such a patient. All rooms should be cleaned at the end of each day and the ease of this is determined by the endoscopy room design.

SEDATION

Although intravenous sedation has been used by endoscopists for over 30 years, quite wide variations in practice and, potentially, safety have only become apparent relatively recently by audit. As in all medicine, any course of action is a balance of risk and benefit. Some patients may tolerate diagnostic endoscopy without any sedation, while others require a sedative if a careful and thorough examination is to take place at all. Sedation significantly increases the hazard of endoscopy, principally by reduced airway protection, respiratory depression with hypoxic injury and hypotension.

Midazolam has become the drug of choice over the previously used diazepam-based preparations – it has a shorter half-life, relatively greater amnesic properties and a milder respiratory depressant effect compared with diazepam. The fundamental principle of sedation in this setting is that the patient remains conscious – i.e. you can still verbally communicate with the, albeit drowsy, patient. If the patient loses consciousness this becomes general anaesthesia, which requires a magnitude increase in patient monitoring and is no longer safe in the standard endoscopy setting.

All trainee and established endoscopists should have received formal supervised training for the use of these drugs. It should be remembered that benzodiazepines have no analgesic properties so, where potentially painful procedures will be carried out, opioid analgesics should be used (generally pethidine or fentanyl). Analgesics should be given before sedatives as they potentiate benzodiazepines by a factor of 4–10 times. The standards and principles of safe sedation are listed in Box 11.1.

Box 11.1. Safe sedation practice

- Two nurse assistants are needed, one fully qualified
- Assess the risk to each patient (see text)
- Oxygen, suction and tipping trolley used
- Full resuscitation equipment available immediately
- Reversal agents flumazenil and naloxone available immediately
- Continuous pulse oximetry in all patients
- Oxygen supplementation in all sedated patients
- Secure venous access in all patients with a 'venflon'
- Give any analgesics first and allow distribution
- Slow titration of sedative to patient response
- Recovery in a properly staffed recovery zone
- Clear and precise instructions for observations if a complication is suspected

All staff need regular resuscitation training and simulation. Some patients are not fit for sedation (or indeed any endoscopy), for example in severe lung disease, vascular disease or clinically significant hypotension. Where benefit/risk ratio is deemed to allow endoscopy in a high-risk case, further monitoring is required as blood pressure and ECG display. Twenty-four per cent oxygen supplementation is universally safe, even for advanced lung disease. Diagnostic upper endoscopy can be safely carried out without any sedative, which only highlights the importance of not adding unnecessary risk for a patient by unsafe practice. Patients may become restless or aggressive and further sedation just makes the situation worse and dangerous. Here it may be better to stop, reverse the sedation and repeat another time. It may be necessary to arrange for a general anaesthetic for a small number of patients. Some patients with induced liver enzymes (alcohol or patients on benzodiazepines) may need an opioid before sedation to potentiate the midazolam. These are the minimum standards permissible for safe conscious sedation and should be an important part of audit and governance in every endoscopy unit.

CONSENT

Another key area in modern endoscopy unit governance is the practice of informed consent. Good medical practice demands that patients undergoing any invasive procedure must be able to take a decision in a calm and considered manner, given sufficient information to make a valid judgement. Treatment or investigation without this is assault. Practice in the NHS has been tightened up by the introduction of standardized consent forms and guidance. This was prompted by public concern following incidents such as the Bristol inquiry where parents of children undergoing major heart surgery were not made aware of the true risks (i.e. local post-operative mortality data) involved.

Over the last 10 years there has necessarily and thankfully been a swing away from the 'quick consent' practice for endoscopy where a patient would arrive in the endoscopy room and be told to 'sign here'! Good consent practice starts with the patient being able to understand why an endoscopy is being recommended and what it involves. Often a complete explanation is required using simple language. Consent includes the ability to recognize the benefits, risks and alternatives to any treatments or tests, with the patient being able to retain this information to make a decision without coercion. This process, ideally, starts at the time of the decision to refer for endoscopy, backed up with information booklets that the patient can read at home at leisure. It is the final responsibility of the endoscopist performing the procedure to ensure that proper informed consent has been given.

The use of information booklets allows the long list of material a patient needs to bear in mind to be absorbed. This includes statements about the procedure, alternative tests or treatment options and not only the potential gains from undergoing the test or treatment, but also the potential complications (giving local complication rates). The options not to undergo the test or treatment should be mentioned and the potential consequences of taking this option. Patients need to be reminded that they can withdraw consent at any time and have free access to a second opinion. If they have any particular concerns or beliefs these must be incorporated in the consent and treatment plan, e.g. Jehovah's Witnesses.

A consent form can be included with the booklet to allow perusal of the document they will eventually sign. Only when a patient has been properly informed will their signature actually mean they have consented. Provision must be made for information in other languages. The standard Department of Health consent forms have two parts. The front page has a top copy to be retained by the patient and includes areas for the name of the procedure, complications with rates, and a list of the information that the patient has been provided with, as well as an interpreter's section if that is required. The consent form must have the name of the consultant in overall responsibility for the patient and the front page is signed by the practitioner to confirm the patient is now fully informed. The top copy should be signed at least 24 h before the test is performed. On the day of the test, the patient should be taken through the details again by the admitting nurse, before a final opportunity for any questions. The final consent is signed on the final page by both the patient and the practitioner again. It is useful to provide individualized books and pre-printed consent forms for standard diagnostic upper and lower endoscopy, endoscopic retrograde cholangiopancreatography (ERCP), endoscopic ultrasound (EUS), percutaneous endoscopic gastrostomy (PEG), and oesophageal stenting and dilatations. Supplementary pages can be added for particular patient groups for extra information such as diabetes, anti-coagulation, etc.

There is less time for an in-patient to consider a proposed endoscopy and this group is, of course, often much more unwell and infirm. Clearly in dire emergencies an experienced endoscopist should make an assessment quickly in the patient's best interests and proceed to potentially life-saving therapeutic endoscopy if appropriate. For less urgent diagnostic in-patient endoscopy, the patients should at least be provided with similar information to out patients to read. It is prudent in urgent elective therapeutic in-patient endoscopy, such as ERCP or PEG, to discuss the proposed therapy in advance with the patient, as such interventions can be considered to have similar risks to a 'mini-laparotomy'.

If a patient is unable to understand the proposed investigation, or weigh the risks and benefits, or has such a poor memory that information cannot be retained, then the endoscopist needs to make a value judgement as to whether to proceed in the patient's best interests. This consent should be recorded on the form for mentally incapacitated adults. Although relatives have no legal power to give consent for an adult, it is helpful and good practice to seek their opinions to arrive at a 'best interest' judgement. If there are any advance directives from a time when the patient was mentally competent, then these should be followed. There is a section to record if relatives or second medical opinions have been sought, as well as a statement as to why a patient is not able to give consent.

OTHER GUIDANCE FOR SAFE ENDOSCOPY: PATIENT FACTORS

All endoscopy units should have readily available advice for medical and nursing staff to follow to deal with common complicating factors affecting safety and preparation for procedures. Most scenarios for elective procedures involve patients on anticoagulants, diabetic patients, prophylaxis from infections (principally endocarditis) and the best form of bowel preparations. Seriously ill patients, for example the anticoagulated patient with acute GI bleeding, are discussed in Chapter 7.

Anticoagulation

This is a balance of risk: what are the risks of inducing excess bleeding by performing a procedure if anticoagulation is continued, versus the risk of thromboembolism if anticoagulation is temporarily discontinued. These are determined by the invasiveness of the procedure and the condition for which anticoagulation is given. Table 11.3 classifies each procedure according to bleed risk and Table 11.4 list the risks of reversing anticoagulation according to the original indication for anticoagulation. Having decided on the balance of these risks the management in Figure 11.1 can be followed.

Antibiotics

Systemic infection after endoscopy is very rare. Nevertheless, although rare, bacterial endocarditis is a life-threatening complication of endoscopy. Studies of bacteraemia and audit of complications suggest a higher incidence of local or systemic infections following:

- oesophageal stricture dilatation
- sclerotherapy for oesophageal varices
- laser therapy in upper gastrointestinal tract
- biliary procedures/ERCP
- PEG.

Analogous to the anticoagulated patient, there is a balance of risk of giving unnecessary antibiotics against preventing post-procedure infection, some lesions being more prone to

Table 11.3 Endoscopy procedure hazard for bleeding

Low risk*	High risk
Diagnostic upper gastrointestinal (GI) endoscopy	Polypectomy
Diagnostic lower GI endoscopy	PEG
Diagnostic ERCP	ERCP sphincterotomy
Diagnostic enteroscopy	EUS FNA or biopsy
Diagnostic EUS	Variceal therapy
	Dilatation
	Argon Beam or Laser therapy

*Standard mucosal biopsies are allowed if INR is known to be <3.0. ERCP, endoscopic retrograde cholangiopancreatogram; EUS, endoscopic ultrasound; FNA, fine-needle aspiration; GI, gastrointestinal; PEG, full term?

Table 11.4 Hazard of reversal of anticoagulation (risk of thrombosis)

Low risk	High risk
Lone atrial fibrillation (AF) or paroxysmal AF	AF due to valvular heart disease
Deep vein thrombosis	Pulmonary embolism
Bioprosthetic valve	Mechanical valve replacement

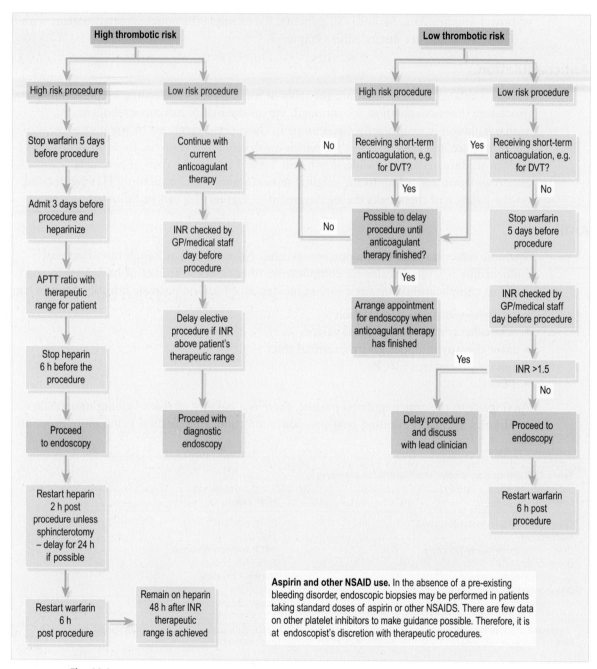

Fig. 11.1
Guidelines for the management of anticoagulated patients having elective endoscopy

Table 11.5 Risk of endocarditis

High risk Always need antibiotics	Prosthetic cardiac valves, including bioprosthetic and homograft valves Previous bacterial endocarditis Complex cyanotic congenital heart disease Surgically constructed systemic pulmonary shunts or conduits
Moderate risk Require antibiotics for procedures listed in text only	Most other congenital cardiac malformations Acquired valvular dysfunction (e.g. rheumatic heart disease) Hypertrophic cardiomyopathy Mitral valve prolapse with valvular regurgitation and/or thickened leaflets
Low risk Generally do not require antibiotics	Isolated secundum atrial septal defect Surgical repair of atrial septal defect, ventricular septal defect, or patent ductus arteriosus (without residua beyond 6 months) Previous coronary artery bypass graft surgery Mitral valve prolapse without valvular regurgitation Previous Kawasaki disease without valvular dysfunction Previous rheumatic fever without valvular dysfunction Cardiac pacemakers (intravascular and epicardial) and implanted defibrillators Physiologic, functional, or innocent heart murmurs (individual cardiologists may request antibiotic cover for heart murmurs) All other patients

endocarditis than others (Table 11.5). In immunocompromised patients the incidence of opportunistic infections is potentially much higher and requires alternative agents. Each hospital will set local antibiotic guidance depending on local conditions, for example, in Nottingham cephalosporins are avoided if at all possible to reduce the incidence of *Clostridium difficile* colitis. Our guidelines are synthesized from opinions from American and European societies for gastroenterology and cardiology. Having assessed the risk for infection, guidance can be followed for non-neutropenic patients in Figure 11.2. Neutropenic patients should receive ampicillin/gentamicin/metronidazole or vancomycin/gentamicin/metronidazole for all procedures. Amoxicillin can substitute for ampicillin. Suggested doses are given in Table 11.6.

Care of diabetic patients

As 1–2% of the population are diabetic, patients and staff often require advice on how to avert significant failures in glycaemic control pre- and post-endoscopy. Factors influencing this include the type of diabetes, the procedure required, the likely recovery time and the history of diabetic control in that individual. Thus, greater problems can be expected for an insulin-dependent patient undergoing bowel preparation for colonoscopy than for a non-insulin-dependent patient having a diagnostic endoscopy with no sedation. If there is any doubt about the management, the diabetes team should be consulted.

All patients are advised to bring their own tablets or insulin and should not drive to or, especially, from the hospital, in case glycaemic control has significantly changed. Patients with difficult control of diabetes, or who are elderly and/or frail should be admitted

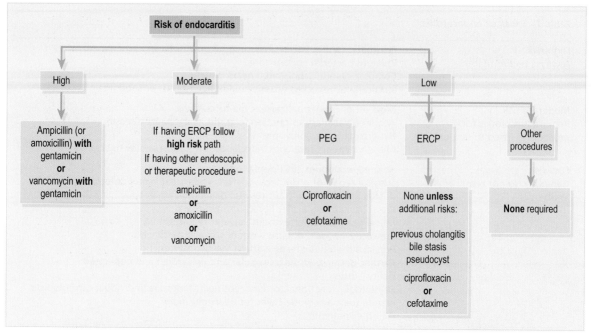

Fig. 11.2
Antibiotic prophylaxis for non-neutropenic patients (>1.5 x 10⁹/l)
ERCP, endoscopic retrograde cholangiopancreatography; PEG, percutaneous endoscopic gastrostomy

Table 11.6 Antibiotic doses for adults

Agents	Dosing
Ampicillin (or amoxicillin) plus gentamicin (patients not allergic to these, and not received these in the previous month)	Ampicillin or amoxicillin 2.0 g intravenously (iv) plus Gentamicin 1.5 mg/kg (not to exceed 120 mg) within 30 min of starting procedure Ampicillin 1 g iv or amoxicillin 1 g orally 6 h post procedure
Vancomycin plus gentamicin (patients allergic to ampicillin/amoxicillin or who have received penicillin within a month)	Vancomycin 1.0 g iv over 2 h plus gentamicin 1.5 mg/kg iv (not to exceed 120 mg); complete injection/infusion within 30 min of starting procedure For urgent endoscopies teicoplanin 400 mg iv bolus can be given instead of vancomycin
Amoxicillin or ampicillin (patients not allergic to these and not received these in the previous month)	Amoxicillin 2.0 g orally 1 h before procedure, or ampicillin 2.0 g iv within 30 min of starting procedure
Vancomycin (patients allergic to ampicillin/amoxicillin or who have received penicillin within 1 month)	Vancomycin 1.0 g iv over 1–2 h Complete infusion within 30 min of starting procedure
Metronidazole	If neutropenic (<1.5 × 10⁹/l) add metronidazole 7.5 mg/kg iv to any of the above steps as appropriate
Ciprofloxacin or cefuroxime (For PEG or ERCP as appropriate)	750 mg ciprofloxacin orally 60–90 min before the procedure OR Cefuroxime 750 mg iv Complete within 30 min of starting procedure

Box 11.2 The GKI protocol for glycaemic control during and after procedures. Alternatively a standard insulin sliding scale can be used

Morning procedure only: omit breakfast

- GKI infusion = 500 ml 10% dextrose + actrapid insulin dose = 1 g KCl
  - Actrapid dose – average build and insulin requirements (40–50 units per day), start with 12 units of actrapid in the bag. If evidence of increased insulin resistance (obesity, steroid therapy, infection or high insulin requirements), start with 16 units actrapid in the bag. If evidence of increased insulin sensitivity (underweight, treated hypopituitarism, etc.) or low insulin requirements – start off with 8 units actrapid.
- Infuse at 80 ml/h (must be via a pump)
- Perform blood glucose test and check hourly: aim is to keep blood glucose between 7 and 12 mmol/l
  - If blood glucose <4 mmol/l – stop the infusion, give 200 ml of 10% dextrose over 5–10 min. Change the infusion to one containing 4 units less actrapid insulin in 500 ml 10% dextrose, infused at the same rate. Reassess in 15 min and then hourly
  - If blood glucose <7 mmol/l and falling, replace infusion with one containing 4 units less actrapid in 500 ml of 10% dextrose at same rate and reassess hourly
  - If blood glucose >12 mmol/l and rising, replace infusion with one containing 4 units more actrapid in 500 ml 10% dextrose. Infuse at same rate and reassess hourly

beforehand. Ideally, patients should be endoscoped first on a morning list. If local anaesthetic to the throat is used, patients may not be able to swallow for 2 h after the procedure and bowel preparation may well upset glycaemic control. Where intravenous insulin is to be used, the patient may need a hospital bed, although with capable patients this is not essential. Insulin can be given in the form of a standard sliding scale or as an infusion of glucose/potassium/insulin (GKI), which is our preferred method. This is less commonly employed than a sliding scale so it is summarized in Box 11.2.

Guidance for diabetics having upper GI endoscopy and ERCP is summarized in Figure 11.3. A simpler scheme would be to halve the insulin dose the previous evening if using a slower acting preparation and omit the next morning insulin of any sort. They should bring their insulin, dextrose tablets, sandwiches and blood glucose testing equipment. They should test their blood glucose in the morning and take a dextrose tablet or clear sugary drink if <4. The blood glucose should be monitored hourly whilst in the unit and, if <4, glucose should be given orally, or intravenously if not able to drink. As soon as they have recovered, they should take their sandwiches and half their usual morning insulin. For patients on very quick acting insulin (e.g. Novorapid or Humolog) they could take their usual dose with their food. Patients on once daily slow-acting insulin, such as glargine, can also take their usual dose.

Guidance for patients having full bowel preparation (colonoscopy and some flexible sigmoidoscopies) is given for non-insulin-dependent diabetes mellitus (NIDDM) in Figure 11.4 and for patients with insulin-dependent diabetes mellitus (IDDM) in Figure 11.5. The latter is a fairly fail-safe scheme. However, many fit insulin-dependent patients can be treated as out-patients. On the day before colonoscopy they could substitute equivalent amounts of clear sugary drinks for their normal meals and snacks, if the special bowel preparation diet doesn't contain sufficient carbohydrate. They should halve their evening insulin dose if it is a slower-acting preparation, check their blood

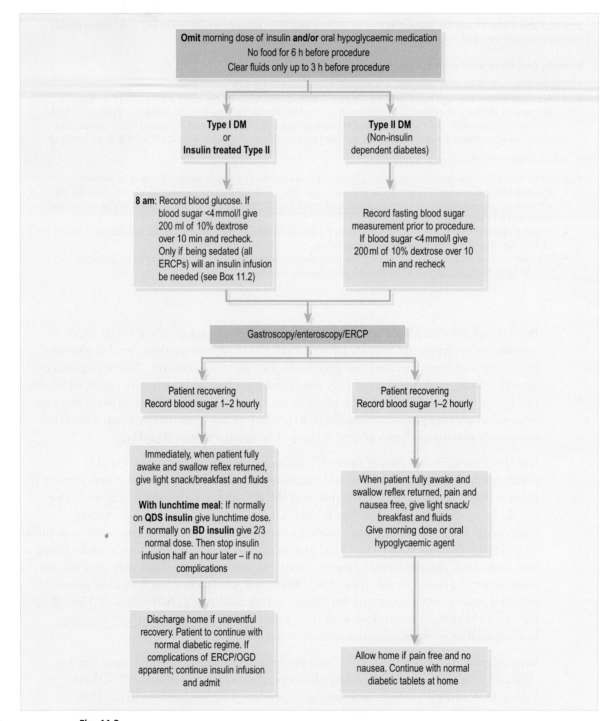

Fig. 11.3
Guidance for diabetic patients having upper gastrointestinal endoscopy including endoscopic retrograde cholangiopancreatography (ERCP). To be done in the morning list

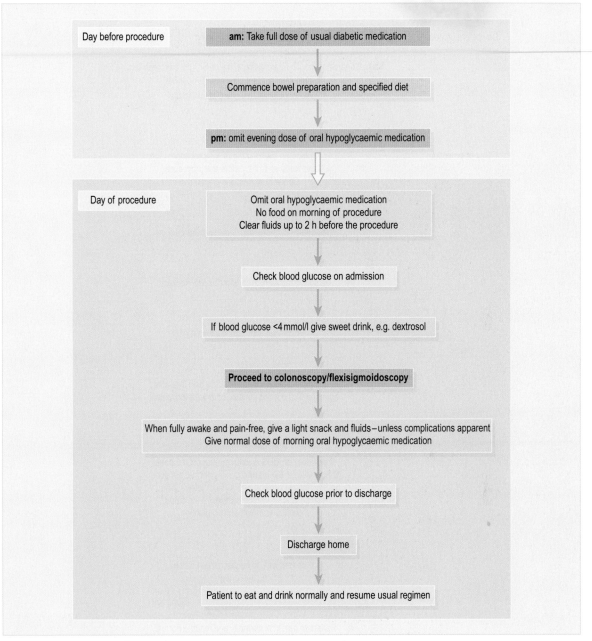

Fig. 11.4
Guidance for non-insulin-dependent diabetes mellitus (NIDDM) patients undergoing full bowel preparations. To be done on the morning list

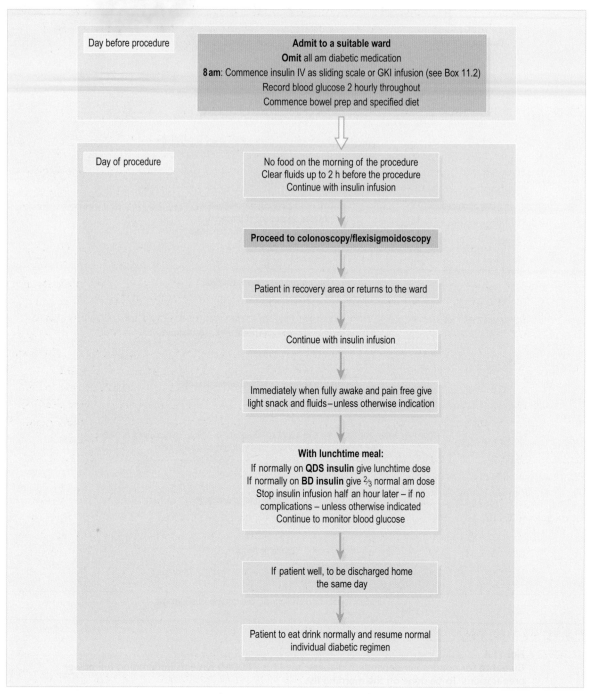

Day before procedure

> **Admit to a suitable ward**
> **Omit** all am diabetic medication
> **8 am**: Commence insulin IV as sliding scale or GKI infusion (see Box 11.2)
> Record blood glucose 2 hourly throughout
> Commence bowel prep and specified diet

Day of procedure

> No food on the morning of the procedure
> Clear fluids up to 2 h before the procedure
> Continue with insulin infusion

> **Proceed to colonoscopy/flexisigmoidoscopy**

> Patient in recovery area or returns to the ward

> Continue with insulin infusion

> Immediately when fully awake and pain free give
> light snack and fluids – unless otherwise indication

> **With lunchtime meal:**
> If normally on **QDS insulin** give lunchtime dose
> If normally on **BD insulin** give ⅔ normal am dose
> Stop insulin infusion half an hour later – if no
> complications – unless otherwise indicated
> Continue to monitor blood glucose

> If patient well, to be discharged home
> the same day

> Patient to eat drink normally and resume normal
> individual diabetic regimen

Fig. 11.5
Guidance for insulin-treated patients undergoing full bowel preparation. To be done on the morning list

sugar in the morning and take a sugary drink if too low. Their morning meal and insulin should be delayed until after the procedure which should be first on the list. If just a flexible sigmoidoscopy is to be performed either unprepared or with an enema only, no special diabetic or dietary advice is required.

Bowel preparation for lower gastrointestinal endoscopy

Safe and accurate flexible sigmoidoscopy or colonoscopy depends on good bowel preparation. The patient should be passing clear fluid before the procedure commences. There is no clear advantage to secretory forms of bowel preparation over lavage agents in terms of efficacy, but possible advantages for some groups of patients. Patients with suspected bowel obstruction, toxic megacolon, severe dysmotility, profuse rectal bleeding or pregnant patients should not be given bowel preparation.

All patients require clear instructions and encouragement if bowel prep is to work well. Standard forms of preparation are given in Box 11.3 and Box 11.4. Patients with colostomies and previous colon resections require normal preparation. Some patients need to be admitted to hospital for assistance, fluid balance monitoring and sometimes intravenous saline – principally frail elderly patients and those with renal failure, some insulin-treated diabetics, severe cardiac failure or ascites. Patients with profuse diarrhoea (assuming not due to faecal overflow) and patients with ileostomies should just follow the dietary advice for bowel preparation but NOT have laxatives. Patients with acute exacerbation of inflammatory bowel disease should be endoscoped with caution – often only limited, unprepared, inspections may be permissible to just obtain a diagnosis. Only when the patient has improved can they have normal bowel preparation for assessment of the extent of disease. Although picolax can be given to inflammatory bowel disease patients, lavage may be preferred because of case reports of exacerbation of disease and obstructive symptoms in some cases of Crohn's disease with the former.

A phosphate enema 20 min before a flexible sigmoidoscopy is acceptable if it is certain that views of the more proximal colon will not be required (e.g. for rectal bleeding). In some centres totally unprepared flexible sigmoidoscopies are undertaken. However, we have a low threshold for formal bowel preparation as often the finding of left-sided polyps prompts the search for more proximal lesions, assuming one has sufficient colonoscopes (as opposed to shorter flexible sigmoidoscopes) available.

GOVERNANCE IN ENDOSCOPY

All of the above sections relate to the maintenance of standards within endoscopy units. It is imperative that all endoscopists and endoscopy units regularly re-appraise their performance individually and collectively. This starts on the day of learning to endoscope and continues life long.

Training in modern endoscopy is no longer dependent on observing a few endoscopies and then being 'thrown in at the deep end'. While experience and apprenticeship are still

Box 11.3 Bowel preparation instructions: key advice to patients for medicines, diet and fluid intake

7 days before procedure
Stop taking any iron tablets

4 days before procedure
Stop taking any constipating agents, e.g. codeine, etc.

The day before procedure
Diet instructions
9 am – Breakfast
Boiled or poached egg with white bread and a scraping of butter or margarine (eat your usual amount of bread). Tea or coffee without milk. Unlimited soft drinks (not fizzy). Unlimited meat extract drinks. No cereals, jam or marmalade.

11.30 am
Tea or coffee without milk. Have a 'Rich Tea' biscuit if usually have a snack.

12–12.30 pm – Lunch
A small portion of steamed, poached or grilled white fish or chicken. White rice or pasta (not wholemeal) or white bread. Plain yoghurt or ice cream, clear jelly. Tea or coffee without milk. Unlimited soft drinks (not fizzy). Unlimited meat extract drinks.

NO FURTHER SOLID FOOD UNTIL AFTER EXAMINATION

6 pm – Evening meal
Clear soup (i.e. soup without milk and any solids). Clear jelly may be taken for dessert. Tea or coffee with a dash of milk. Unlimited clear fluids. Unlimited meat extract drinks.

10.30 pm – Bedtime
Tea or coffee without milk

Fluid and drinks instructions
Continue to drink plenty of clear fluids (i.e. tea, coffee, squash, clear soups, Bovril) until 2 h before the procedure. Diabetics should use sugar-free squash and have glucose tablets or similar sugary drinks if symptoms of hypoglycaemia. Ask them to write down all the cups and glasses of fluids they take. Warn them to expect frequent bowel motions and eventually diarrhoea, starting within 3 h of the first dose. Some stomach discomfort is normal. Suggest use of barrier cream if peri-anal soreness and to stay within easy reach of the toilet.

They may eat normally once the examination is over. A high-fibre diet (e.g. wholemeal bread, All Bran, etc.) will help restore normal bowel habit, which will usually return within a day or two.

important in training, it is no longer acceptable for trainees to be left endoscoping on unsupervised lists. Endoscopy is a practical skill that some learn faster than others. All trainees require a structured programme consisting of information and practical based teaching, including all of the above sections. Training has been standardized with the development of approved training courses developed under the wing of the 'Joint Advisory Group', JAG, with the Royal Colleges and now the Modernisation Agency. A number of national and regional training centres have been set up to supervise SpR training and courses. Centres are themselves regulated to ensure quality teaching by suitably trained teachers in practical skills, with standardized methods and involvement in these will be essential for all trainees registered. There is no longer any place for 'part time' endoscopists where endoscopy skills are not required for future careers.

Box 11.4 Sample instructions for the successful use of laxatives in the preparation of the bowel for colonoscopy

The day before the procedure
Picolax and senna
If having a morning colonoscopy the next day, take senna (senokot) granules at 8 am BEFORE BREAKFAST, one sachet of picolax at 11 am and the second picolax at 4 pm.

If having an afternoon colonoscopy the next day, take senna granules at 9 am AFTER BREAKFAST, one sachet of picolax at 12 pm and the second picolax at 7 pm.

Senokot granules are mixed with half a cup of warm water. Stir for 2–3 min. Solution may be hot, wait for drink to cool.

Half sachets can be used on frail patients.

Polyethylene glycol (Klean-prep)
To prepare the laxative, fill a jug or bowl with 1 l (or 2 pints) of water. Empty the contents of one Klean-prep sachet into it. Stir until the powder is completely dissolved and the solution is clear. Drink one glassful (250 ml or ½ pint) of the Klean-prep drink about every 15 min until all consumed (about 1 h). Suggest patients take their time, no need to rush.

For a **morning** colonoscopy, start one sachet at 4 pm and a second at 5 pm. Wait until 7 pm or later until bowels have opened before taking the third sachet. A fourth sachet needs to be taken at 8 pm unless the bowels are passing absolutely clear fluid.

For an **afternoon** colonoscopy, start one sachet at 6 pm and a second at 7 pm. Wait until 8 am the day of the procedure or later until the bowels have opened before taking the third sachet. A fourth sachet needs to be taken at 9 am unless the bowels are passing absolutely clear fluid.

As discussed above, information is paramount to being able to provide an efficient endoscopy service. It is also essential for governance. What is really required is an outcomes analysis for all that we do, but such information is difficult to obtain. It is relatively easy for endoscopists to know what complications have resulted from procedures performed if they occur immediately, but recording of complications requires ongoing surveillance. All forms of outcomes should, ideally, be analyzed, not just the technical result of an endoscopic procedure. For example, have guidelines been adhered to, what near-misses have occurred, what do patient surveys indicate, is decontamination effective, are all the endoscopies performed indicated, and what are the caecal intubation rates for endoscopists? This requires quite some effort to maintain, but is essential for modern practice.

Information technology will play an increasing role in endoscopy. There are several database systems commercially available to record endoscopy results, images, provide analysis on findings, schedule patients and send results electronically. However, no system yet can provide a true endoscopy management tool, using standardized endoscopy terminology (although draft minimal datasets do exist) which requires true integration into electronic patient records. Such a system could aid all aspects of clinical governance in endoscopy, with anything from helping endoscopists plan the correct follow-up for given findings, seamless onward booking to further tests, measuring changes in capacity of the unit as a whole, suggesting alterations to booking diaries to help manage demand and so on. Such a system is still some way off, although development of electronic records is now a priority in the NHS.

Table 11.7 Drugs used in the modern endoscopy suite (alphabetical order)

Drug	Form and dose	Comments
Adrenaline	1:10 000 via injection needle 1 ml volumes up to 10 ml	Standard 10 ml vials as found in resuscitation trolleys Inject around base of bleeding ulcers or into polyp stalk prior to polypectomy High first-pass metabolism generally prevents systemic side effects
Fentanyl	50–200 µg intravenous (iv)	Opioid analgesic for ERCP or colonoscopy Give before any benzodiazepines May potentiate sedatives by 4–10 times Care in liver disease and hypotension
Flumazenil (Anexate)	200 µg slow iv injection and subsequent infusion	For reversal of benzodiazepines 200 µg over 15 s followed by 100 µg every 60 s to 1000 µg Short half-life compared to benzodiazepine – review frequently after administration May cause hypertension, panic attack, vomiting
Terlipressin (Glypressin)	2 mg iv QDS	Adjunct to control of variceal bleeding Nitrate patch can be applied to chest wall to prevent angina pectoris in ischaemic heart disease, but less frequent than vasopressin infusions
GTN spray	Two sprays sublingually	Pre-ERCP at intubation, improves access to papilla May potentiate hypotension
N-butyl-2-cyanoacrylate (HistoAcryl Glue)	Mix 1:1 with lipiodol 1–2 ml via injection needle	For sclerosis of gastric varices Requires good co-ordination with flushes of lipiodol to prevent damage to endoscope, pre-lubricated with silicone oil
Hyoscine (Buscopan)	20–40 mg iv	Pre ERCP to prevent peristalsis during ERCP or after maximum insertion of enteroscope or colonoscope to allow full inspection of mucosa Often causes tachycardia Care in elderly, ischaemic heart disease
Indigo carmine	5–10 ml 0.1% solution down biopsy channel or submucosal injection needle	For chromoendoscopy of upper or lower gastrointestinal (GI) tract to improve contrast when visualizing mucosal irregularities by collecting in crevices Requires good bowel preparation Helps stain muscularis propria while performing SMR
Lignocaine spray (Xylocaine)	5 sprays to oropharynx. Max 20 applications	For analgesia to throat to aid patient comfort Systemic absorption has rarely been reported (hypotension, dysrhythmias, convulsions)
Lugol's iodine	5–10 ml 2% solution down biopsy channel	For chromoendoscopy of oesophagus to improve contrast when visualizing mucosal dysplasia Squamous epithelium stains dark – abnormal areas do not stain
Methylene blue	3–10 ml 1% solution down biopsy channel	For chromoendoscopy of Barrett's oesophagus Wash mucosa with 10 ml 10% acetylcysteine solution before to remove mucus

Table 11.7 Drugs used in the modern endoscopy suite (alphabetical order) (cont'd)

Drug	Form and dose	Comments
Metoclopramide (Maxolon)	10 mg slow iv	Useful to prevent retching during upper GI endotherapy Stated to be contraindicated in GI haemorrhage, but benefit may outweigh risk if retching is preventing effective endotherapy
Midazolam (Hypnovel)	0.5–5 mg iv	For conscious sedation Slowly titrate dose increments May cause disinhibition and agitation Hiccoughs Often causes hypotension, extreme care needed with respiratory disease
Naloxone	100–200 µg iv, repeated every 2 min until response	Opiate antagonist used if opioid suspected to cause hypoventilation May need further doses after 1–2 h as shorter half-life Can cause dysrhythmias
Omeprazole (Losec)	80 mg iv STAT 8 mg/kg/h iv infusion for 72 h post endoscopy	Possible use to reduce re-bleeding post-therapeutic endoscopy for lesions likely to bleed again. Oral proton pump inhibitors may be as effective
Polyethylene glycol with electrolytes (Movicol, Klean-Prep)	One sachet per litre of water 4 l generally required over 4–6 h	Lavage solution for full bowel prep May be flavoured, but bitter due to electrolytes added To be used with suitable low residue diet and encouragement
Pethidine	25–100 mg iv	Analgesic for ERCP or colonoscopy Give before any benzodiazepines May potentiate sedatives by 4–10 times Potentiates hypotension
Phosphate enema (Fleet, Fletcher's)	1 application PR	For bowel prep pre-flexible sigmoidoscopy Avoid in inflammatory bowel disease
Sodium citrate (Microlette)	5–10 ml PR (1–2 vials)	For bowel prep pre flexible sigmoidoscopy
Sodium picophosphate (Picolax)	2 sachets taken 6 h apart, dissolved in water PO	For bowel preparation pre-colonoscopy Patient needs to drink plenty of fluid, and advice on suitable low residue diet
Sodium tetradecyl sulphate (STD, Fibro-Vien)	1% solution into injection needle in varix	For sclerotherapy of oesophageal varices 1–2 ml per varix Largely superseded by banding kits, but useful where banding not possible

DRUGS COMMONLY USED IN ENDOSCOPY

Endoscopists should be familiar with the few agents used in the peri-procedure period and are summarized in Table 11.7 for reference. It is better to be familiar with a small selection of agents and local hospital practice may favour alternatives. Some agents (e.g.

diazemuls, some sclerosants, vasopressin) have been largely replaced by safer alternatives, but may still be used by some endoscopists. Endoscopists should always enquire about drug allergies prior to proceeding. Antibiotics are discussed above.

SUMMARY

It is hoped that the topics introduced in this chapter demonstrate how modern endoscopy is not just learning how to perform an ever expanding range of techniques, but represents a microcosm of good medical practice, maintaining standards and giving patients the best possible service given available resources.

Further Reading

Cotton P, Williams C. Practical Gastrointestinal Endoscopy, 4th Edn. Blackwell Science Limited, 1996.
Mainly concerned with a thorough description of how to endoscope, but includes some aspects of unit management.
Sivak MV Jr. Gastroenterologic Endoscopy, 2nd Edn. Saunders, 2000.
Superb and comprehensive double volume text covering all aspects of endoscopy with an American bias. No colour photos. Also available as CDRom (June 1999).

Useful Websites

www.bsg.org.uk Website for the British Society for gastroenterology with guidelines for various aspects of endoscopic safety.
www.asge.org Website for American Society for Gastrointestinal Endoscopy, with links to American guidelines. Access to the related Gastrointestinal Endoscopy journal site is by subscription which publishes papers on safety and management issues.
www.omed.org Organisation Mondiale d'Endoscopie Digestive site. Has links to version 2 of a minimum standard dataset for endoscopy records.
www.modern.nhs.uk/endoscopy Lists background to the drive to improve endoscopy services with practical tips on how to improve efficiency. Describes history of the booked appointments system and links to other NHS plan sites.

Statistics and epidemiology for the gastroenterologist

12

INTRODUCTION

Statistical analysis of data is not, in general, a conscious function of day-to-day delivery of care. However, many clinicians will have some statistical knowledge, either taught at undergraduate or 'membership' level, or acquired to help with research projects, critical review writing, etc. The purpose of this chapter is to outline the importance of a good understanding of statistical analysis, draw together important statistical concepts and explain the principles that underlie these concepts.

The vast majority of practising clinicians will not need to have a rigorous understanding of the mathematics per se, particularly as much of the analysis of data may be performed by computer, but will need to understand the principles underlying statistical analysis in certain circumstances.

Clinical medicine evolves and changes rapidly and is populated with many conflicting opinions and data, resulting in a need for all clinicians to go back to original reports and to assess their impact on their own practice – there is of course no one definitive source where the answers to a clinical problem may be found. Many clinicians are stimulated into setting up their own studies and also have an obligation to look critically at their own practice as part of clinical governance. Finally, all clinicians use a form of statistical analysis (albeit often unconsciously) when they request an investigation or interpret the result of an investigation.

Therefore, clinicians need to understand statistics to perform the tasks shown in Box 12.1, and specifically they need to understand the concepts outlined in Box 12.2.

HISTORY

Pierre CA Louis (1787–1872) is considered to be one of the founding fathers of modern medical statistics. Prior to the 19th century, medicine was interested primarily in individual patients, rather than the quantification and description of groups of patients with similar conditions. Louis, however, performed a retrospective analysis of blood letting as a treatment for pneumonia and concluded that, contrary to opinion current at that time, it

Box 12.1 Tasks requiring a knowledge of statistics

- Designing a study or experiment
- Analyzing the results of a study or experiment they have performed
- Reviewing the design of other published work
- Critically reviewing the analysis of data derived from other studies
- Analyzing audit data in the context of other published information
- Understanding the clinical meaning of tests and their results.

Box 12.2 Statistical concepts

- Sources of data, nature of variables and the process of measurement
- Descriptive techniques in statistics
- The difference between a sample and a population
- Probability and hypothesis generation or testing
- The applicability of the various statistical tests available.

was not as effective as commonly believed. In fact delayed or no blood letting reduced mortality and, although his paper would not have stood up to the modern test of peer review and the results did not reach our current definition of statistical significance, they were reported as being 'startling and apparently absurd'. Although many commentators rejected his analysis and accused him of 'substituting mathematical for logical analysis, to make arithmetic take the place of induction and calculation that of reason', his work did have a profound effect, with French imports of leeches falling from 42 million to just a few thousand per year. Over the following 180 years medical statistical analysis has grown to dominate medical research and investigators who fail to apply it rigorously may be subject to the reverse accusation; namely of allowing logic or reasoning to distort the truth as revealed by statistics. In reality, induction and reasoning remain vital components of research and the practice of medicine and, by having a clear understanding of the principles of statistical analysis, it can be applied appropriately and with an understanding of its limitations.

DATA, VARIABLES AND MEASUREMENT

In order to understand complex biomedical systems and problems, it is necessary to measure or count something to generate the raw material (data) for analysis. A characteristic, which takes on different values when assessed in different persons, places, things or at different times, is known as a variable. To understand which statistical method to use to analyze sets of data, the process of data acquisition and the nature of the variables to be assessed must be known.

Box 12.3 Scales for the measurement of statistics

- Nominal – items are named or classified, but with no rank order
- Ordinal – items are classified, with a rank, e.g. below average, average, above average
- Interval – items are put in order and the number assigned relates to a distance between items, e.g. °C: the difference between 20 and 30 is the same as the difference between 40 and 50, but zero does not necessarily mean an absence of temperature
- Ratio – as interval measurements, but with a true zero, e.g. height, weight, °Kelvin.

Sources of data

Sources of data may be:

- routine records
- surveys
- experiments
- external sources.

The statistical methods described in this chapter are most valid when applied to an experiment of some description, rather than any of the other sources of data.

Variables

Variables may be:

- quantitative – can be measured, e.g. height
- qualitative – belong to a particular group, can be counted to give frequency of occurrence
- random – their value cannot be predicted, e.g. adult height cannot be predicted at birth
- discrete, e.g. number of bowel movements per day
- continuous, e.g. weight.

Measurements

Measurements may be made on any of the scales shown in Box 12.3.

In general, when gathering data the aim is to understand the behaviour or characteristics of a population of entities (the largest possible collection of entities for which there might be an interest), which may be people, cells, departments, or any thing else under investigation. In an ideal world, observations of all the entities in the population would be made and then it would not be necessary to use statistics to make inferences. Practically, however, measurements are made on subsets of a population (i.e. a sample) and the way in which a sample is selected and studied influences the type of analysis that should be applied and the inferences which can be made about the total population.

TYPES OF EXPERIMENT

For statistical purposes an experiment may be any method of gathering data, but usually implies some sophistication in the way in which data are acquired. Analyzing data taken from non-experimental sources (routine records, surveys and external sources) may be done in a similar way provided that heed is taken of the method of acquisition of those data and the potential for bias.

Observation

A simple observation may be the starting point for progression in medicine, but is quite clearly open to misinterpretation. The sequence of events shown in Figure 12.1 may be noted.

With no prior knowledge of the interaction between that drug and gastrointestinal bacteria it would not be possible to conclude anything in particular about causation or, indeed, any form of relationship between the two events (other than the time order, i.e. the latter event cannot be the cause of the former).

Case series

Evidence of an association (whether causative or not) between two events may be obtained from multiple observations, as shown in Figure 12.2.

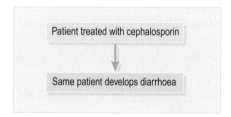

Fig. 12.1
Simple observation

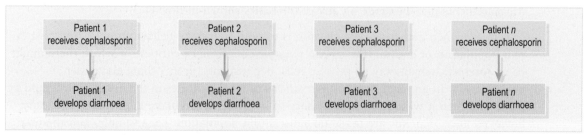

Fig. 12.2
Case series

Box 12.4 Case-control study

- Retrospective
- Look for exposure to risk in cases
- Look for exposure to risk in controls
- Determine odds ratio where:

$$O.R = \frac{\text{exp to risk in cases}}{\text{exp to risk in controls}}$$

Box 12.5 Cohort study

- Observes future events
- Determine group exposed to risk
- Determine control group
- Calculate relative risk where:

$$R.R = \frac{\text{incidence in cases}}{\text{incidence in controls}}$$

In this example the data can be analyzed in a simplistic way. The number of occurrences of this event can be counted. Intuitively, it may seem that this is happening often, indeed, more often than would be expected by chance only, but it cannot be said with any certainty, nor can inferences about causation be made.

Case-control and cohort studies

To move beyond this stage of uncertainty, experiments of one form or another can be performed. Two experiments, which may help to demonstrate a real association between these events, are case-control and cohort studies. The simplest way to differentiate these types of study is to look at the direction in time of the observation (see Boxes 12.4 & 12.5).

Note that in either of these cases the 'risk' can be a positive or negative risk. In this example the risk would be exposure to a cephalosporin. For a case-control study it would be necessary to compare the frequency of exposure to cephalosporins (in a pre-determined time-scale) in patients with new-onset diarrhoea and compare that with the exposure to cephalosporins in a suitably matched control sample (similar age, sex, co-morbidity, exposure to other potential risks, etc.). For a cohort study it would be necessary to identify those patients treated with a cephalosporin and determine the onset of diarrhoea in those and compare that with a matched group of patients not treated with a cephalosporin – note the importance of matching; the matched group might be expected to have, for example, a similar underlying condition treated with an alternative antibiotic.

In this example the risk is clearly a negative one. As has been stated, the 'risk' could be a positive one. An example would be exposure to aspirin and myocardial infarction:

$$O.R = \frac{\text{previous aspirin use in cases (MI)}}{\text{previous aspirin use in controls}}$$

$$R.R = \frac{\text{incidence of MI in aspirin takers}}{\text{incidence of MI in controls}}$$

Confounding factors

The problem with case-control and cohort studies is fundamentally one of confounding factors. Assuming cases and controls are adequately matched, a result may still be affected greatly by a confounding factor. These are by definition unknown (since if known they could be accounted for in the matching process) and, therefore, may seem obscure. The question that might be asked in the current example is 'could there be anything else which happens to (or is an attribute of) a patient who receives a cephalosporin which could be theoretically related to diarrhea and which doesn't apply to the controls?' Since most biological mechanisms are, at best, poorly understood, then this is a difficult question to answer.

The confounding factor may be totally unrelated to the disease process. For example, in a hospital-based case-control study it may be that clinicians who have a preference for cephalosporins over quinolones for the treatment of respiratory infections work on a ward where hygiene standards are lower. A simple, but overlooked, association such as this will lead to a 'positive' result in a case-control or cohort study even if cephalosporins have no effect on the gastrointestinal (GI) tract. If the study designers were aware of this 'confounding factor' then it could be removed. However, it is the unanticipated confounding factors that are going to be critical.

Bias

Bias may occur in any study as part of the selection process of cases and controls. Bias results from selecting out a particular group of patients with certain characteristics related to the attribute being measured within a study. In a case-control or cohort study, biases are most common when it comes to the method of selecting cases or controls. These biases are most likely to be unconscious and difficult to detect. An example of study design that may introduce a bias is as shown in Figure 12.3.

In this example, suppose half the ward patients had been given a cephalosporin and 20% of all patients developed diarrhoea independent of their exposure to a cephalosporin, but for every 100 patients, the nurses reported all 10 of the patients who developed diarrhoea on a cephalosporin, because they were aware of the nature of the study, but fewer (say 5) of the 10 patients who developed diarrhoea whilst not on a cephalosporin. This would give a result substantially different from the correct one as shown in Table 12.1.

This fairly straightforward example clearly shows how bias may arise – clearly in most experiments simple bias such as this can be designed out, but more subtle bias may easily be overlooked in the design of any study.

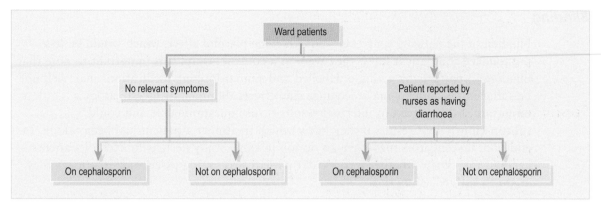

Fig. 12.3
Bias in an observational experiment

Table 12.1 Bias in an observational experiment			
The expected answer	**Diarrhoea (cases)**	**No-diarrhoea (controls)**	
Cephalosporin	10	40	
No-cephalosporin	10	40	
Exposure to risk	0.5	0.5	O.R=1
The answer obtained	**Diarrhoea (cases)**	**No-diarrhoea (controls)**	
Cephalosporin	10	40	
No-cephalosporin	5	45	
Exposure to risk	0.6667	0.471	O.R=1.42

Interventional studies

In order to overcome problems related to confounding factors and some sources of bias, interventional studies may be performed of which there is a clear hierarchy:

- Uncontrolled (no comparison group, of little value statistically)
- Controlled (but not randomized – susceptible to problems of bias)
- Randomized
- Blinded (patients not aware of treatment received)
- Double-blinded (investigator and patient not aware of treatment)
- Cross-over (subjects receive both treatment and placebo).

In an interventional study (the commonest types being randomized-controlled studies with varying degrees of blinding), a patient is allocated to a specific pathway with the intention of following them and recording their outcome in a predetermined way. By setting up a study with controls and then intervening on the treatment group, many biases may be avoided. A more superior study is likely to result if the patients are randomized to either treatment or control groups, which should (if numbers are high enough) result in similar characteristics on average in each group.

Blinding

Blinding of the patients is necessary to overcome placebo effect, which would be less pronounced if a patient knew they were in a control group. It is important to note that blinding of patients by giving unlabelled and similar-looking medications may well not be sufficient as patients may recognize side effects. Blinding of investigators is important, as they need to interpret results or use questionnaires and could subconsciously bias results if they knew which treatment a patient had been taking. In addition, investigators may have an option in some study designs to exclude patients – again–if they knew whether a particular patient was taking placebo or treatment they might be influenced by this.

ANALYSIS OF RESULTS OF INTERVENTIONAL STUDIES

Variability in biological systems

In most biological systems there is huge variability. It would not be suspected that there would be a 100% correlation of bowel symptoms with previous antibiotic exposure. Thus, in a hypothetical study comparing the incidence of diarrhoea after treatment of a respiratory infection with a quinolone or a cephalosporin, it would not be expected to see diarrhoea in all the cephalosporin-treated patients and none of the others, in which case statistical analysis would be redundant.

Predicting the behaviour of a 'population'

When an experiment or study is performed, the purpose is to use the information to say something useful about a population (a group of things, people, events, etc.). If patient X develops diarrhoea on drug A and patient Y doesn't develop diarrhoea on drug B, the only thing this observation shows is what has already happened. It doesn't predict whether the same thing will happen again, nor does it predict what will happen in a population. This is because the episode of diarrhoea may have happened by chance. If a patient is chosen at random from a population it will not be possible to predict their bowel activity in advance – it is a random variable.

In the analysis of an experiment it is necessary to consider some background information about the population the experimental subjects are drawn from. It would be useful to know what the average distribution of bowel habits was in the background population – this would make it easier to understand whether any study group deviated from that background. However, it is not possible to know exactly the bowel habit of an entire population, unless it is measured in everyone, but it is possible to select a sample of individuals and make some inferences about the population from measurements performed in that sample.

There are a number of different ways of measuring this diarrhoea. To illustrate the concepts underlying hypothesis testing, stool weights will be used – a continuous

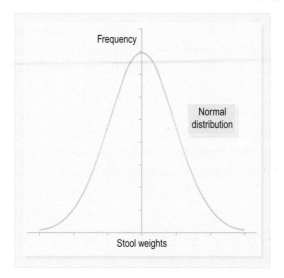

Fig. 12.4
Normal distribution

(random) variable, as opposed to stool frequency – a discrete variable. In reality, stool is rarely weighed, but using a variable like this makes the principles easier to understand.

Determining the mean and distribution of a population

It is likely that a population of in-patients has varying stool weights. If they didn't, statistical analysis would not be necessary to answer the question about the effect of diarrhoea. The question is – in what way do they vary?

To perform statistical analysis, an assumption is made that weights of stool are distributed according to the 'normal' distribution. Most readers will be familiar with the typical bell-shaped curve of the normal distribution (Fig. 12.4).

In this example the x-axis represents stool weights and the y-axis represents the frequency of occurrence. The standard normal distribution has a mathematical formula to describe its shape, is centred about zero and stretches to infinity in both directions. This 'standard' normal curve can be transformed mathematically to have a non-zero centre (or mean, represented by μ) and its degree of spread can be changed – the defining variable being the standard deviation (s.d. represented by σ). However, any normal curve is still symmetrical about its centre point and stretches to infinity in both directions.

Distributions such as the normal distribution can be used to determine the proportion of a population in whom the variable in question will lie between defined points. Thus, in Figure 12.5 the area under the curve coloured pink divided by the total area under the curve represents the proportion of the population for whom the x-variable will lie between A and B.

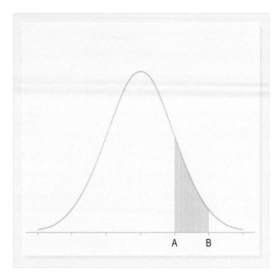

Fig. 12.5
Normal distribution – characteristics 1

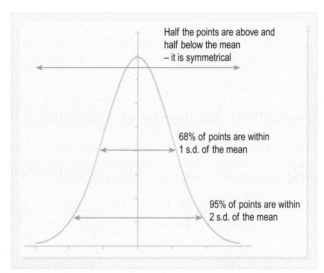

Fig. 12.6
Normal distribution – characteristics 2

In the normal distribution, 95% of the population lies within approximately 2 standard deviations of the mean and 68% lies within 1 standard deviation (Fig. 12.6).

With this knowledge about the normal distribution it can then be asked whether stool weights would, indeed, be normally distributed. Of course, the actual distribution of stool weights would not be normal as there could be asymmetry about the mean and the distribution would not extend to infinity in both directions. However, for statistical purposes the normal distribution remains a reasonable approximation.

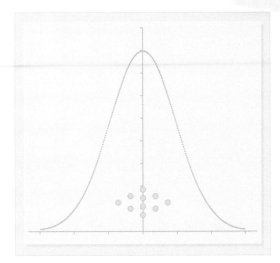

Fig. 12.7
Repeated samples – distribution of means

Once this assumption is made, it would be useful to determine the parameters of the normal distribution, which approximates to the overall population of stool weights (note that in this example the focus is on in-patient symptoms and, therefore, the 'population' is the group that contains all possible in-patient stool weights, rather than referring to a particular population of people). The only practical way to determine the mean stool weight of in-patients would be to measure a sample of stool weights and try to use that information to say something about the population.

Samples, their means and the distributions of their means

It is possible, for example, to measure stool weights from 50 consecutive patients and calculate the mean for that sample. The question then is how does this relate to the population mean, which remains unknown? If it is assumed that the population of stool weights are normally distributed and the sample of 50 is a random sample, then each one of the sample is just as likely to come from the lower half of the distribution as the upper half and, on average, the most likely value of the sample mean will be the population mean. However, the chance of the sample mean being exactly the population mean is small, since, although the 50 patients are taken at random, by chance it could easily occur that in this particular sample there were some extreme values or one or two more from above the mean than below.

Another question that could be asked, therefore, is what would happen if repeated samples of 50 random patients were collected. The result is likely to appear as in the Figure 12.7.

In this example each red dot represents a sample mean and it intuitively seems likely that, most commonly, the sample mean will be fairly close to the population mean and

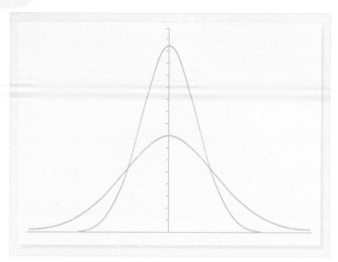

Fig. 12.8
Distribution of population vs sample mean

that, occasionally, a sample mean will deviate from the population mean, but it is unlikely that a sample mean is out towards the periphery of the population distribution as this would require extreme values in the sample, not counterbalanced by others. These features of distributions of sample means can be described mathematically. If the population is normally distributed with mean μ and s.d. σ, then the sample means will be distributed normally with mean μ and an s.d. of $\sigma/\sqrt{n}$, where n is the number of entities in the sample. This can be expressed graphically as in Figure 12.8.

In this graph the blue curve represents the distribution of the population and the red curve represents the distribution of sample means for a given sample size.

Confidence interval for a population mean

With theoretical information about the distribution of sample means, some inferences about a population mean can be made by taking a single sample and calculating the mean of that sample. It has already been stated that for any normal curve, 95% of the values will lie within 2 s.d. of the mean (approximately, the exact formula being $\mu \pm 1.96\ \sigma$). The means of repeated samples of size n should follow a normal distribution whose centre is the population mean (μ) and whose s.d. is that of the population divided by $\sqrt{n}$ (i.e. $\sigma/\sqrt{n}$) – this value being known as the standard error of the mean (s.e.m.). Therefore, even if nothing is known about the background population, it can be said 95% of the time a random sample will have a mean that is within 2 s.e.m. of the population mean – as illustrated in Figure 12.9 – the graph shows a theoretical population in blue and the expected distribution of sample means (with a given sample size n) in red. The vertical bars are 2 s.e.m. away from the centre of curves, i.e. the area between them represents 95% of the area under the red curve.

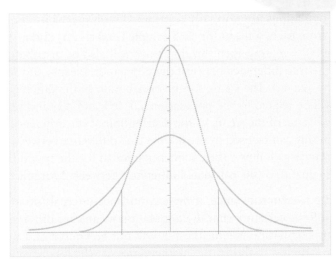

Fig. 12.9
Predicting the sample mean

Obviously it will not normally be possible to 'see' the blue curve, or the red curve. It will, however, be possible to calculate a sample mean and if enough is known about the variability of the population it will be possible to calculate the s.e.m. It is clear that for every 100 sample means calculated, 95 are expected to lie within 2 s.e.m. of the population mean (the centre of the distribution of sample means will be the same as the centre of the population distribution as discussed above). Therefore, for any one sample mean it is 95% certain that the population mean is no 'further away' than 2 s.e.m., although the direction will not be known. Logically, therefore, it can be said with 95% confidence that the population mean lies between (sample mean − 2 × s.e.m) and (sample mean + 2 × s.e.m.).

Thus the 95% confidence intervals for a population mean are:

the sample mean ± 2 × s.e.m.

A method of calculating a 95% confidence interval for a population mean has, therefore, been derived, using the parameters of a sample. It should be noted, however, that one major assumption has been made. It has been assumed that the s.d. of the population (σ) was already known, which allowed calculation of the s.e.m. (s.e.m. = $\sigma/\sqrt{n}$). In practice, that will not be the case, but the population s.d. can be estimated from the s.d. of the sample. This introduces error (and hence uncertainty, making the confidence interval wider) and changes the mathematics, but does not alter the fundamental principle illustrated above.

Confidence interval for the difference between two means

Before returning to the original example the confidence interval for the difference between the means of two populations will be considered. This is calculated very much as above.

If two populations are normally distributed with means μ_1 and μ_2 and a sample of size n is taken from each, a mean for each sample is taken (m_1 and m_2) and a difference (d) is calculated ($d = m_1 - m_2$) then this difference will also be distributed normally, centred on $\mu 1 - \mu 2$ (the true difference between the population means) and with a predictable variability (s.e.m.). The s.e.m. for the distribution of the difference between two sample means will be related to the population s.d. ($\sigma 1$ and $\sigma 2$) and proportional to $1/\sqrt{n}$. The calculated value of the s.e.m. of the distribution of the difference between two random sample means can be used to predict the true difference between population means with 95% certainty as follows: the confidence interval for the true difference between population means is equal to d (the calculated difference between 2 sample means) $\pm\ 2 \times$ s.e.m.

This is a powerful tool since, if these confidence intervals do not overlap zero, it can be said with 95% certainty that the population means are different. As before with predicting population means, the s.d. will not be known and will need to be estimated from the sample variability, the mathematics of which is beyond the scope of this chapter. Nonetheless, although this may widen the confidence intervals it does not alter the fundamental principle outlined.

Generating and testing a hypothesis

Returning to the original example, it has been illustrated that by taking a sample of the entity of interest it is possible to derive information about a theoretically infinite population. It is possible to predict stool weights in a group of patients, measure them and determine whether they are different from those expected. The principles outlined can now be used to try and answer the clinically important question. To do this, it is necessary to go through a number of stages:

- Define the clinically important question
- Set some hypotheses to be tested
- Define how to measure the clinical variables
- Design and perform the experiment
- Analyze the data to determine the answer.

One possible experiment is illustrated in Figure 12.10.

This experiment may help clinical practice by giving two alternative courses of action to compare assuming that both courses are equally valid in other respects.

For the scenario in the figure above it can be assumed that the patients are drawn from the same population, randomly allocated to each treatment arm, followed through treatment with no withdrawals and are in all other ways similar within the two arms.

What is required of the statistical analysis is a comparison of the two theoretical populations of stool weights following antibiotic treatment for all (past, present and future) patients. This information is needed to predict future outcomes and the experiment is simply giving a sample of those theoretical populations. It can be assumed that the stool weights from each arm of the trial will be normally distributed with means and s.d. that are unknown.

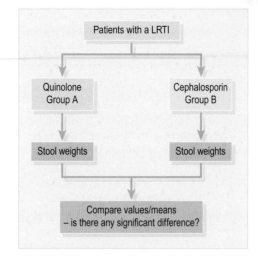

Fig. 12.10
Experimental design: comparing two groups

The clinical question must now be rephrased in a way that relates to the data generated. It is easier to disprove a hypothesis than to prove one, therefore, it is necessary to generate a hypothesis that would be more interesting if it were disproved, e.g.

'There is no difference in stool weights (a marker of acquisition of diarrhoea) between patients treated with a quinolone or a cephalosporin for a lower respiratory tract infection.'

This is a useful hypothesis because, if disproved, then there is at least some difference between these antibiotics as regards bowel function. A hypothesis such as this is known as a null hypothesis (NH) and the logical alternative is the alternative hypothesis (AH). The NH can be expressed in terms of the numerical data, i.e. 'there is no difference between the population means for stool weights for patients in group A or B', or:

$$\mu \, (\text{grpA}) - \mu \, (\text{grp B}) = 0$$

It has been stated that sample means are, in general, distributed normally, with a mean equal to the population mean. Statistical theory also states that the difference between two sample means is distributed normally and that this distribution is centred on the actual difference between the population means.

The NH states that the population means are identical. If that NH were true then, theoretically, each time this experiment is performed and the difference between the sample means is calculated, a result will be obtained that will be normally distributed, centred on zero. This is illustrated in Figure 12.11.

This seems intuitively correct – the difference between sample means will not always be zero, but it will tend to cluster around zero and there is no reason for it to go higher rather than lower, i.e. it will be symmetrical.

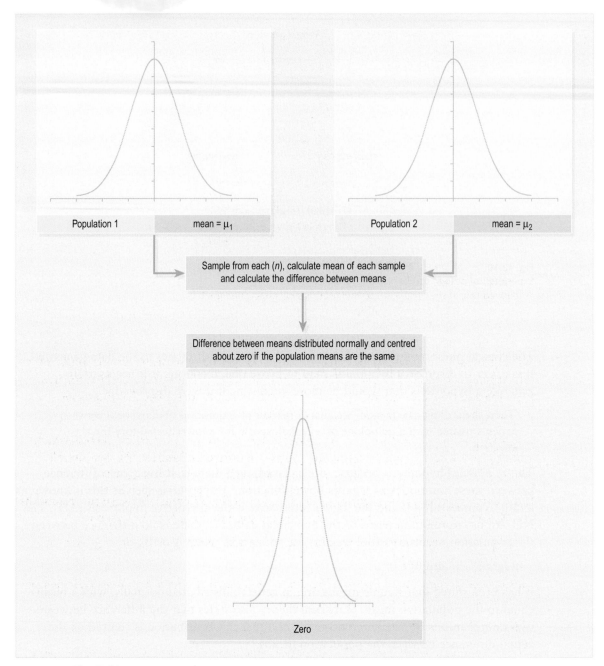

Fig. 12.11
Difference between two sample means

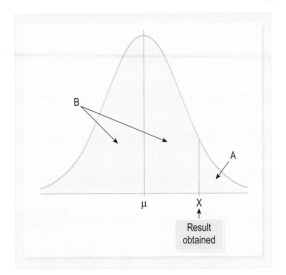

Fig. 12.12
One-tailed test. If the type of antibiotic used has no effect then $\mu = 0$

It is not possible to fully define the distribution for population means, as the spread of this normal curve is not known. However, just as the population s.d. can be estimated from the sample s.d., then so can the s.d. of the curve that describes the difference between the means (the formula is not important).

It is now possible to perform the experiment. It is known from statistical theory exactly what to expect if the NH were true. In practice, a difference between the two sample means will be obtained (it is highly unlikely to be exactly zero) (Fig. 12.12).

If the curve represents the theoretical distribution of the difference between sample means and X is the actual result obtained, then the question that needs to be asked is:

> 'What is the probability of getting this (non-zero) result or one more extreme, given that the NH is true ($\mu = 0$)?'

The answer to that question should be clear – it is the area under the curve A divided by the total area under the curve (A + B).

This will give a number that can be indicated by the letter '*P*'.

The above example has shown the principles underlying the calculation of a '*P*'-value. It is of fundamental importance to realize that whenever a '*P*'-value is seen, it gives an answer to the question above – if the NH isn't known or the meaning of 'this result or one more extreme' isn't clear, then a '*P*'-value has no meaning.

If *P* is small, then the chance of getting the observed result is small and there is evidence against the NH. If *P* is very small, then the NH is rejected. The level at which that decision is made is entirely arbitrary (and is usually referred to as α), but traditionally is set at 1 in 20, i.e. if $P<0.05$ then the NH is rejected. There is nothing exceptional about

311

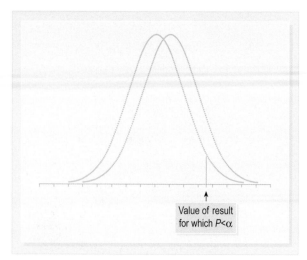

Value of result
for which $P<\alpha$

Fig. 12.13
Type II error because actual difference is small

this figure and the fact that P falls below it doesn't make an alternative hypothesis true – it just adds weight to that idea.

Type I error

A type I error is rejecting the NH when it is in fact true.

It is clear that P could be small just by chance. Suppose a cut-off is set for P of <0.05 to reject the NH. The NH will be rejected for any result (X) of the experiment that exceeds the value that will generate a P value of <0.05. The probability of X falling into that zone is by definition 1:20, therefore, the cut-off for P ($= \alpha$) is the probability for any one experiment of making a type I error.

Type II error

A type II error is failing to reject the NH when it is not actually true.

A type II error depends on four variables:

1. The value of α
2. The s.d. of the population
3. The sample size
4. The actual effect of the treatment.

Suppose there is a small difference in stool weights between the global population of patients treated with one antibiotic compared to another. The difference between sample means will, therefore, be normally distributed about the *actual* difference between the two populations. There will be two overlapping normal populations (Fig. 12.13).

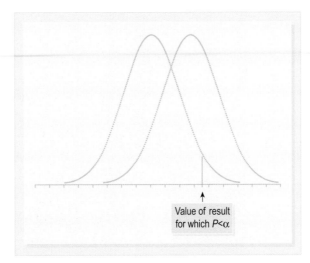

Fig. 12.14
No type II error of actual differences large

The blue curve is the theoretical distribution of differences between the sample means if the NH were true and the red sample is the actual distribution with a small non-zero difference between means. The NH will only be rejected if the value obtained exceeds the line indicated (this is derived from the NH – blue – curve and the chosen value of α: usually 0.05). The actual chance of getting a value high enough to do that is defined by the red curve (the true distribution of differences between population means). As can be seen if the red curve is close to the blue curve (the true difference between treatments is small) it would be rare to get an experimental result within the critical area. If the true difference is bigger – represented in Figure 12.14 – then the result (i.e. a random value from the red curve) is more likely to be greater than the critical value, making the probability of a type II error less.

If either the s.d. within the population is lower or the sample size is greater, a type II error is less likely, since in either case the normal curves will be 'taller' and 'narrower' (Fig. 12.15).

In either or these cases, there is a higher probability of getting a result from the red curve, which is greater than the critical value defined by the blue curve, i.e. more likely to get a true positive result.

Clearly if in any of these cases the value of α is changed to a larger value (e.g. redefine statistical significance as a 1:10 chance of getting that result by chance) then the critical value will go down and a type II error is less likely (but a type I error is more likely).

Power of a study

The power of a study is simply:

1 minus the probability of a type II error

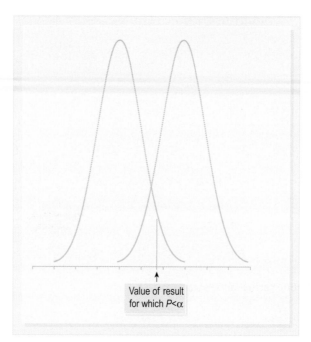

Fig. 12.15
No type II error if sample size larger, or less variability in population

Therefore, the same variables that affect the probability of a type II error occurring, affect the power in the opposite direction. For most studies the degree of background variability is fixed, but any experimental design that can reduce it will increase the power. It is also usually accepted that α will be fixed, although it could be argued in some circumstances that a cut-off of 1:20 is too stringent, or not stringent enough.

The 'actual effect' of any treatment cannot be altered, but some treatment effects are so small that they are not clinically relevant even if they can be demonstrated to be statistically significant. If the other variables are fixed, an experiment or study has to have a large sample size to detect a small effect, but a smaller sample size to detect a larger effect. It is, therefore, possible to ask the question:

> 'What sample size is needed to detect 80% of the time (probability of type II error = 20%) at a significance level α = 0.05 an effect of at least X (a clinically relevant level of difference)?'

For any given level of clinical relevance, a different required sample size can be determined. The value of 80% power is arbitrary and arguably too low, but it depends on whether there is more concern about making a type II or a type I error.

t-test

The above description of using a normal distribution to describe the likelihood of getting a particular sample mean given a stated NH in fact only applies if the

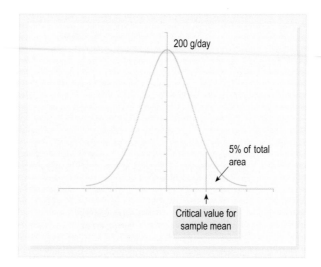

Fig. 12.16
One-tailed test

population s.d. is known. Given that this is rarely the case the population variability is estimated from the sample variability. This changes the mathematics slightly in that it is necessary to use a different distribution – the *t*-distribution, which takes on a different shape depending on the sample size (from which is derived the no. of 'degrees of freedom').

'One-tailed' vs 'two-tailed' *t*-tests

When testing a sample mean for significant difference from that predicted by a particular NH, it is necessary to determine whether large or small values are to be considered equally. This depends on the question being asked. For example, the question of diarrhoea really pertains to a large stool weight. Therefore, it could be said that the NH is that the population in question has a stool weight no greater than 200 g/day and the alternative hypothesis is that the average stool weight exceeds this value:

NH: μ = 200 g/day
AH: stool wt >200 g/day

This is illustrated in Figure 12.16.

Although the NH represents an infinite number of hypotheses it can be shown mathematically that if it is rejected for 'equality' it will also be rejected for the other values, therefore, only one test needs to be performed for NH: μ = 200 g/day.

In other circumstances it may be necessary to test two conditions for the alternative hypothesis:

NH: μ = 200 g/day
AH: μ >200 g/day or μ <200 g/day

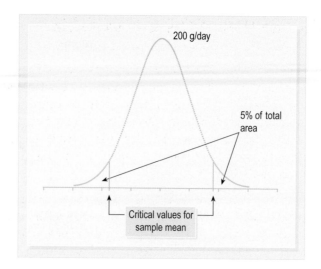

Fig. 12.17
Two-tailed test

In this case, the question for testing becomes 'what is the probability of getting the result obtained or one more extreme *in either direction* given the NH' and the graph for obtaining the critical value is as shown in Figure 12.17.

If the result of the experiment falls outside the area bounded by the two lines for the critical value then the NH will be rejected.

A one-tailed test is statistically more powerful (less likely to make a type II error), but it relies on some assumptions that may not be valid. Thus, if little is known about the effect of a drug and it could possibly cause constipation as well as diarrhoea, then a one-tailed test might not be appropriate. In general if either question is valid (even if not clinically interesting) then a two-tailed test should probably be performed.

Central limit theorem

The above discussion has shown how predictions about the distribution of a sample mean made on the basis of a NH can be used to determine whether, given a particular experimental result, the NH is likely to be true. It has been assumed (and it can be mathematically shown) that if within a particular population a variable is normally distributed, then the sample means will be normally distributed. In practice, most variables under scrutiny will not be normally distributed. The central limit theorem states that even if the variable is not normally distributed in a population, provided the sample size is large enough the sample mean will be distributed normally and the above analysis is valid. A reasonable cut-off for the sample size is generally taken to be 30.

HYPOTHESIS TESTING FOR CATEGORIES

In this example stool weights have been used as a variable to be tested. In practice, it may not be appropriate to do this and it may be easier to define patients as having diarrhoea or not and test whether diarrhoea is more likely to occur in patients treated with a particular antibiotic. To do this it is necessary to define (arbitrarily) diarrhoea, e.g. more than three loose stool movements per day. It is possible to look at patients treated with one or another antibiotic and count the number with diarrhoea. Results could be expressed as in Table 12.2.

As with the analysis for stool weights it is necessary to define what would have happened if there was no relationship between exposure to an antibiotic and the development of diarrhoea. To do this the expected frequencies for each part of the table can be calculated (Table 12.3). Their row and column totals are first calculated.

The expected values for each cell are then calculated by assuming that the number in each column is distributed in the proportions defined by the row totals (Table 12.4).

Table 12.2 Hypothesis testing for categories 1

	No antibiotic	Cephalosporin	Quinolone	Row total
Normal	86	37	42	
Diarrhoea	14	13	8	
Total				

Table 12.3 Hypothesis testing for categories 2

	No antibiotic	Cephalosporin	Quinolone	Row total
Normal	86	37	42	165
Diarrhoea	14	13	8	35
Total	100	50	50	

Table 12.4 Observed and expected values

	No antibiotic	Cephalosporin	Quinolone	Row total
Normal	86	37	42	165
	$100 \times 165/200 = 82.5$	41.25	41.25	
Diarrhoea	14	13	8	35
	$100 \times 35/200 = 17.5$	8.75	8.75	
Total	100	50	50	

Values in italics are the expected values for each cell

Table 12.5 Calculation of chi-squared

	No antibiotic	Cephalosporin	Quinolone	Row total
Normal	86	37	42	
	82.5	*41.25*	*41.25*	165
	(86–82.5)²/82.5 = 0.148	0.438	0.014	
Diarrhoea	14	13	8	
	17.5	*8.75*	*8.75*	35
	(14–17.5)²/17.5 = 0.7	2.064	0.064	
Total	100	50	50	

Values in italics are the expected values for each cell, bold values are O–E squared divided by E

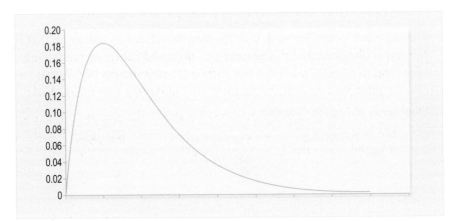

Fig. 12.18
χ^2 distribution

NH and AH have been defined to calculate these values:

- NH: The development of diarrhoea is independent of the type of antibiotic used
- AH: The development of diarrhoea is not independent of the type of antibiotic used.

As before, it is necessary to perform a calculation to answer the question: what is the probability of getting the results obtained even if the NH is true? To do this, it is required to have a measure of how far from the expected values (E) the observed ones (O) are. For each cell the difference between observed and expected is calculated, then squared and divided by the expected value (Table 12.5).

All these values are added together (note that all are positive because of the squared term) to give the test statistic known as Chi-squared (χ^2) – in this case it is 3.428 (approx).

If the NH is true, then larger values of χ^2 are unlikely and smaller values are more likely – χ^2 has a probability distribution as in Figure 12.18.

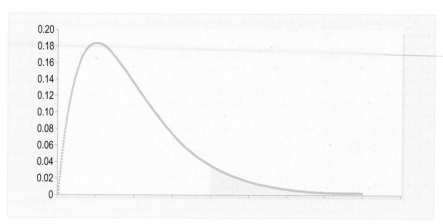

Fig. 12.19
χ^2: critical value

The value obtained for χ^2 is plotted as below and the question – 'what is the probability of getting this result (or one more extreme) assuming the NH is true?' – is answered, i.e. it is the pink area divided by the total area under the curve (Fig. 12.19).

Thus, a *P*-value for the data has been obtained – the probability that this could occur given the NH and one can proceed as above, rejecting or accepting the NH at a certain level of significance (α) – with the same definitions for errors.

2×2 tables

Note that in this example there is a 3×2 table. This depends on the experimental design and if there wasn't a no-treatment group then there would be a 2×2 table. In this case the mathematics is different – there are two possible solutions: one is the Yates, continuity correction and the other is to use Fisher's exact test. The latter is controversial, as it requires fixed marginal totals, which, in practice, are rarely seen, but as detailed discussion of both of these options is outside the scope of this chapter, the reader is referred to Daniel (1995). Some statistical computer programmes will use the Yates, continuity correction where required, but it is worth checking before running any analysis.

Small expected values

The χ^2 test is not appropriate if the calculated expected value falls below 5 in any one cell. This problem can occasionally be overcome by combining columns or rows if it is appropriate and logical to do so. χ^2 analysis where expected frequencies are low may be inappropriate, but can be seen not infrequently in published literature.

LINEAR REGRESSION AND CORRELATION

Another way of examining data is to look for correlation between two variables.

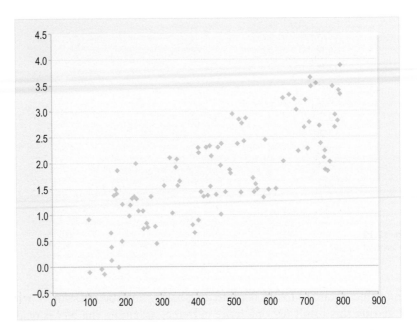

Fig. 12.20
Scatter plot

Scatter plots and correlation

Moving on from the example above there may be a desire to look for correlation between daily stool weights for the patients and weight loss over a particular defined period. This should allow determination as to whether there is some correlation between diarrhoea and clinical harm. Results might occur as in Figure 12.20 with weight loss on the y-axis and stool weight on the x-axis.

Regression lines

There appears to be some correlation between these two variables and a best-fit line can be calculated – this assumes that a linear correlation is being sought; otherwise the data could be transformed in some way. The mathematics involved is beyond the scope of this chapter, but, essentially, the equation for a line is sought that minimizes the sum of the squares of the vertical distance of each point from that line as shown in Figure 12.21.

Like any straight line, this takes the equation:

$$y = ax + b$$

Correlation coefficients

There is another important variable for this situation – the correlation coefficient. This is r, which may take on a value from −1 to +1 and is a measure of how closely the two

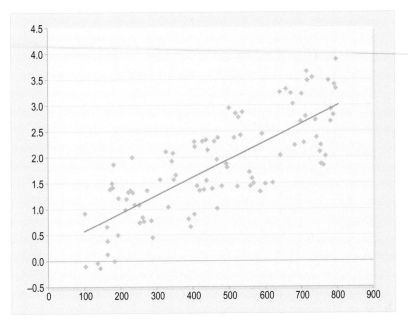

Fig. 12.21
Scatter plot: best-fit line

variables are related, i.e. how closely the points are clustered around the best-fit line. The calculation of r is outside the remit of this chapter. The value of r does not directly relate to the slope of the regression line, but as r approaches zero, then the slope of the line is also zero. The further r is from zero, the more likely the correlation observed between two variables is going to be statistically significant.

Hypothesis testing for a correlation coefficient

A NH and an AH can, therefore, be set for this situation:

- NH: changes in the y variable are random and unrelated to the value of the x variable ($r = 0$; x and y variables are independent)
- AH: changes in the y variable are at least in part dependent on the x variable.

It is possible to predict the behaviour of r for random samples of independent x and y variables of a size *n*. If a large value of r is obtained, it is possible to calculate the probability of this occurring given the NH, thus generating a *P*-value, to be interpreted as in the previous examples. Note, that a significant value of r may be obtained with a large sample even with a small value for a (in the equation y = ax + b), thus even though there is a statistically significant correlation between the variables, this may not be particularly clinically relevant – most of the differences seen between y values are still due to other factors, or y values don't actually vary that much at all. Clearly as before, the smaller interdependence of interest, the larger the sample size required to avoid type II errors.

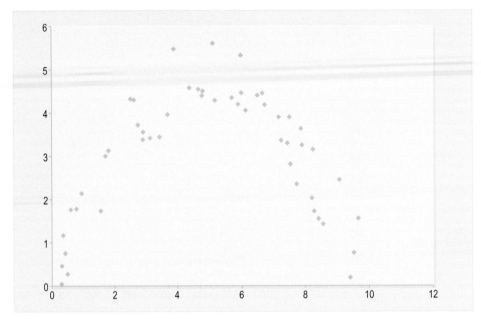

Fig. 12.22
Non-linear correlation

Errors in hypothesis tests for correlation coefficients

Type I and type II errors occur with hypothesis testing for the correlation coefficient just as with other hypothesis tests. It should be noted that there are further sources of a type II error in this case. In particular, the NH may not be rejected because of a low value of r when, in fact, there is correlation but it is non-linear. This is illustrated in the Figure 12.22. The scatter plot clearly shows a relationship between the x and y variables (in this case y is related to sin x), but when a regression line is fitted the slope is near zero and r is small and not statistically significant (Fig. 12.23).

This chapter has looked at the theory underlying three important statistical models that allow the testing of hypotheses about population means, categories and correlation. There are numerous statistical methods that rely on these fundamental concepts, but allow the testing of data when one of the methods described above is not applicable.

NON-PARAMETRIC TESTS

Parametric tests (of which the *t*-test and linear regression are two examples) have two characteristics:

1. They test statements about population parameters
2. They require some knowledge or assumption about the distribution of the variable concerned in the population.

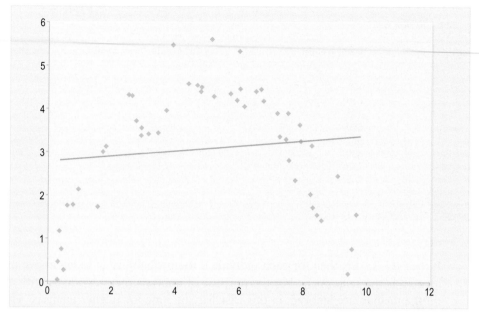

Fig. 12.23
Non-linear correlation: attempt at best-fit line

Tests that do not meet the first criteria are known as non-parametric, whilst those that don't meet the second are called distribution-free. In reality, all these other tests are usually grouped together under the 'non-parametric' heading. The χ^2 test for independence as discussed under 'Hypothesis testing for categories' is one example. Others are discussed below.

Sign test

This test relies only on having a continuous variable to test. There are no assumptions about the distribution of the variable in the population. It can be used to test whether a sample is consistent with a specified value for the population median (equal to the mean if the distribution is symmetrical).

Supposing it was necessary to test whether the median stool weight for a population, from which a sample of 10 individuals had been assessed, was 200 g per day. The results could be analyzed as shown in Table 12.6.

The NH would be set as:

NH: Median = 200

Alternative hypothesis:

AH: Median <> 200

Table 12.6 The sign test

Patient	Stool weight	+ for greater than median; – for less than median
A	180	–
B	200	0
C	650	+
D	435	+
E	280	+
F	385	+
G	680	+
H	270	+
I	245	+
J	275	+

If the NH is true, then for each individual the probability of being above or below the median is the same (0.5). For the purpose of analysis the individuals with a score exactly on the median are ignored, in this case leaving nine for further analysis. The binomial theory can then be used to answer the question – 'what is the probability of getting a result like this or one more extreme, given the NH'. To do this, it is necessary to calculate the probability of this distribution (only 1/9 below the hypothesized median), the more extreme possibility (0/9 below) and also the equivalent extremes (8/9 and 9/9) occurring to have a two-tailed test (the alternative hypothesis made no assumptions about which way the result might go). The mathematics is unimportant, but the binomial theory will give an exact probability in the same way as it will give an answer to the question 'what is the chance of tossing a coin and getting the same result three times in a row?' (answer = 1/4, i.e. 1/8 for the probability of three heads and 1/8 for the probability of three tails).

The above example gives a *P*-value of 0.039, which can be used as before.

The sign test does not make full use, however, of the data. In this example there is equal weight given to patients G and I even though they have very different stool weights.

Wilcoxon Signed Rank Test for Location

This test is appropriate where a non-parametric test is required, e.g. the sample size is less than 30 and the population is not normally distributed (central limit theorem not applicable).

It requires that:

- the sample is random
- the variable is continuous
- the population is symmetrical
- the measurement scale is interval.

It can be used to test the hypothesis that the mean is a given value and also to test the alternative hypotheses that the mean is not equal to, or is less than or greater than this value.

Table 12.7 Wilcoxon Signed Rank Test

Patient	Stool weight	Weight –270	Absolute value	Rank (ignoring zero value)	Signed rank (+)	Signed rank (–)
A	180	–90	90	5		–5
B	200	–70	70	4		–4
C	650	+380	380	8	+8	
D	435	+165	165	7	+7	
E	280	+10	10	2	+2	
F	385	+115	115	6	+6	
G	680	+410	410	9	+9	
H	270	+0	0			
I	245	–25	25	3		–3
J	275	+5	5	1	+1	
				Total	+33	–12

Using the above data, a new hypothesis that the mean stool weight is 270 g/day can be tested. For each subject the difference is calculated between the value and the hypothesized mean, these differences are ranked in order (according to their absolute value), then re-assigned the direction (+,–) for that rank as in Table 12.7.

If the NH were true, it would be expected that the totals (on average) would be the same. The probability of getting the difference observed can be calculated (or more usually looked up in a table) using the smaller value (in this case 12) and the number of items tested (in this case nine) in a table. This gives the probability of this result or one more extreme (a *P*-value), which in this case is >0.05, therefore, it cannot be said that the NH is false – from this sample there is no conclusive evidence that the mean stool weight is different from 270.

Median test and the Mann–Whitney *U* test

These tests are similar to the sign and Wilcoxon tests above, but allow comparisons of medians. Both test data obtained by measuring a continuous variable, the measurement scale being at least ordinal.

The simpler median test allows determination of whether two samples come from a population with the same median (and distribution). The alternative hypothesis is that the populations differ with respect to their medians. In this test the samples are pooled and a median for the pooled data is determined. If the samples were from the same population then it would be expected that each sample would have a similar number of values above and below this pooled median. If the number in each group above and below the pooled median is calculated, a 2×2 table can be constructed (Table 12.8).

If the samples were from the same populations the values in the above table would be independent of their column. Applying a χ^2 test can test the hypothesis that they come from the same population or two populations with the same median.

Table 12.8 The median test

	Sample 1	Sample 2	Total
Number of values above pooled median	a	b	
Number of values below pooled median	c	d	
Total			

Table 12.9 Mann–Whitney U Test

Subject (treatment group one represented by letters, group two by numbers)	Treatment group 1 – stool weights	Rank	Treatment group 2 – stool weights	Rank
A	180	1		
B	210	2		
C	260	3		
1			275	4
2			290	5
D	310	6		
E	340	7		
3			400	8
4			415	9
F	445	10.5		
G	445	10.5		
H	525	12		
I	545	13		
5			600	14
6			625	15
7			655	16
J	670	17		
8			685	18
9			690	19
10			700	20
Total		82		128

The Mann–Whitney U test uses more of the information available when comparing the medians of two samples (in the same way that the Wilcoxon test uses more information than the sign test). To compare medians of two samples, all the information from both samples is placed in rank order keeping track of which sample it came from as in Table 12.9.

Sufficiently high values or low values of the totals are inconsistent with the NH. A test statistic can be calculated for each total:

$$\frac{\text{Total} - n(n+1)}{2}$$

[where n is the number of observations in that sample]

and an approximate P value can be obtained form a statistical table.

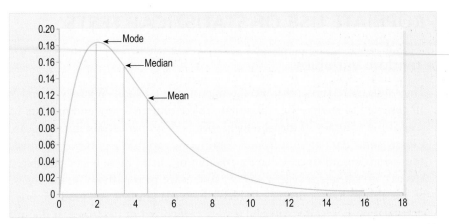

Fig. 12.24
Positively skewed distribution

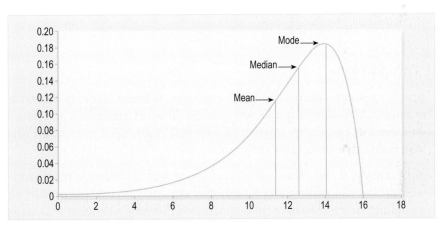

Fig. 12.25
Negatively skewed distribution

Further notes on non-parametric tests

The Mann–Whitney U and median tests are suitable for testing samples taken from populations with a skewed distribution, whereas the Wilcoxon test requires a symmetrical population. Skewed populations may be positive or negatively skewed as in Figures 12.24 and 12.25 (one may well expect stool weights to be positively skewed).

If the populations are symmetrical then the median and mean are the same and the conclusions drawn from the Mann–Whitney U test will also apply to the means.

INAPPROPRIATE USE OF STATISTICAL TESTS

Discrete random variables

The t-test, correlation tests and the sign, median, Mann–Whitney U and Wilcoxon tests are all designed to analyze variables that are continuous – any intermediate value is possible, even if the accuracy of measurement means that only certain intervals can be measured. Clearly some data are not from a continuous variable, e.g. bowel actions/day, number of admissions/month since to have a fraction of one of these is not possible. Some variables are less easy to categorize, e.g. a scoring system for histopathological changes. Intuitively, it may be possible to have a degree of fibrosis between grade 4 and grade 5, but in reality, for statistical purposes, if it can't be readily recognized or described, it doesn't exist. Frequently, however, the above statistical tests will be used to analyze integer data. For a small number of integers, e.g. bowel action/day, it is clearly appropriate to use χ^2 approach, combining data if needed into ranges. For situations where the numbers are large (and, therefore, the smallest interval is tiny compared to the numbers being compared), tests such as those described may not give a result too far from the truth – an example of this may be number of admissions/month. However, mathematically this method is not valid and care needs to be made when reviewing integer data that have been analyzed in this way.

Multiple comparisons

Another common error is multiple comparisons being made on one set of data. For example, there may be a unit that uses 10 different antibiotics and data could be collected on a number of patients treated with each. It is not valid to compare sets of these data with each other using tests such as the t-test.

For example, if there was one control group and 10 different treatments were compared with the control group using a t-test and one came out as 'statistically significant', it would not necessarily be a valid conclusion that this treatment was statistically different from the control group. The reasoning is as follows. The hypothesis test answers the question 'what is the chance of this result (or one more extreme) occurring if the NH (no difference between groups) is true?' If a cut off for significance is set at $P<0.05$, then, on average, a 'significant' result would occur 1:20 times. Since the most different treatment is chosen retrospectively, then (as this could equally be any of the 10 treatments) the chances of any one coming up as significant is 0.05×10 (assuming all the antibiotics are different and the treatments are independent), i.e. a 'significant result' would be seen every other time that experiment is performed even if the NH is true.

Another example would be comparing four different groups (without any being set aside as a control). Again this would lead to multiple comparisons (six in total) and increases the probability of a type I error by a factor of six if a standard t-test is used on the largest difference.

The correct method of analysis is to use the Analysis of Variance (ANOVA) (or its non-parametric equivalent the Kruskal Wallis Analysis of Variance by Ranks). A detailed discussion of ANOVAs is not possible, but the purpose of these tests is to determine whether the degree of variability seen between groups is significantly larger than would be expected by chance, given the overall degree of variability in the data. A good discussion of ANOVAs and particularly the experimental design required to make them valid, is given by Montgomery (1997).

Use of statistical tests to compare groups post-randomization

Following randomization to a treatment and control group, potential confounding factors, e.g. age, weight, smoking, etc., are identified and then compared using statistical tests to see if there is a 'significant' difference between the groups that would invalidate any differences found in the response to treatment. The flaw in this technique can easily be seen by repeating the hypothesis question: 'what is the chance of seeing a difference as large as or greater than the one observed if the two groups are actually random samples from the same population?' Clearly, this is nonsense since, assuming there was no flaw in the randomization process, it is known the two groups came from the same population at random. The question that needs answering is: 'is the observed difference between the groups large enough to give a biologically plausible explanation for the subsequent difference in response to treatments?' Statistical analysis alone will not be of use in answering this question.

Primary outcome analysis and sub-group analysis

To be statistically valid, the hypothesis being tested should be defined prior to performing an experiment and analysis should be directed towards this primary outcome. If, alternatively, an experiment is performed and statistical analysis is performed retrospectively on other outcomes, then, essentially, the same error is occurring as using these tests for comparing multiple groups. It is potentially even less valid since the number of potential comparisons being performed is not even clear, as the experimenters concentrate on the outcomes with the largest difference seen retrospectively.

UNDERSTANDING AND INTERPRETING TEST RESULTS

Most tests used in clinical medicine are not 100% accurate. Some might argue that none are, since even an objective test result could be assigned to the wrong patient. Confusion exists, however, as to how to interpret the sensitivity and specificity of a test in routine practice.

For a definition of the terms used see Box 12.6.

Pre-test and post-test probability

It is clear that in most cases when a test is performed, the patient already has indicators (symptoms, signs, other test results, demographics, etc.) pointing towards a particular

---

Box 12.6 Test result definitions

- Sensitivity – the probability of a positive result if the disease is present
- Specificity – the probability of a negative result if the disease is absent
- Gold standard – a diagnostic test or *set of conditions* which, if met, have a sensitivity/specificity of (as near as possible) 100%
- False-positive – a positive result in the absence of disease
- False-negative – a negative result in the presence of disease
- Pre-test probability – the likelihood the patient has the condition given the information already known: equivalent to the population prevalence of a condition if the patient is selected at random

---

condition. However, it is rare to have a precise idea of the pre-test probability. For example, a patient in hospital who develops diarrhoea has a higher pre-test probability of having pseudomembranous colitis than one out of hospital and the pre-test probability is even higher if they have already had a related antibiotic, but the exact numbers are hard to define.

The importance of understanding pre-test probability prior to performing a test is illustrated by the examples given below.

Example 1

A screening test for a condition with a prevalence of 1% has a 99% sensitivity and specificity. If a person has a positive result, what is the chance they have the condition?

To answer this, suppose 10 000 were tested. Of these, 100 would have the condition and 99% of those a positive result. Nine thousand nine hundred would be disease free and 99% (9801) would have a negative result. This can be expressed as in Table 12.10.

Therefore, if the test is positive, then the chance of the disease being present or absent is exactly 0.5 (50%)!

Example 2

If it is highly likely that a patient has a particular condition on clinical grounds (e.g. 95% certain) but to 'confirm' this, a test with 90% sensitivity and 85% specificity is performed, a table can be constructed for 100 such patients (Table 12.11).

Although a positive test will fairly much confirm the suspicion, the disease is still more likely to be present (9.5/(9/5+4.25) = 70% approx) than not, even if the test is negative, questioning the usefulness of this test.

Tables such as these are easy to construct for any hypothesized pre-test probability, test with known sensitivity and specificity and shed useful light on whether to perform a test. Clearly, the 'mental calculation' of pre-test probability is the most critical part of the process of determining the appropriate use of tests in particular clinical scenarios.

Table 12.10 Sensitivity and specificity in a screening test

	Disease present	Disease absent
Positive test	99 (sensitivity = 99%, therefore: 99% of those with the disease have a positive test)	99
Negative test	1	9801 (specificity = 99%, therefore: 99% of those without the disease have a negative test)

Table 12.11 Sensitivity (90%) and specificity (85%) with high pre-test probability

	Disease present	Disease absent
Positive test	85.5 (i.e. 90% of 95)	0.75
Negative test	9.5	4.25 (i.e. 85% of 5)

Likelihood ratios

If the pre-test probability (or prevalence) of a condition is known or estimated, then another useful way of determining the usefulness of a test is to calculate and use the likelihood ratio. The likelihood ratio for a positive test is the ratio of true-positive rate (sensitivity) to the false-positive rate (100–specificity). Conversely, the likelihood ratio for a negative test is the ratio of false-negative rate (100–sensitivity) to true-negative rate (specificity), i.e.:

$$L.R \text{ (+ve test)} = \frac{sens}{(1-spec)}$$

$$L.R. \text{ (−ve test)} = \frac{(1-sens)}{spec}$$

These values are useful because they give a direct indication of how much the chance of having a condition is increased by a positive test, or decreased by having a negative test. It is not possible, unfortunately, to simply multiply the prevalence by the likelihood ratio. It is necessary to calculate firstly the pre-test odds (the ratio of prevalence to absence):

$$pre\text{-}test\ odds = \frac{prevalence}{(100-prevalence)}$$

for a given test (positive or negative) then the post-test odds can be calculated:

post-test odds = pre-test odds × likelihood ratio (using the appropriate one whether the test was +ve or −ve)

Finally, this can be converted back to a post-test probability:

$$post\text{-}test\ probability = \frac{post\text{-}test\ odds}{(100-post\text{-}test\ odds)}$$

This is clearly cumbersome to use routinely, but a normogram is available (Fagan's Likelihood Ratio Normogram: from Fagan TJ 1975 NEJM 293:257) that allows pre-test probabilities to be converted directly to post-test probabilities using the appropriate likelihood ratio for a positive or negative test.

ANALYZING PUBLISHED DATA

With a good understanding of the principles underlying the acquisition of data and statistical analysis, it is possible to analyze published reports critically to inform the practice of clinical medicine. There are many texts covering evidence-based medicine and its practice, but the following should serve as a reminder of the important factors when analyzing papers. Some points refer to all clinical papers, others to particular subsets as indicated.

Randomization of patients in therapeutic trials

This avoids bias inherent in non-randomized trials. The randomization process should not be able to be influenced.

Per-protocol vs intention-to-treat analysis

In most trials not all patients complete treatment. There may be exclusions for reasons associated with, or independent of the treatment, but it is often impossible to reliably distinguish between these. An intention to treat analysis compares outcomes between the groups assigned to treatments at randomization regardless of whether they complete treatment. Since the purpose of a trial is often to inform decisions to embark on treatment or not, then this is a superior analysis (since the 'drop-outs' will occur in real clinical practice as well) and the overall outcome is what is important. This is especially true where failure to complete the study is due to side effects of the treatment, etc. However, if failure to complete a study occurred more frequently in one arm than another owing to reasons not related to the drug, then errors may occur with an intention-to-treat analysis and per-protocol (i.e. only comparing patients who completed both arms) is likely to yield better information. Whichever analysis is performed, all patients in a study must be accounted for.

Blinding of the study

Un-blinding leads to bias because the placebo effect is likely to be higher in patients who suspect they are receiving an active treatment and subjective assessment of these patients may be different if the clinician is un-blinded. Causes of possible un-blinding, e.g. obvious side effects of a drug, should be sought to determine whether this played a role.

Similarity of groups treated

Despite randomization, differences may occur between the treatment groups. As discussed above a *t*-test comparing parameters between groups is inappropriate. A judgement needs to be made as to whether the differences noted between groups are biologically significant enough to account for observed differences in outcome.

Gold standards

In any study evaluating a test, the validity of the gold-standard needs to be assessed, e.g. endoscopic retrograde cholangiopancreatography (ERCP) is often considered the gold-standard for comparison when new methods of identifying common bile duct (CBD) stones are evaluated. In reality, even ERCP has an error rate and this needs to be taken into account when looking at the other tests' performance, e.g. are false-positives of a new test in fact false-negatives of the 'gold-standard'?

Applicability to a particular patient

Trials of new treatments or tests are usually performed on sub-sets of patients with fairly strict inclusion and exclusion criteria. Firstly, it is important to evaluate whether these criteria (even if applied pre-randomization) could affect the outcome of a study. Secondly, a judgement then needs to be made as to whether the treatment or test can be reliably applied to a patient type not included in the original study, e.g. elderly, co-morbidity, etc.

Comparing prognosis/screening strategies

A study that looks at prognosis can be subject to many biases. Many studies of prognosis compare groups that are not randomized, or compare with historical controls. Particular problems occur when considering malignancy and early diagnosis.

Lead-time bias

If a test diagnoses a tumour earlier and a longer mean survival is reported, this can all be due to the fact that the tumour was found the same amount of time earlier in its natural history – a slow-growing tumour diagnosed 2 years earlier with a new test will result in 2 years more 'survival' without any improvement in the patient's overall prognosis (they just knew about their disease longer).

Length-time bias

Tumours that would never have become clinically apparent during a patient's lifetime may be diagnosed by a more sensitive test, giving an apparent significant increase in survival that is clearly spurious. This partly may be because the definition of what is a malignant tumour is unclear. One particular example being the diagnosis of early gastric cancer/high-grade dysplasia, which may be associated with an excellent prognosis following treatment; however, had it remained undiagnosed, no ill effects might have been seen.

These problems may be overcome by performing a large randomized control-led trial, allocating one group to screening and keeping the other as a control. Caution needs to be exercised when interpreting these studies. All cause mortality is probably of more

> **Box 12.7 Points to consider when reading a systematic review**
>
> - Are all the relevant trials included?
> - Have unpublished trials been sought?
> - Are the trials similar enough to warrant evaluation together?
> - Were similar outcome measures used in the different trials?
> - Is publication bias playing a role – look for the use of tools such as funnel-plots?
> - Are trials excluded on subjective or objective grounds?
> - Is the exclusion of some trials valid – are reasons stated within the paper?
> - Is the conclusion supported by large randomized studies?

importance to a patient than disease specific mortality, but studies are often underpowered to detect the former and quote only the latter. Furthermore, it is vital that, apart from the screening test and subsequent treatment, the groups were treated and followed up identically and that large numbers are not lost to follow-up.

These comments about prognostic trials clearly apply to conditions other than malignancy.

Systematic reviews and meta-analyses

A complete discussion of systematic reviews and meta-analyses is outside the scope of this chapter. However, when considering a systematic review, a number of points should be borne in mind (see Box 12.7).

It should be remembered that the conclusions of systematic reviews are frequently overturned by subsequent large randomized controlled trials and are far from a 'gold-standard' for evaluating clinical practice.

Further Reading

Banerjee A. Medical statistics made clear – an introduction to basic concepts. Royal Society of Medicine Press Ltd, London, 2003.

Daniel WW. Biostatistics: a foundation for analysis in the health sciences. John Wiley & Sons inc., New York, 1995.

Montgomery DC. Design and Analysis of Experiments. John Wiley & Sons inc., New York, 1997.

Sackett DL, Straus SE, Richardson WS, Rosenberg W, Haynes RB. Evidence Based Medicine: How to practice and teach EBM 2nd Edn. Churchill Livingstone, Edinburgh, 2000.

Index

W